Fever of Unknown Origin

INFECTIOUS DISEASE AND THERAPY

Series Editor

Burke A. Cunha

Winthrop-University Hospital
Mineola, New York
and
State University of New York School of Medicine
Stony Brook, New York, U.S.A.

Fever of Unknown Origin

edited by

Burke A. Cunha

Winthrop-University Hospital
Mineola, New York
and
State University of New York School of Medicine
Stony Brook, New York, U.S.A.

informa

healthcare

New York   London

Informa Healthcare USA, Inc.
52 Vanderbilt Avenue
New York, NY 10017

© 2007 by Informa Healthcare USA, Inc.
Informa Healthcare is an Informa business

No claim to original U.S. Government works
Printed in the United States of America on acid-free paper
10 9 8 7 6 5 4 3 2 1

International Standard Book Number-10: 0-8493-3615-5 (Hardcover)
International Standard Book Number-13: 978-0-8493-3615-7 (Hardcover)

Library of Congress Cataloging-in-Publication Data

Fever of unknown origin / edited by Burke A. Cunha.
    p. ; cm. -- (Infectious disease and therapy ; v. 42)
  Includes bibliographical references and index.
  ISBN-13: 978-0-8493-3615-7 (hb : alk. paper)
  ISBN-10: 0-8493-3615-5 (hb : alk. paper)
  1. Fever. 2. Physical diagnosis. 3. Diagnosis, Laboratory. I. Cunha, Burke A. II. Series.
  [DNLM: 1. Fever of Unknown Origin--diagnosis. W1 IN406HMN v.42 2007 / WB 152 F4286 2007]

RB129.F4845 2007
616'.047--dc22   2006101893

Visit the Informa Web site at
www.informa.com

and the Informa Healthcare Web site at
www.informahealthcare.com

For Marie,
who, more than any other,
personifies grace, beauty, and virtue.

Foreword

Almost 100 years ago, Richard Cabot of the Massachusetts General Hospital, in a book titled *Differential Diagnosis*, discussed "long fevers," which were found to be most often caused by tuberculosis, typhoid fever, abscesses, and endocarditis (1). Twenty years later, Alt and Barker of the Peter Bent Brigham Hospital added tumors as an important cause (2). Thirty years after that, in 1961, Petersdorf and Beeson, in the first prospective study, defined the criteria for fever of unknown (or unexplained) origin and added collagen disease as another major cause, responsible for 20% of their 100 cases (3). Their criteria—fever for at least three weeks, reaching 101°F at least some of the time—remains the standard today, although there are now different definitions for certain specific clinical subgroups.

Today, diagnosis in medicine is all too often a technologic challenge. Not so with fever of unknown origin, which has always been and continues to be a challenge to the mind, with the two major diagnostic tools a meticulous history and a very thorough physical examination, supplemented as indicated by appropriate use of our technologic cornucopia. As Petersdorf noted in 1969, from the intellectual point of view, the diagnosis of fever of unknown origin remains a challenge and is "one of the things that make medicine fun" (4). In part, the satisfaction results from the fact that the overwhelming majority of fevers of unknown origin are eventually solved.

Because the fever of unknown origin is both challenging and rewarding, it has attracted marvelous and adroit clinicians ever since it was first defined as an entity in 1931. There is permanence to the approach to these vexing enigmas and, at the same time, there are always substantial new developments—new diseases, new patient subgroups, new supporting technologies. When I was in medical school in the early 1950s, the lectures on fever of unknown origin were given by an extraordinary diagnostician, Louis Weinstein, of Tufts Medical School, and, in large part, they are wonderfully relevant to approaching the fever of unknown origin of today.

Another member of that pantheon of superb clinicians who devoted a great deal of effort to fevers of unknown origin, Philip A. Tumulty, of Johns Hopkins University School of Medicine, wrote in 1967 that "while laboratory, X-ray and other procedures may be helpful, and I do not minimize the importance of laboratory tests, the mainstay of the clinical approach to the problem of the patient with "Fever of Unknown Origin" remains an analysis of the data derived from an accurate, complete history and physical examination, and hence, meticulous collection of such data should be the primary concern of the physician ... in obtaining the history of the present illness, it is imperative to pay strict attention to even the smallest details of the exact mode of its onset, for even trivial details may hold the answer" (5).

Every clinician experienced in tackling fevers of unknown origin has personal "pearls" or specific simple laboratory tests in which he or she is particularly interested. My own are: (*i*) the sedimentation rate, which may help separate benign from more serious entities, and may also support certain infections, brucellosis for example, as the cause of the fever of unknown origin; (*ii*) the alkaline phosphatase; if substantially elevated, an explanation must be sought and this often leads to the diagnosis; (*iii*) the platelet count; if elevated, it suggests mycobacteria, lymphoma, a few other tumors, and inflammatory bowel disease; and (*iv*) whether there are nucleated red blood cells in the periphery which, in the absence of hemolysis, suggests marrow-invasive disease.

In the end, after all the lists of entities and diagnostic approaches are compiled, fever of unknown origin is, to some extent, a series of instructive anecdotes strung together to inform and help successive generations of physicians. With that in mind, and to whet the reader's appetite for this excellent and useful monograph, I am going to share six instructive cases from my own experience. The first three cases illustrate the importance of a careful history or, alternatively, of asking the question in the correct way.

Case 1: A 24-year-old man was hospitalized with three weeks of fever and shaking chills. The history and physical examination were unrevealing. He had mild hepatic function test abnormalities and appeared to have a large right adrenal gland. A tentative diagnosis of infected adrenal cyst was made, but, at surgery, he was found to have a ruptured appendix with surrounding infection. He had been asked whether he had abdominal pain at the time of hospital admission and also whether he experienced any pain at the onset of or a few days before he developed fever and chills. He denied both. When the diagnosis was established, he was asked if he had experienced abdominal pain in the weeks prior to the onset of fever. He denied any pain "except for that one night." He reported that, two weeks prior to the onset of fever, he woke up at night with peri-umbilical pain, which then moved to his right lower quadrant. He called his physician, who told him to take a cathartic, assuring him the pain would disappear by the next morning. It did indeed because, of course, he perforated. Annoyed at missing the classic presentation of acute appendicitis, I asked him why in the world he had not told us of this bout of pain two weeks prior to the ostensible onset of his complaints. His prompt and apt answer was "Hey, doc, why didn't you ask me?"

Case 2: A 42-year-old man was hospitalized with a six-month history of intermittent fever. History and physical examination, both done repeatedly, were unrevealing, as were the laboratory tests. He had a very extensive world-wide travel history, so an extensive and fruitless search was made for entities such as an amebic liver abscess. Finally, I decided to take another history (the fourth I had taken), starting with his hair and moving systematically towards his toes. Actually, it didn't take long to discover the problem. We had previously asked him about pain in his neck at the onset of the fever, as well as before and after he became febrile. He again denied any pain, but, when we asked what turned out to be the correct question, namely, had he experienced discomfort on swallowing, he remembered a 10-day period at the start of his illness when he did have relatively mild pain on swallowing. This had been six months ago and had been so mild he had completely forgotten about it until the question jogged his memory. That was the clue we had been looking for. Thyroid function tests were not particularly abnormal, but a thyroid biopsy showed clear and impressive evidence of subacute thyroiditis.

Case 3: A 64-year-old woman was hospitalized with fever of six weeks duration. History, physical examination, and laboratory tests were unrevealing. We had done repeated histories and physical examinations, to no avail. We had repeatedly asked her if she had experienced diarrhea. She had not. We had asked her how many bowel movements she had each day. The answer was one. Finally, we asked a simple question that solved the diagnostic dilemma. We asked how many bowel movements a day she used to have in the year before her fever started. The answer was one every three days. This patient, with her single bowel movement a day, was experiencing what, for her, was diarrhea. Subsequent radiology studies showed what appeared to be mild ileoculitis, but a biopsy showed florid disease.

Case 1 is an example of inadequate history taking. Cases 2 and 3 are more subtle and show the value of taking repeated histories and changing or expanding the way questions are asked. In Case 2, the difference between asking about neck pain as opposed to discomfort on swallowing meant the difference between a continuing enigma and an easily established diagnosis. Case 3 is a perfect illustration of the value of the Tumulty advice—pay attention to the smallest detail of the patient's history.

The next two cases illustrate the value of repeating the physical examination as many times as needed and not overlooking subtle findings.

Case 4: In this case, we knew the microbial cause of the fever, but not the origin. A 42-year-old man experienced three discrete episodes of enterococcal bacteremia over a six-month period, with interval intermittent fever. As a consultant during each episode, I had performed a "thorough" physical examination, focusing particularly on examining the heart for murmurs and listening for bruits that would suggest an intravascular source of the bacteremia. Each of the examinations was unrevealing. The third, comprehensive, physical examination, like the other two, was quite negative. The patient, who had taken off his undershirt during my cardiac examination, was sitting in bed, and, as I prepared to leave, I noticed a small round lesion under his right breast that I had obviously overlooked. We consulted a dermatologist, who elected to remove the lesion, which turned out to be an epithelial tumor in the center of which was an enterococcal abscess. After its extirpation, there was no more fever or bacteremia. That tiny superficial lesion, easy to overlook, was the key to solving the case.

Case 5: A 72-year-old woman was hospitalized after six weeks of intermittent fever. History and physical examination were unrevealing. Because, in this age group, the biliary tract is often the site of infection, a biliary ultrasound was performed, as was a computed tomography scan of the abdomen. Both appeared normal, as were liver function tests. On the fifth hospital day, the third complete physical examination was performed. For the first time, she felt mild, but reproducible discomfort during palpation of the right upper quadrant. That was enough for surgical consultation and abdominal exploration which revealed empyema of the gallbladder. In older persons, gallbladder infection is often an incredibly treacherous disease. Even with no history suggesting gallbladder disease, no leukocytosis, right upper quadrant pain or tenderness, and with negative scans, gangrene or empyeme of the gallbladder is often found at surgery. In this case, the third physical examination provided a subtle, but critical, finding.

The final case illustrates the importance of paying attention to the temperature pattern.

Case 6: A 64-year-old woman had been hospitalized with six weeks of fever of up to 104°F to 105°F. At the time of the consultation, she had been in the hospital for

10 days, with no diagnosis other than fever of unknown origin. Her temperature pattern was striking, with a consistent daily maximum at 8 A.M. Before seeing the patient, that information alone narrowed the likely diagnoses to: tuberculosis, salmonellosis, periarteritis hepatic abscess, and endocarditis. The studies already performed made salmonellosis, liver abscess, and endocarditis unlikely. Although tuberculosis was a possibility, in this wealthy, suburban recluse, periarteritis made much more sense. This seemed even more likely after I saw the patient and observed muscle wasting. Actually, I talked myself out of that diagnosis and into gallbladder disease, but, fortunately, the listing of periarteritis prominently in the differential diagnosis prompted a muscle biopsy which showed florid vasculitis.

The daily fever pattern is often overlooked as a potential diagnostic clue; in particular, the importance of reversal of the diurnal pattern is usually ignored or its usefulness downplayed in infectious diseases texts and articles on fever. As pointed out by one of the clinical giants in the field of fevers of unknown origin, Theodore Woodward, of the University of Maryland School of Medicine, in an article titled *The Fever Pattern as a Clinical Diagnostic Aid* (6), it can be enormously helpful, as it was in this case.

Fevers of unknown origin are always challenging, they are fun and their solution is rewarding. The bedrock of meeting that challenge is a combination of a meticulous history, a thorough physical examination, and a thoughtful differential diagnosis list followed by a specifically targeted set of laboratory studies and tests. To that bedrock approach, the information in the chapters that follow should markedly enhance the ability of every clinician to meet that challenge.

Donald B. Louria, MD
New Jersey Medical School,
Department of Preventive Medicine,
Newark, New Jersey, U.S.A.

REFERENCES

1. Cabot R. Differential Diagnosis. Philadelphia, PA: W.B. Saunders, 1911.
2. Alt HL, Barker MH. Fever of unknown origin. JAMA 1930; 94:1457–1460.
3. Petersdorf RG, Beeson P. Fever of unexplained origin: report of 100 cases. Medicine 1961; 40:1–30.
4. Petersdorf RG. Fever of unknown origin. Ann Intern Med 1969; 70:864–866.
5. Tumulty PA. Topics in clinical medicine. The patient with fever of undetermined origin. Johns Hopkins Med J 1967; 120:95–106.
6. Woodward TE. The fever pattern as a clinical diagnostic aid. In: Mackowiak PA, ed. Fever: Basic Mechanisms and Management. New York: Raven Press, 1991:83.

Preface

Fever of unknown origin is one of the most challenging diagnostic dilemmas in the field of infectious diseases. Since antiquity, fever has been a cardinal manifestation of infectious disease. In ancient medicine, the early descriptions of fever were concerned with acute, life-threatening infectious diseases. Through the ages, different fever patterns have been recognized, and their associations with various infectious disease disorders appreciated. The diagnostic significance of the relationship of pulse to temperature has been studied and remains an important way to assess the diagnostic significance of acute fevers. Yet, it was only during the 20th century that prolonged, unexplained, febrile disorders were given the emphasis they deserve in the medical literature. The fever patterns and characteristics of prolonged, febrile illnesses due to such infections as typhoid fever, chronic malaria, tuberculosis, and so on were studied in great detail. Gradually, the notion of acute versus prolonged fevers emerged in writings about the diagnostic approach to patients with fever.

In the modern era, prolonged, unexplained fevers were first put forth by Elliot Kieffer in his seminal work *"Prolonged and Perplexing Fevers."* While the characteristics of fevers and their associated infectious disorders had been well characterized by Osler in his classical textbook in 1894, Kieffer was the first to dedicate an entire work to prolonged fevers, which subsequently became known as fevers of unknown origin, or FUOs. Petersdorf published his classic study of fevers of unknown origin in 1961 and updated his findings 20 years later. Other important individuals who specialized in and wrote about diagnosing fevers of unknown origin included Weinstein, Wolff, and Louria. Medical as well as infectious disease textbooks now include entire chapters on fevers of unknown origin. Prior to the present volume, the most recent book was *Fever of Undetermined Origin*, edited by Henry W. Murray, and was published in 1983. Murray's accompanies Kieffer's as the only two textbooks devoted entirely to the subject of fever of unknown origin. The distribution of infectious and noninfectious disorders causing fever of unknown origin have changed as a result of an aging population, devices associated with medical procedures, and sophisticated diagnostic tests and radiologic procedures. While some newly recognized disorders presenting as fever of unknown origin have been described, in the main, there is a difference in distribution of disorders, both infectious and noninfectious that have been previously described in the fever of unknown origin literature and books.

So what is the rationale for a millennium book on fever of unknown origin? The answer is quite simple. There is a great need for a single sourcebook that utilizes the newer diagnostic tests that are important in diagnosing fevers of unknown origin. Not only has the distribution of disorders causing fevers of unknown origin changed, but new entities presenting as fever of unknown origin need to be addressed in a current treatise. This book on fevers of unknown origin is current and written by clinicians for clinicians. Accordingly, its perspective is distinctly clinical. The clinical diagnostic approach is emphasized throughout, as therapy has a minor role in the clinical approach to fevers of unknown origin. The tried and true principles of a pertinent history and physical examination are stressed, particularly a focused history and physical examination, which are especially important in the fever of unknown origin patient. Laboratory tests should not be ordered in a shotgun fashion, but selectively, and should reflect the likely diagnostic possibilities, as well as the clinical clues ascertained from the history, physical exam, or routine laboratory tests. Because fevers of unknown origin are such a common clinical problem, today's clinicians need an up-to-date and comprehensive book length reference to assist them in their clinical approach to patients. This book should become the standard reference text on fever of unknown origin for clinicians and remain useful for many years.

Burke A. Cunha

Contents

Contributors

Ariff Admani Department of Medicine, Saint Michael's Medical Center, Newark, New Jersey, U.S.A.

Anastasia Antoniadou Fourth Department of Internal Medicine of Athens University Medical School, University General Hospital ATTIKON, Athens, Greece

Wendy S. Armstrong Division of Infectious Diseases, Department of Medicine, Cleveland Clinic Foundation, Cleveland, Ohio, U.S.A.

Emilio Bouza Servicio de Microbiología Clínica y E. Infecciosas, Hospital General Gregorio Marañón, University of Madrid, Madrid, Spain

Charles S. Bryan Department of Medicine, University of South Carolina, School of Medicine, Columbia, South Carolina, U.S.A.

Burke A. Cunha Infectious Disease Division, Winthrop-University Hospital, Mineola, New York, U.S.A.

Lucinda M. Elko Department of Medicine, University of South Carolina, School of Medicine, Columbia, South Carolina, U.S.A.

Helen Giamarellou Fourth Department of Internal Medicine of Athens University Medical School, University General Hospital ATTIKON, Athens, Greece

Tonya Jagneaux Department of Medicine, Louisiana State University Health Sciences Center, New Orleans, Louisiana, U.S.A.

Douglas S. Katz Department of Radiology, Winthrop-University Hospital, Mineola, New York, U.S.A.

Powel Kazanjian Division of Infectious Diseases, Department of Internal Medicine, University of Michigan Medical Center, Ann Arbor, Michigan, U.S.A.

Daniel C. Knockaert Department of General Internal Medicine, Gasthuisberg University Hospital, Leuven, Belgium

Aaron R. Kosmin Section of Infectious Diseases, Department of Medicine, Temple University School of Medicine, Philadelphia, Pennsylvania, U.S.A.

Leonard R. Krilov Division of Pediatric Infectious Disease, Winthrop-University Hospital, Mineola, New York, U.S.A.

Belén Loeches Servicio de Microbiología Clínica y E. Infecciosas, Hospital General Gregorio Marañón, University of Madrid, Madrid, Spain

Fred A. Lopez   Department of Medicine, Louisiana State University Health Sciences Center, New Orleans, Louisiana, U.S.A.

Bennett Lorber   Section of Infectious Diseases, Department of Medicine, Temple University School of Medicine, Philadelphia, Pennsylvania, U.S.A.

Patricia Muñoz   Servicio de Microbiología Clínica y E. Infecciosas, Hospital General Gregorio Marañón, University of Madrid, Madrid, Spain

Dean C. Norman   UCLA Geffen School of Medicine and VA Greater Los Angeles Healthcare System, Los Angeles, California, U.S.A.

Charles V. Sanders   Department of Medicine, Louisiana State University Health Sciences Center, New Orleans, Louisiana, U.S.A.

Leon G. Smith   Department of Medicine, Saint Michael's Medical Center, Newark, New Jersey, U.S.A.

Yogi Trivedi   Department of Radiology, Winthrop-University Hospital, Mineola, New York, U.S.A.

Megan Bernadette Wong   VA Greater Los Angeles Healthcare System, Los Angeles, California, U.S.A.

Elizabeth Yung   Department of Radiology, Winthrop-University Hospital, Mineola, New York, U.S.A.

Section I: General Concepts

1   Fever of Unknown Origin: Clinical Overview and Perspective

Burke A. Cunha

Infectious Disease Division, Winthrop-University Hospital, Mineola, New York, U.S.A.

OVERVIEW

The term fever of unknown origin (FUO) was originally meant to describe perplexing fevers of prolonged duration (1). Petersdorf, in his classic 1961 paper, was the first to define criteria for the diagnosis of FUO. The criteria for classic FUO includes a fever lasting three weeks or more, accompanied by temperatures that are >101°F (38.3°C) (2). This definition has been modified over the years to take into account the change in diagnostic modalities and the proportion of patients evaluated for FUO in the ambulatory versus the inpatient setting. Different definitions have been put forward to describe the difference in length of diagnostic workup taking into account the outpatient setting (3–10).

Because there is no general agreement on these new nonclassic criteria for FUO, it is probably better, and certainly more clinically useful, to simplify the current criteria for FUO. FUO at the present time should signify prolonged fevers with temperatures of at least 101°F (38.3°C), that remain diagnosed after a focused and appropriate laboratory workup. This clinical definition is useful and eliminates two of the major diagnostic problems in using the term FUO as a diagnostic term. Many clinicians diagnose patients with FUO who have had an inadequate laboratory workup or who have not had prolonged, undiagnosed fevers for three or more weeks.

Therefore, the workup should be focused and based on the clues provided by the history, physical exam, and laboratory tests that suggest an organ system involvement or category of disorder causing the FUO, such as collagen vascular disease, malignancy, infection, and so on. It makes little sense to order tests for every conceivable cause of an FUO when there is nothing to suggest the diagnosis in the history and physical exam or basic laboratory tests (11–15).

CAUSES OF FUO

In the classic article on FUO by Petersdorf, infectious diseases were the single largest category responsible for FUOs (2). Years later, Petersdorf again reported on the relative incidences of disorders causing FUOs and found that neoplasms had replaced infections as the most common category causing FUOs (9). Since the 1990s, there have been further changes in the relative distribution of causes responsible for FUOs. Differences in the literature on the proportion of disorders ascribed to infection, noninfectious inflammatory disorders, malignancy, and so on, vary according to the geography and demographics of the patients described. Series that describe FUO in pediatrics have a very different distribution of disorders than reviews of elderly patients with FUOs (16–20). The relative proportion of inpatients versus outpatients in a series also bears somewhat on the distribution. Geography is also important, depending on the geographical location. Various diseases associated with FUO, for example, Q fever, may be disproportionately represented in a series coming from areas where certain infectious diseases are endemic. Therefore, in approaching the patient with FUO, the clinician must take into account the different demographic and geographic factors in the literature and adjust those for the particular locality where the physician is located (8,10,16).

The changes in the relative distribution of entities responsible for FUO are primarily due to changes in diagnostic testing rather than to a major shift in the relative incidence of general categories, for example, infection, malignancy, collagen vascular diseases, and so on. The biggest change in diagnostic categories is related to a decrease in the relative proportion of collagen vascular diseases causing FUO. The reason for this change is the increase in sophisticated serological tests that render the diagnosis of collagen vascular diseases more accurate. Because of accurate, early diagnostic testing for collagen vascular diseases, those accompanied by fevers of prolonged duration do not remain undiagnosed, and therefore do not fulfill the criteria of an FUO. The collagen vascular diseases that have remained important causes of FUO are those for which no serological tests are available, that is, polymyalgia rheumatica (PMR)/temporal arteritis, late onset rheumatoid arthritis (LORA), and juvenile rheumatoid arthritis (adult Still's disease). Today, because of the tremendous increase in polypharmacy, the number of medications patients are on make the diagnosis of drug fever as a cause of FUO relatively more common. In addition, as the general population ages, the relative incidence of malignancy increases with age, and this is reflected in the series on FUOs (21–26).

Infectious disease causes that were important in early FUO series were subacute bacterial endocarditis (SBE). At the present time, SBE is a relatively uncommon cause of FUO because most patients seen by a physician with fever and heart murmur have blood cultures drawn and/or cardiac echocardiography done, thereby diagnosing SBE and eliminating this category as an FUO. Obscure intraabdominal abscesses remain an important component of the infectious category in the FUO literature. Perforation of the retrocecal appendix, pericolonic abscess resulting from a perforation from an otherwise unsuspected colon tumor, occult liver or splenic abscesses, and prosthetic graft infections may easily be missed and eventually present as an undiagnosed prolonged fever, fulfilling the criteria of FUO (4,15,27) (Table 1).

FUO IN SPECIAL POPULATIONS

Aside from the classic definition of FUO, FUOs have been described in selected subgroups. Such FUO special populations include nosocomial FUOs, FUOs in HIV/AIDS, FUOs in children, FUOs in the elderly, and so on. These classifications are not substantially different from a classic FUO. Rather, it is that they recognize a different distribution of disorders in different patient subsets. The disadvantage of such a system is that it may create confusion that there is something special about FUOs in a certain category, such as pediatrics or the elderly. Age difference changes the relative distribution but does not affect the actual causes of FUO (8,15). Similarly, in patients with human immunodeficiency virus (HIV), the distribution is skewed by opportunistic pathogens as well as by geography. Visceral leishmaniasis in endemic areas is a major diagnostic consideration with FUO,

TABLE 1 Diseases Causing Classical Fever of Unknown Origin

Type of disorder	Common	Uncommon	Rare
Malignancy	Lymphomas	Preleukemias	Atrial myxomas
	Metastases to liver/CNS	Hepatomas	tumors
	Hypernephromas	Myeloproliferative disorders	Pancreatic carcinoma
		Colon carcinomas	Multiple myeloma
Infections	Miliary TB	SBE	Periapical dental abscesses
	Extrapulmonary TB (Renal TB, TB meningitis)	CMV	Chronic sinusitis
		Toxoplasma gondii	Subacute vertebral osteomyelitis
	Intra-abdominal/ pelvic abscesses	Typhoid (enteric) fevers	Listeria
		Intra/perinephric abscess	Yersinia
		Splenic abscess	Brucellosis
			Relapsing fever
			Rat bite fever
			Chronic Q fever
			Cat scratch fever
			HIV
			EBV
			Leptospirosis
			Blastomycosis
			Histoplasmosis
			Coccidioidomycosis
			Infected aortic aneurysms
			Infected vascular grafts
			Trypanosomiasis
			LGV
			Permanently placed central IV-line infections
			Prosthetic device infections
			Relapsing mastoiditis
			Leishmaniasis (Kala-azar)
Rheumatologic	Still's disease (adult JRA)	PAN	SLE
			Takayasu's arteritis
	Polymyalgia rheumatica/ temporal arteritis	Rheumatoid arthritis (elderly)	Felty's syndrome
			Pseudogout (CPPD)
			Behçet's disease
			FMF
Miscellaneous causes	Drug-fever	Granulomatous hepatitis	Regional enteritis
	Cirrhosis		Whipple's disease
			Fabray's disease
			Hyperthyroidism
			Pheochromocytomas
			Addison's disease
			Subacute thyroiditis
			Cyclic neutropenia
			Polymyositis
			Wegener's granulomatosis
			Weber-Christian disease
			Sarcoidosis (e.g., basilar meningitis, hepatic granulomas)

(Continued)

TABLE 1   Diseases Causing Classical Fever of Unknown Origin (*Continued*)

Type of disorder	Common	Uncommon	Rare
			Pulmonary emboli (multiple/ small)
			Hypothalamic dysfunction
			Habitual hyperthermia
			Factitious fever
			Pseudolymphomas
			Kikuchi's disease
			Hyper IgD syndrome

Abbreviations: CMV, cytomegalovirus; CNS, central nervous system; EBV, Epstein-Barr virus; FMF, familial Mediterranean fever; HIV, human immunodeficiency virus; JRA, juvenile rheumatoid arthritis; LGV, lymphogranuloma venereum; PAN, periarteritis nodosa; SBE, subacute bacterial endocarditis; SLE, systemic lupus erythematosus; TB, tuberculosis.
Source: Adapted From Ref. 15.

whereas in nonendemic areas, visceral leishmaniasis should not be considered in the differential diagnosis of FUO in HIV patients (27,28). Similarly, patients with nosocomial FUOs have a higher incidence than do the classic FUO general population of infected arteriovenous (AV) grafts, nosocomial endocarditis, obscure abscesses, obscure procedure-related abscesses, and so on. The use of FUO subsets has the advantage of focusing HIV doctors on the differential diagnosis in their specialty, but serves little or no purpose in doctors not taking care of HIV patients. Similarly, pediatricians do not need to be familiar with the causes of FUO in the elderly, as it has little relevance in children and vice versa with elderly patients (4,15) (Tables 2–4).

Therefore, the use of FUO subsets in various circumstances helps the physicians seeing patients in the various FUO population subsets to adjust diagnostic possibilities accordingly. FUOs in subsets are really a variation on a theme and do not represent different causes responsible for FUO in the subset but rather a difference in distribution of disorders seen in the general population (6,9,16).

Clinicians should use the frequency distribution of disorders causing an FUO to guide their diagnostic approach in patients with prolonged, unexplained fevers meeting the definition of FUO. Demographic/geographic considerations need to be factored into the diagnostic approach to avoid needless or misdirected diagnostic testing. With FUO patients, there are almost always one or, more clues from the history and physical examination or nonspecific laboratory tests that suggest a disease category in general, or more specifically, a number of diagnostic possibilities. The diagnostic workup should be focused and directed by clues suggesting a diagnostic category or a particular diagnosis. The point of the history, physical examination, and nonspecific laboratory clues in the diagnostic workup is to prompt the clinician to order further tests based on the pattern of organ system involvement to make a definitive diagnosis (10–12,15,16,) (Table 5).

Empiric therapy of FUO should be discouraged except as related to very few clinical entities. By treating the fever of an FUO, important diagnostic clues, that is, fever curves, the relationship of pulse to temperature, and so on are eliminated, depriving the clinician of potentially important diagnostic information. Decreasing the fever may make the patient feel better, but it does not answer the fundamental question of what is causing the patient's prolonged, elevated temperatures. The empiric therapy for FUOs is best limited to patients where the possibility of

TABLE 2 Fever of Unknown Origin in Special Populations: HIV

Infectious causes	Noninfectious causes
Common	Common
Mycobacterium tuberculosis	Drug fever
Mycobacterium avium-intracellulare	Thrombophlebitis
Visceral leishmaniasis (Kala-azar)	
Histoplasmosis	
Uncommon	Uncommon
Nontuberculous Mycobacterium	Non-Hodgkin's lymphoma
Pneumocystis (carinii) jiroveci pneumonia	
Toxoplasmosis	
Cryptococcus	

Abbreviation: HIV, human immunodeficiency virus.
Source: Adapted from Ref. 15.

TABLE 3 Fever of Unkown Origin in Special
Populations: Children

Infectious causes	Noninfectious causes
Common	Common
Chronic mastoiditis	Leukemias
Chronic sinusitis	Lymphomas
Subdiaphragmatic abscess	JRA
CMV	
EBV	
Visceral larva migrans	
Uncommon	Uncommon
Perinephric abscess	PAN
Renal abscess	Neuroblastomas
Psittacosis	
Rare	Rare
Histoplasmosis	Drug fever
Toxoplasmosis	
SBE	
Brucella	
Leptospirosis	

Abbreviations: CMV, cytomegalovirus; EBV, Epstein-Barr virus;
JRA, juvenile rheumatoid arthritis; PAN, periarteritis nodosa;
SBE, subacute bacterial endocarditis.
Source: Adapted from Ref. 15.

TABLE 4 Fever of Unknown Origin in Special Populations:
Neutropenic Fever

Infectious causes	Noninfectious causes
Common	Common
Invasive/disseminated fungal infections	CNS metastases
Hepatosplenic candidiasis	Hepatic metastases
Perirectal/ischiorectal abscess	
Semipermanent central IV lines	
Uncommon	Uncommon
Bacteremia (fastidious organism)	Drug fever

Abbreviation: CNS, central nervous system.
Source: Adapted from Ref. 15.

TABLE 5 Organ-System Involvement in Classical Fever of Unknown Origin

CNS	Heart
TB meningitis	SBE
Sarcoid meningitis	Atrial myxomas
Tumors	Takayasu's arteritis
Chronic encephalitis	
Brain abscess	Kidneys
SBE	SBE
Takayasu's arteritis	Hypernephroma
	Intra/perinephric abscess
Neck	PAN
Subacute thyroiditis	Renal TB
Adult JRA	HIV
Relapsing mastoiditis	Lymphomas
Kikuchi's disease	SLE
	Leptospirosis
Lymph nodes	Brucellosis
Lymphomas	
CSF	Spleen
TB	SBE
LGV	Splenic abscess
EBV	Lymphomas
CMV	CMV
Toxoplasmosis	HIV
HIV	
Adult JRA	Liver
Brucellosis	Hepatoma
Whipple's disease	Metastatic carcinoma
Kikuchi's disease	Cirrhosis
Joints	Liver abscess
Whipple's disease	Sarcoidosis
Rat bite fever	Granulomatous hepatitis
Brucellosis	Brucellosis
FMF	Q fever
LGV	EBV
Hyper IgD syndrome	CMV
Small intestine	Rat bite fever
FMF	Adult JRA
Lymphomas	Kikuchi's disease
Regional enteritis	Drug fever
Whipple's disease	
Pelvis	No localizing signs
Pelvic abscess/tumors	Preleukemias
	Myeloproliferative diseases
Biliary tract	SBE
Subacute cholangitis	Miliary TB
PAN	Brucellosis
Gallbladder wall abscess	Q fever
	Colon cancer
Bone marrow	HIV
Lymphomas	Lymphomas
Carcinomas	Typhoid fever
Miliary TB	Drug fever
Histoplasmosis	Factitious fever
Brucellosis	Infective aortic aneurysm
Typhoid fever	

Abbreviations: CMV, cytomegalovirus; CNS, central nervous system; CSF, cat scratch fever; EBV, Epstein-Barr virus; FMF, familial Mediterranean fever; HIV, human immunodeficiency virus; JRA, juvenile rheumatoid arthritis; LGV, lymphogranuloma venereum; PAN, periarteritis nodosa; SBE, subacute bacterial endocarditis; SLE, systemic lupus erythematosus; TB, tuberculosis.
Source: Adapted from Ref. 15.

miliary tuberculosis (TB) is high. Empiric anti-TB therapy in this setting is not only justifiable but also reasonable and may be lifesaving. The other situation in which empiric therapy may be useful in the FUO setting is in the treatment of PMR/temporal arteritis. Low-dose steroids for PMR in the appropriate clinical setting may confirm the diagnosis. If temporal arteritis is suspected and visual symptoms appear, it is critical that high-dose steroids be given to prevent blindness. The most common error in the therapy of FUO is to give prolonged courses of antipyretics or antibiotics to the patient without a definite diagnosis. Such an approach masks the problem, losing valuable time in the diagnostic workup, and does nothing to determine the root cause of the patient's FUO (10,12,15,30).

REFERENCES

1. Keefer CS, Leard SE. Prolonged and Perplexing Fevers. Boston: Little Brown and Co, 1955.
2. Petersdorf RG, Beeson PB. Fever of unexplained origin: report on 100 cases. Medicine (Baltimore) 1961; 40:1–30.
3. Vanderschueren S, Knockaert D, Adrienssens T, et al. From prolonged febrile illness to fever of unknown origin: the challenge continues. Arch Intern Med 2003; 163:1033–1041.
4. Brusch JL, Weinstein L. Fever of unknown origin. Med Clin North Am 1988; 72: 1247–1261.
5. Bryan CS. Fever of unknown origin. Arch Intern Med 2003; 163:1003–1004.
6. Gleckman R, Crowley M, Esposito A. Fever of unknown origin: a view from the community hospital. Am J Med Sci 1977; 274:21–25.
7. de Kleijn EM, Vandenbroucke JP, van der Meer JW, for the Netherlands FUO Study Group. Fever of unknown origin (FUO), I: a prospective multicenter study of 167 patients with FUO, using fixed epidemiologic entry criteria. Medicine (Baltimore) 1997; 76:391–400.
8. Kazanjian PH. Fever of unknown origin. Review of 86 patients treated in a community hospital. Clin Infect Dis 1992;15:968–973.
9. Petersdorf RG. Fever of unknown origin: an old friend revisited. Arch Intern Med 1992; 152:21–22.
10. Knockaert DC, Vanneste LJ, Vanneste SB, et al. Fever of unknown origin in the 1980s: an update of the diagnostic spectrum. Arch Intern Med 1992;152:51–55.
11. Louria DB. Fever of unknown etiology. Del Med J 1971; 43:343–348.
12. Murray HW, ed. FUO: fever of undetermined origin. Mount Kisco, NY: Futura Publishing, 1983.
13. Cunha BA. Diagnostic significance of nonspecific laboratory abnormalities in infectious diseases. In: Gorbach SL, Bartlett JG, Blacklow NE, eds. Infectious Diseases. 3rd ed. Philadelphia: Lippincott Williams and Wilkins, 2004:158–165.
14. Cunha BA. Fever of unknown origin. Infect Dis Clin North Am 1996;10:111–128.
15. Cunha BA. Fever of unknown origin (FUO). In: Gorbach SL, Bartlett JB, Blacklow NR, eds. Infectious Diseases in Medicine and Surgery, 3rd ed. Philadelphia: WB Saunders, 2004:1568–1577.
16. Cunha BA. Fever of unknown origin (FUO): focused diagnostic testing and simplified diagnostic criteria. Scand J Infect Dis (in press 2007).
17. Cunha BA. Fever of unknown origin in the elderly—a commentary. Infect Dis Clin Pract 1993; 2:380–383.
18. Esposito AL, Gleckman R. Fever of unknown origin in the elderly. J Am Geriatric Soc 1978; 26:498–505.
19. Kauffman CA, Jones PG. Diagnosing fever of unknown origin in older patients. Geriatrics 1984; 39:46–51.
20. Knockaert DC, Vanneste LJ, Bobbears HJ. Fever of unknown origin in elderly patients. J Am Geriatr Soc 1993; 41:1187–1192.

21. Malmvall BE, Bengtsson BA, Alestig K, et al. The clinical pictures of giant cell arteritis. Temporal arteritis, polymyalgia rheumatica, and fever of unknown origin. Postgrad Med 1980; 67:141–150.
22. Weinberger A, Kessler A, Pinkhas J. Fever in various rheumatic diseases. Clin Rheumatol 1985; 4:258–266.
23. Calamia KT, Hunder GG. Giant cell arteritis (temporal arteritis) presenting as fever of undetermined origin. Arthritis Rheum 1981; 24:1414–1418.
24. Cunha BA, Parchuri S, Mohan S. Fever of unknown origin: temporal arteritis presenting with persistent cough and elevated serum ferritin levels. Heart Lung 2006; 35:112–116.
25. Cunha BA. Fever of unknown origin caused by adult juvenile rheumatoid arthritis: the diagnostic significance of double quotidian fevers and elevated serum ferritin levels. Heart Lung 2004; 33:417–421.
26. Calabro JJ, Marchesano JM. Fever associated with juvenile rheumatoid arthritis. N Engl J Med 1967; 267:11–18.
27. Bujak JS, Aptekar RG, Deck JL, et al. Juvenile rheumatoid arthritis presenting in the adult as fever of unknown origin. Medicine (Baltimore) 1973; 52:431–434.
28. Cunha BA. Fever of unknown origin in HIV/AIDS patients. Drugs Today 1999; 35: 429–434.
29. Bissuel F, Leport C, Perrone C, et al. Fever of unknown origin in HIV-infected patients: a critical analysis of a retrospective series of 57 cases. J Intern Med 1994; 236:529–535.
30. Manfredi R, Calza L, Chiodo F. Primary cytomegalovirus infection in otherwise healthy adults with fever of unknown origin: a 3-year prospective survey. Infection 2006; 34: 87–90.

2 Fever of Unknown Origin: A Focused Diagnostic Approach

Burke A. Cunha

Infectious Disease Division, Winthrop-University Hospital, Mineola, New York, U.S.A.

OVERVIEW

Disorders presenting as fevers of unknown origin (FUO) are varied and extensive (1–11). Clinicians often order every conceivable test to try to diagnose all of the myriad causes of FUO that are part of the differential diagnosis of FUO in general, but are not sign/symptom-related. The main difficulty with diagnostic testing in patients with FUO is that it is unfocused. All disorders have a specific pattern of organ involvement. The pattern of organ involvement, in turn, determines the history, physical findings, and nonspecific laboratory abnormalities associated with various diseases. In a patient with FUO, there are almost always one or more clues from the history, physical examination, or nonspecific laboratory tests that suggest a particular diagnosis or at least limit diagnostic possibilities. History, physical, and laboratory tests are usually helpful in defining the pattern of organ involvement as well as eliminating entire categories from further diagnostic consideration. In a patient with a history of diverticulitis presenting with left lower quadrant pain and FUO, it is not cost effective or clinically useful to order tests for collagen vascular diseases, thyroid function tests, and so on, which have no bearing on the clinical presentation (12–15).

FOCUSED DIAGNOSTIC APPROACH

After the history, physical exam, and nonspecific laboratory tests, further tests should be based on localizing the disease process anatomically to determine its organ system distribution, which in turn is critical in defining differential diagnostic possibilities. With an FUO, general features of the disorder apparent from the history, physical, and nonspecific laboratory tests usually suggest a general disease category, that is, infection, malignancy, or rheumatic disease. The clinical presentation features should suggest a particular category of disorders may be further refined by both nonspecific and specific laboratory testing, leading ultimately to a definitive diagnosis. If an inflammatory noninfectious disorder is suspected, then the test battery for rheumatic disorders should be focused and complete. If the clinical presentation suggests a malignancy, then diagnostic efforts should be directed to rule in or rule out a malignancy with further focused testing or imaging studies. Similarly, with infectious diseases, tests should be focused and based on the most likely diagnostic infectious etiologies based on the patient's age, geography, and clinical presentation (2,4,9, 10,12–15).

    The greatest errors in FUO workup relating to the diagnostic evaluation are related to overtesting and undertesting. Ordering tests that have no potential clinical usefulness is wasteful and unnecessary. Alternately, too few diagnostic tests,

TABLE 1   Fever of Unknown Origin: Nonspecific Laboratory Clues as a Guide to Further Focused Laboratory Testing

For all FUO categories
  CBC
  ESR
  LFTs
  Chest X ray
  ANA
  UA
  Routine blood cultures
CBC
  Leukocytosis → neoplastic and infectious panels
  Leukopenia → neoplastic infections, and RD panels
  Anemia → neoplastic, infections, and RD panels
  Myelocytes/metamyelocytes → neoplastic panel
  Lymphocytosis → neoplastic and infectious panels
  Lymphopenia
  Atypical lymphocytes
  Eosinophilia → neoplastic, RD, and infectious panels
  Basophilia → neoplastic panel
  Thrombocytosis → neoplastic, infectious, and RD panels
  Thrombocytopenia → neoplastic, infectious, and RD panels
ESR
  Highly elevated → neoplastic, infectious, and RD panels
LFTs
  ↑ SGOT/SGPT → RD panel
  ↑ all phosphatases → neoplastic and RD panels
ANA
  Increased ANA → RD panel
  Increased RF → infectious and RD panels
Chest X ray
  Any lung parenchymal abnormality/adenopathy/pleural effusion → neoplastic, infectious, or RD panels
Blood cultures
  Imaging studies

Abbreviations: ANA, antinuclear antibodies; CBC, complete blood count; ESR, erythrocyte sedimentation rate; LFTs, liver function tests; RD, rheumatic disease; SGOT/SGPT, serum glutamic-oxaloacetic transaminase/serum glutamic pyruvate transaminase; UA, urine analysis.

particularly those that are necessary and appropriate, not relevant to the clinical setting, prolong a misdirected diagnostic FUO workup. The key to the diagnostic approach with FUOs is a focused and complete clinically relevant workup. Using a focused approach, physicians can arrive at a definitive diagnosis more quickly, less expensively, and less invasively than using the "shotgun" approach (9,10,15).

Clinicians often fail to appreciate the diagnostic significance of subtle or nonspecific findings in the history/physical examination and laboratory tests, which often provide important clinical clues to the diagnosis. Sometimes, subtle findings are the only clues that are available and must be pursued. Subtle clues often suggest the pattern of organ involvement, which will further focus and direct the diagnostic workup (14–19).

NONSPECIFIC LABORATORY ABNORMALITIES

Besides subtle abnormalities in nonspecific tests, certain tests are relatively underutilized in the FUO workup. For example, the erythrocyte sedimentation rate (ESR),

TABLE 2 A Focused Diagnostic Approach

Infectious panel	Neoplastic panel	Rheumatic panel
Blood tests	Blood tests	Blood tests
Special blood cultures	Ferritin	DS DNA
(↑ CO_2/6 weeks)	SPEP	SPEP
Q fever serology	Radiologic tests	Ferritin
Brucella serology	CT/MRI abdomen/ pelvis[a]	CPK
Bartonella serology	Gallium scan	ACE
Salmonella serology	BM biopsy	Radiologic tests
Viral serologies	(if myelophthistic	Head/chest CT/MRI
EBV	anemia/abnormal	Temporal artery biopsy
CMV	RBCs/WBCs)	(if ESR >100,
HHV-6	TTE (if heart murmur	without alternate
Radiologic tests	with negative	diagnosis)
CT/MRI	blood cultures)	Low-dose steroids
Abdomen/pelvis[a]	Other tests	(prednisone 10 mg/day
Gallium scan	Naprosyn test	if PMR likely)
Panorex films of		
jaws (if all else		
negative)		
Other tests		
Naprosyn test		
Anergy panel/PPD		

[a]Chest/head CT/MRI (if head/chest infectious etiology suspected).
Abbreviations: ACE, angiotensin converting enzyme; BM, bone marrow; CMV, cytomegalovirus; CPK, creatine phosphokinase CT, computed tomography; DS DNA, double-stranded DNA; EBV, Epstein-Barr virus; MRI, magnetic resonance imaging; PMR, polymyalgia rheumatica. SPEP, serum protein electrophoresis; TTE, transthoracic echocardiography.

if very highly elevated, that is, >100 mm/hr, quickly limits diagnostic possibilities to relatively few disorders. Another commonly underutilized test is the serum protein electrophoresis (SPEP), useful and may suggest a variety of infectious disorders, common collagen vascular diseases, or even lymphoma (15–20). SPEP is usually only thought of as useful to diagnose or rule-out multiple myeloma, but clearly other abnormalities may be much more helpful in an FUO workup (14,19) (Tables 1–2).

Perhaps the most underutilized test in FUO patients is serum ferritin levels. Elevations of serum ferritin levels are often ignored or explained away as being due to ferritin acting as an "acute phase reactant." In a patient with FUO, by definition, the process is no longer acute, and elevations in the serum ferritin level take on a very different significance. Elevated serum ferritin levels may suggest certain collagen vascular diseases, for example, systemic lupus erythematosus (SLE), juvenile rheumatoid arthritis (JRA), or temporal arteritis. Ferritin levels may also be elevated in a variety of myeloproliferative disorders as well as with any malignancy. Importantly, elevated ferritin levels in the FUO context strongly argue against an infectious etiology (21–25).

The value of the nonspecific tests mentioned is enhanced when combined with other history/physical examination findings to further direct the diagnostic work up in the FUO patients. Nonspecific tests are often helpful in suggesting an otherwise unsuspected diagnosis and are useful in eliminating entire diagnostic categories from further consideration.

The diagnostic specificity of nonspecific laboratory tests is enhanced when results are combined. For example, increases in α_1/α_2 on serum protein

TABLE 3 Focused Diagnostic Approach to Fever of Unknown Origin: Clues to Infectious Diseases

History
  Fatigue (any chronic infection)
  Weight loss (abscesses, HIV, TB, SBE)
  Night sweats (abscesses, HIV, TB, SBE)
  Headache (typhoid fever, TB, brucellosis, HIV)
  Mental confusion (brucellosis, TB, chronic viral/parasitic CNS infections, HIV, CSF)
  Sudden vision loss (SBE, brain abscess)
  CVA (TB, SBE)
  Tongue pain (relapsing fever)
  Shoulder pain (subdiaphragmatic abscess)
  Arthralgias (LGV, Whipple's disease, rat bite fever, brucellosis, HIV)
  Cough (TA, TB)
  Heart murmur (SBE)
  Back pain (TB, brucellosis, SBE)
  Thigh pain (brucellosis)
  Early satiety (brucellosis, splenic abscess, typhoid fever)
  Animal contact (brucellosis, typhoid fever, Q fever, CSF, psittacosis, rat bite fever)
  IVDA/blood transfusions (CMV, HIV)
Physical findings
  Relative bradycardia (typhoid fever, leptospirosis, psittacosis, brucellosis, malaria)
  Epistaxis (psittacosis, relapsing fever)
  Conjunctivitis (TB, CSF)
  Conjunctival suffusion (relapsing fever)
  Subconjunctival hemorrhage (SBE)
  Uveitis (TB)
  Adenopathy
    Localized (toxoplasma, CSF, HIV)
    Generalized (HIV, EBV, CMV, TB, LGV, brucellosis)
   Heart murmur (SBE)
  Trapezius tenderness (subdiaphragmatic abscess)
  Spinal tenderness (SBE, brucellosis, typhoid fever)
  Hepatomegaly (relapsing fever, typhoid fever, Q fever)
  Splenomegaly (TB, SBE, brucellosis, EBV, CMV, psittacosis, relapsing fever, typhoid fever)
    Thigh tenderness (brucellosis)
    Thrombophlebitis (psittacosis)
    Epididymoorchitis (TB, brucellosis, leptospirosis, EBV)
    Arthritis (rat bite fever, brucellosis, osteomyelitis, typhoid fever, Whipple's disease)
Nonspecific laboratory findings
CBC
  Leukopenia (HIV, TB, brucellosis, typhoid fever)
  Lymphopenia (HIV, TB)
  Lymphocytosis (TB, EBV, CMV, toxoplasmosis)
  Monocytosis (SBE, TB, brucellosis, CMV)
  Atypical large/bizarre lymphocytes (toxoplasmosis, CMV, EBV)
  Thrombocytopenia (HIV, CMV, RSV, relapsing fever)
  Thrombocytosis (abscess, osteomyelitis, SBE, TB)
ESR
  Highly elevated ESR >100 mm/hr (abscess, osteomyelitis, SBE)
Rheumatoid factor
  Increased rheumatoid factors (SBE)
SPEP
  Polyclonal gammopathy (HIV)
  Increased SGOT/SGPT (EBV,CMV, Q fever, psittacosis, toxoplasmosis, relapsing fever, brucellosis)
  Increased alkaline phosphatase (TB)

Abbreviations: CBC, complete blood count; CMV, cytomegalovirus; CNS, central nervous system; CSF, cat scratch fever; CVA, cardiovascular accident; EBV, Epstein-Barr virus; ESR, erythrocyte sedimentation rate; HCV, hepatitis C virus; HIV, human immunodeficiency virus; LGV, lympho-granuloma venereum; RSV, respiratory syncytial Virus; SBE, subacute bacterial endocarditis; SGOT/SGPT, serum glutamic-oxaloacetic transaminase/ serum glutamic pyruvate transaminase; SPEP, serum protein electrophoresis; TA, temporal arteritis; TB, tuberculosis.

electrophoresis (SPEP) plus an otherwise unexplained isolated explanation of the alkaline phosphatase may be the only clue pointing to a lymphoma. Either finding by itself would be not very helpful, even in the FUO context. The more nonspecific-test-abnormalities present in an FUO patient, the more likely it is that a specific diagnosis will be suggested. For example, in a patient with an elevated ferritin level and an ESR >100 mm/hr the differential is large and primarily related to neoplasms, but primarily restricted to the general categories of malignancy and collagen vascular disease. If, in addition to an elevated serum ferritin level and a highly elevated sedimentation rate, the patient also has basophilia, then collagen vascular diseases are eliminated and the diagnosis is in the general category of a neoplasm (12,15) (Tables 3–5).

TABLE 4 Focused Diagnostic Approach to Fever of Unknown Origin: Clues to Malignant Disorders

History
    Fatigue (any neoplastic disorder)
    Decreased appetite/weight loss (any neoplastic disorder)
    Headache (primary/metastatic CNS neoplasms)
    Cough (pulmonary neoplasms)
    Night sweats (any neoplastic disorder)
Physical findings
    Relative bradycardia (lymphomas)
    Sternal tenderness (preleukemias, myeloproliferative disorders, lymphoreticular malignancies)
    Pleural effusion (lymphomas, pulmonary neoplasms, metastases)
    Heart murmur (atrial myoma)
    Hepatomegaly (hematoma, metastases, lymphomas)
    Splenomegaly (leukemias, lymphomas)
    Ascites (peritoneal/omental metastases)
    Lymphadenopathy (lymphomas, CLL)
    Epididymoorchitis (lymphoma)
Nonspecific laboratory tests
CBC
    Leukocytosis (MPD, CLL)
    Leukopenia (lymphoreticular malignances)
    Anemia (any malignancy)
    Myocytes/melamyelocytes/nucleated RBCs/ "teardrop RBCs" (neoplastic bone marrow
      involvement)
    Atypical (small/uniform) lymphocytes (CLL)
    Eosinophilia (MPD, leukemias, lymphomas)
    Basophilia (MPD, leukemias, lymphomas)
    Thrombocytopenia (any malignancy with bone marrow involvement)
    Thrombocytosis (any malignancy)
ESR
    Highly elevated ESR >100 mm/hr (any neoplastic disorder)
LFTs
    Increased alkaline phosphatase (hepatomas, lymphomas, liver metastases)
SPEP
    Increased monoclonal gammopathy (multiple myeloma)
    Increased α_1/α_2 globulins (lymphomas)
Serum ferritin
    Increased ferritin levels (MPD, any malignancy)

Abbreviations: CBC, complete blood count; CLL, chronic lymphocytic lymphoma; CNS, central nervous system; ESR, erythrocyte sedimentation rate; LFT, liver function tests; MPD, myeloproliferative disorders; RBC, red blood cells; SPEP, serum protein electrophoresis.

TABLE 5   Focused Diagnostic Approach to FUO: Clues to Rheumatic Disorders

History
  Dry eyes (LORA, SLE)
  Watery eyes (PAN)
  Vision disorders/eye pain (Takayasu's arteritis, TA)
  Headache (temporal pain, TA)
  Neck pain (jaw pain, adult JRA)
  Dry cough (TA)
  Abdominal pain (PAN, SLE)
  Myalgias/arthralgias (PAN, adult JRA, FMF, LORA, SLE)
    generalized
    localized
Physical findings
Eyes
  Band keratopathy (adult JRA)
  Conjunctivitis (SLE)
  Uveitis (adult JRA, sarcoidosis, SLE)
  Dry eyes (LORA, SLE)
  Watery eyes (PAN)
  Fundi ["cytoid bodies" (SLE), "candlewax drippings" (sarcoidosis)]
  Lymphadenopathy (Kikuchi's disease, adult JRA)
  Splenomegaly (SLE, LORA, sarcoidosis, Kikuchi's disease)
  Epididymoorchitis (PAN)
Nonspecific laboratory tests
Blood tests (all rheumatic disorders)
CBC
  Leukopenia (SLE)
  Lymphopenia (sarcoidosis/lymphoma syndrome)
  Eosinophilia (sarcoidosis, PAN)
  Thrombocytopenia (SLE)
ESR
  Highly elevated ESR >100 mm/hr (all rheumatic disorders)
LFTs
  Increased SGOT/SGPT (Kikuchi's disease, adult JRA)
  Increased alkaline phosphatase (PAN)
SPEP
  Polyclonal gammopathy (SLE)
  Increased α_1/α_2 globulins (SLE)
Ferritin
  Increased ferritin levels (adult JRA, SLE, TA)

Abbreviations: ESR, erythrocyte sedimentation rate; FMF, familial Mediterranean fever; JRA, juvenile rheumatoid arthritis; LFTs, liver function tests; LORA, late onset rheumatoid arthritis; PAN, periarteritis nodosa; SGOT/SGPT, serum glutamic-oxaloacetic transaminase/serum glutamic pyruvate transaminase; SLE, systemic lupus erythematosus; SPEP, serum protein electrophoresis; TA, temporal arteritis.

IMAGING TESTS

Imaging tests have an important role in the FUO workup, particularly in identifying malignant versus infectious etiologies. Cardiac echocardiography is helpful in diagnosing endocarditis or atypical myomas (12,15). Gallium/indium scans can identify only malignancy/infection.

As nonspecific laboratory tests should be combined to increase diagnostic specificity, so can aspects of the history and physical examination. The key clinical point is that a syndromic diagnosis based on combining key findings in the history, physical examination, and nonspecific laboratory tests can direct the diagnostic evaluation and prompt specific and definitive testing to determine the cause of the FUO. Computed tomography/magnetic resonance imaging (CT/MRI) scans can provide further anatomical definition of abnormalities detected on gallium/indium/positron emission tomography (PET) scans. Alternately, total body/regional CT/MRI scans can identify/rule out malignancy/infection. Most causes of FUO can be diagnosed by noninvasive means. Some causes of FUO require tissue/pathological confirmation. Nonspecific tests indicate/locate the tissue to be biopsied to arrive at a definitive diagnosis (26–32).

REFERENCES

1. Petersdorf RG, Beeson PB. Fever of unexplained origin: report on 100 cases. Medicine (Baltimore) 1961; 40:1–30.
2. Louria DB. Fever of unknown etiology. Del Med J 1971; 43:343–348.
3. Weinstein L. Clinically benign fever of unknown origin: a personal retrospective. Rev Infect Dis 1985; 7:692–699.
4. Murray HW, ed. FUO: Fever of Undetermined Origin. Mount Kisco, NY, Futura Publishing, 1983.
5. Kauffman CA, Jones PG. Diagnosing fever of unknown origin in older patients. Geriatrics 1984; 39:46–51.
6. Kazanjian PH. Fever of unknown origin. Review of 86 patients treated in community hospital. Clin Infect Dis 1992; 15:968–973.
7. Knockaert DC, Vanneste LJ, Vannester SB, et al. Fever of unknown origin in the 1980s: an update of the diagnostic spectrum. Arch Intern Med 1992; 152:51–55.
8. Knockaert DC, Vanneste LJ, Bobbears HJ. Fever of unknown origin in elderly patients. J Am Geriatr Soc 1993; 41:1187–1192.
9. Cunha BA. Fever of unknown origin. Infect Dis Clin North Am 1996; 10:111–128.
10. Cunha BA. Fever of unknown origin. In: Gorbach SL, Bartlett JG, Blacklow NE, eds. Infectious Diseases. 3rd ed. Philadelphia: Lippincott Williams and Wilkins, 2004: 1568–1577.
11. Brusch JL, Weinstein L. Fever of unknown origin. Med Clin North Am 1988; 72: 1247–1261.
12. Sen P, Louria DB. Noninvasive and diagnostic procedures and laboratory methods. In: Murray HW, ed. FUO: Fever of Undetermined Origin. Mount Kisco, NY, Futura Publishing, 1983:159–190.
13. Ravel R. Clinical Laboratory Medicine. 6th ed. New York: Mosby, 1995.
14. Wallach J. Interpretation of Diagnostic Tests. 7th ed. Philadelphia: Lippincott Williams and Wilkins, 2000.
15. Cunha BA. Diagnostic significance of nonspecific laboratory abnormalities in infectious diseases. In: Gorbach SL, Bartlett JG, Blacklow NE, eds. Infectious Diseases. 3rd ed. Philadelphia: Lippincott Williams and Wilkins, 2004:158–165.
16. Shafiq M, Cunha BA. Diagnostic significance of lymphopenia. Infect Dis Pract 1999; 23:81–82.
17. Sullivan CL, Cunha BA. The significance of eosinophilia in infectious disease. Hosp Pract 1989; 25:21–27.
18. Cunha BA. The diagnostic significance of thrombocytosis and thrombocytopenia in infectious disease. Infect Dis Pract 1995; 19:68.
19. Tietz NW, ed. Clinical Guide to Laboratory Tests. 4th ed. Philadelphia: WB Saunders, 2006.
20. Cunha BA. The diagnostic significance of erythrocyte sedimentation rate. Intern Med 1992; 13:48–51.
21. Krol V, Cunha BA. Diagnostic significance of serum ferritin levels in infectious and non-infectious diseases. Infect Dis Pract 2003; 27:196–197.
22. Beyan E, Beyan C, Demirezer A, et al. The relationship between ferritin levels and disease activity in systemic lupus erythematosus. Scand J Rheumatol 2003; 32:225–228.

23. Cunha BA. Fever of unknown origin caused by adult juvenile rheumatoid arthritis: the diagnostic significance of double quotidian fevers and elevated serum ferritin levels. Heart Lung 2004; 33;417–421.
24. Schwarz-Eywill M, Helig B, Bauer H, et al. Evaluation of serum ferritin as a marker for adult Still's disease activity. Ann Rheum Dis 1992; 51:683–685.
25. Cunha BA, Parchuri S, Mohan S. Fever of unknown origin: temporal arteritis presenting with persistent cough and elevated serum ferritin levels. Heart Lung 2006; 35: 112–116.
26. Peters AM. Nuclear medicine imaging in fever of unknown origin. Q J Nucl Med 1999; 43:61–73.
27. Datz FL, Anderson CE, Ahluwalia R, et al. The efficacy of indium-111 polyclonal IgG for the detection of infection and inflammation. J Nucl Med 1994; 35:74–83.
28. Hilson AJW, Maisey MN. Gallium-67 scanning in pyrexia of unknown origin. Brit Med J 1979; 2:1130–1131.
29. Knockaert DC, Mortelmans LA, De Roo MC, et al. Clinical value of gallium-67 scintigraphy in evaluation of fever of unknown origin. Clin Infect Dis 1994; 18:601–605.
30. Quinn MJ, Sheedy PF II, Stephen DH, et al. Computed tomography of the abdomen in evaluation of patients with fever of unknown origin. Radiology 1980; 136:407–411.
31. Rowland MD, Del Bene VE. Use of body computed tomography to evaluate fever of unknown origin. J Infect Dis 1987; 156:408–409.
32. Blockmans D, Knockaert D, Maes A, et al. Clinical value of [(18)F] fluorodeoxyglucose positron emission tomography or patients with fever of unknown origin. Clin Infect Dis 2001; 32:191–196.

3 Fever of Unknown Origin in Children

Leonard R. Krilov

Division of Pediatric Infectious Disease, Winthrop-University Hospital, Mineola, New York, U.S.A.

Febrile illnesses are much more common in children than adults, but most episodes of fever are short-term and resolve spontaneously, and/or are associated with a detectable source of infection. Considerations of fever of unknown origin (FUO) in childhood are loosely based on Petersdorf and Beeson's 1961 definition in adults of ≥3 weeks of illness with fever >101°F (38.3°C) on several occasions persisting without diagnosis, despite medical evaluation (1). Series of pediatric patients with unexplained fever have used shorter duration (≥8 days) of fever without explanation after initial evaluation (2–6).

There are other, related fever syndromes in children that should be distinguished from FUO in that they present differently and require different approaches to diagnosis and treatment. These include fever without focus, including occult bacteremia, and recurrent fever syndromes. In the former situation, studies suggested that 5% to 10% of nontoxic young children (3 to 24 months of age) with acute onset of fever [temperature >102°F (39.4°C)], leukocytosis [white blood count (WBC) > 15,000 mm^3], and absence of localized findings may be at risk for bacteremia most often secondary to *Streptococcus pneumonia* or *Hemophilus influenzae* Type b (Hib) infection (7,8). This is an acute illness and raises issues about the need for empiric antibiotics in at-risk children. Since the introduction of conjugate Hib and *Streptococcus pneumoniae* (Prevnar) vaccines into the routine childhood immunization schedule, the incidence of this occult bacteremia syndrome has decreased dramatically, suggesting the potential to avoid empiric antibiotic therapy in this setting (9). The risk of these cases of occult bacteremia progressing to sepsis and/ or meningitis was low even in the preconjugated vaccine era.

Children with cyclical or recurrent fevers should also be defined separately from FUO in that different diagnostic considerations apply, and hence, different approaches to the evaluation are employed. Irregular episodes of febrile illnesses raise issues of recurrent infections and possible immune deficiency syndromes, inflammatory bowel disease, or systemic onset juvenile rheumatoid arthritis. Episodes of fever that occur in predictable cyclical intervals, with each episode typically <8 days' duration, might lead to consideration of FAPA (fever, abdominal pain, pharyngitis, adenitis and/or aphthous ulcers) syndrome (10), familial Mediterranean fever (11), cyclical neutropenia (12), and hyper-IgD syndrome (13). Although there are no definite diagnostic criteria for FAPA syndrome, episodes usually occur in three- to four-week cycles that are so regular parents can predict the timing of the next fever. Children with this diagnosis are entirely well between episodes, and no one around them gets ill before or after them, as a rule. This may be the most common recurrent-fever syndrome in otherwise healthy children. The other recurrent-fever syndromes are much less common and beyond the scope of this review.

Evaluation of the child with prolonged fever or FUO begins with a detailed history that includes information on duration of fever, height of fevers, pattern, response to antipyretics, localizing symptoms, nonspecific findings (e.g., irritability, lethargy, per orally intake), ill contacts, travel or visitors from abroad, animal and insect exposures, sexual activity, and medication use.

Physical examination of the child with FUO begins with a definition and documentation of fever. A rectal temperature of up to 101.3°F (38.5°C) in the younger children, especially later in the day and/or after exercise, may be considered normal in the well-appearing child. In addition to a complete general physical examination, certain features of the evaluation should be specifically emphasized in looking for a focus of inflammation. Examples include palpation for a tender tooth, careful observation for oral ulcers, auscultation for a new onset or changing heart murmur, and palpation for lymphadenopathy. A plotting of growth parameters and a review of prior growth curves may also be revealing. Serial examinations may also be helpful in detecting changes over time, as well as in monitoring for weight loss.

In two pediatric studies, abnormal physical findings were reported to contribute to diagnosis in 60% of the cases of FUO analyzed (2,3). Cutaneous changes, significant heart murmur, joint abnormalities, hepatomegaly and/or splenomegaly were the findings that contributed to diagnosis.

Laboratory investigations in the child with FUO are aimed at assessing general measures of inflammation and specific tests (often serologies and/or cultures) are aimed at ascertaining a specific etiology (Table 1). The choice of serologies and cultures may be determined in part by aspects of the history (e.g., travel, animal, or insect exposure) or physical examination (e.g., new heart murmur, swollen joint). General screening tests might include complete blood count (CBC), erythrocyte sedimentation rate (ESR), C-reactive protein (CRP), renal and hepatic profiles, urinalysis, and stool for occult blood and white blood cell analyses.

TABLE 1 Approach to the Laboratory Evaluation in the Child with Fever of Unknown Origin

---

Screening tests
  Complete blood count
  Acute phase reactants (erythrocyte sedimentation rate, C-reactive protein)
  Renal and hepatic profiles
  Stool for occult blood and white blood cells
  Urinalysis
  Abdominal ultrasound
Tests for specific infections
  Urine culture and sensitivity
  Additional cultures (stool, blood)
  Epstein-Barr virus serology; other viral agents
  Mantoux tuberculin skin test
Additional tests based on history (e.g., travel, animal exposure), physical exam, laboratory screening tests
  Thick and thin smears (malaria, babesia)
  Additional serologies (e.g., Lyme, HIV, bartonella)
  Imaging studies (e.g., chest radiograph, CAT scans, MRIs, radionucleotide studies)
  Biopsies (e.g., lymph node, bone marrow)

Abbreviations: CBC, complete blood count; HIV, human immunodeficiency virus; CAT, computed axial tomography; MRI, magnetic resonance imaging.

Imaging studies may be used to localize or better define an abnormality appreciated on physical examination. In the absence of a suspected or detected abnormality, however, routine radiographs are of low yield and are not routinely useful in the evaluation of the child with FUO, with the possible exception of an abdominal ultrasonogram (4). In the more severely ill child, on the other hand additional invasive studies and scans may aid in the diagnosis (14). Computed axial tomography (CAT) scans, magnetic resonance imaging (MRI), and/or nuclear medicine scans should be performed judiciously and in consultation with a radiologist in this setting. Biopsies of bone marrow, abnormal masses, or lymph nodes may be useful in this setting, although in the absence of an ill appearance or hematological abnormalities, bone marrow examination is not generally warranted (15).

The potential causes of FUO in children parallel those observed in series of adults with this diagnosis (Table 2). The distribution, however, is somewhat different in children, with viral infection being the predominant diagnosis in such cases and spontaneous recovery being the usual outcome. Additionally, >50% to 60% of pediatric FUO cases remain without definitive diagnosis. A long-term follow-up (5 plus years after presentation) study showed that these children remained well and that their fevers resolved even in the absence of a specific diagnosis (16). Furthermore, in older studies, infectious diseases such as sinusitis, pyelonephritis, and osteomyelitis were described. These are less common findings in more recent series of pediatric FUO cases. With newer diagnostic modalities and identification of new diseases, cat scratch disease, Epstein-Barr virus infection, and human immunodeficiency virus (HIV) infection have been identified as causes of FUO in children (5,6).

It is also important to consider age-related differences in diagnostic considerations for children with FUO. In children >6 years of age, collagen vascular diseases [most commonly systemic onset juvenile rheumatoid arthritis (JRA)] and inflammatory bowel disease (Crohn's disease and ulcerative colitis) are potentially important considerations. In children with JRA, rheumatoid factor is often not detectable on laboratory examination. Malignancies are less likely to present as FUO in children than those reported in adult series, but consideration of leukemia, lymphoma, neuroblastoma, and other cancers is warranted, especially in the presence of unexplained weight loss, anemia, masses on physical examination, or elevated lactic acid dehydrogenase (LDH) or uric acid.

Thus, FUO in children, as in adults is a challenging condition for the clinician. It is also a prime example of how careful attention to patient history, physical examination, and appropriate use of laboratory studies can be used to make the appropriate diagnosis or to offer reassurance in the absence of diagnosis that the prognosis is generally good.

TABLE 2 Differential Diagnosis of Fever of Unknown Origin in Children

Infections
Systemic—tuberculosis, typhoid fever, viral syndrome (e.g., EBV infection), cat scratch disease
Focal—e.g., dental abscess, urinary tract infection, pyelonephritis, infectious endocarditis, abscess (e.g., perirectal), osteomyelitis, sinusitis
Inflammatory bowel disease (Crohn's disease, ulcerative colitis)
Rheumatologic (systemic onset juvenile rheumatoid arthritis, Kawasaki disease)
Drug fever
Unknown

Abbreviation: EBV, Epstein-Barr virus.

REFERENCES

1. Petersdorf RG, Beeson PB. Fever of unexplained origin: Report on 100 cases. Medicine 1961; 40:1–30.
2. Pizzo PA, Lovejoy FH, Smith DH. Prolonged fever in children: Review of 100 cases. Pediatrics 1975; 55:468–475.
3. Lohr JA, Hendley JO. Prolonged fever of unknown origin: A record of experiences with 521 childhood patients. Clin Pediatr 1977; 16:768–772.
4. Steele RW, Jones SM, Lowe BA, et al. Usefulness of screening procedures for diagnosis of fever of unknown origin in children. J Pediatr 1991; 119:526–530.
5. Jacobs RF, Schutze GE. *Bartonella henselae* as a cause of prolonged fever and fever of unknown origin in children. Clin Infect Dis 1998; 26:80–84.
6. Chantada G, Casak S, Plata JD, et al. Children with fever of unknown origin in Argentina: An analysis of 113 cases. Pediatr Infect Dis J 1994; 13:260–263.
7. McCarthyPL,Grundy GW, Spiegel SZ, et al. Bacteremia in children: An outpatent review. Pediatrics 1976; 57:861–868.
8. Teele DW, Pelton SI, Grant AJ, et al. Bacteremia in febrile children under 2 years of age: Results of cultures of blood of 600 consecutive febrile children in a "walk-in" clinic. J Pediatr 1975; 81:227–234.
9. Stoll ML, Rubin LG. Incidence of occult bacteremia among highly febrile young children in the era of pneumococcal conjugate vaccine. Arch Pediatr Adolesc Med 2004; 158:671–675.
10. Thomas KT, Fede HM, Lawton AR, et al. Periodic fever syndrome in children. J Pediatr 1999; 135:15–21.
11. Ehrenfeld EN, Eliakin M, Rachmilewitz M. Recurrent polyserositis (familial Mediterranean fever, periodic disease): A report of 55 cases. Am J Med 1961; 31:107–123.
12. Wright DG, Dale DC, Fauci AS, et al. Human cyclic neutropenia: Clinical review and long term follow up of patients. Medicine 1981; 60:1–13.
13. Gross C, Schnetzer JR, Ferrante A, et al. Children with hyperimmunoglobulinemia D and periodic fever syndrome. Pediatr Infect Dis 1996; 15:72–77.
14. Opsimos H, Dadiz R, Schroeder SA, et al. Ten-month old boy with persistent fever and a chest mass. J Pediatr 2005; 146:267–272.
15. Hayani A, Mahoney DH, Fernbach DJ. Role of bone marrow examination in the child with prolonged fever. J Pediatr 1990; 116:919–920.
16. Miller LC, Sisson BA, Tucker LB, et al. Prolonged fevers of unknown origin in children: Patterns of presentation and outcome. J Pediatr 1996; 12:419–423.

4 Fever of Unknown Origin in Cirrhosis

Ariff Admani and Leon G. Smith

Department of Medicine, Saint Michael's Medical Center, Newark, New Jersey, U.S.A.

INTRODUCTION

Over 100 years ago, it was reported that fever could be directly attributed to cirrhosis of the liver. The concept of fever attributed solely to cirrhosis, however, has not been universally accepted. Fever in a cirrhotic patient is often a matter of great concern. Numerous diagnostic maneuvers, including cultures, blood tests, imaging studies, and, on occasion, invasive procedures are employed to ascertain the cause of fever.

Cirrhotic fever could be defined as fever of undiagnosed etiology occurring in the patient with cirrhosis in the absence of an identified infection, malignancy, collagen vascular disease, alcoholic hepatitis, pancreatitis, tuberculosis, fungal infection, or drug fever. Fever attributed to cirrhosis is often low-grade, protracted, unaccompanied by focal signs and symptoms, and less likely to be associated with tachycardia and tachypnea than in patients with infections. Biliary cirrhosis and alcoholic cirrhosis tend to produce higher fevers (1).

The pathogenesis of fever of cirrhosis has not been fully elucidated. It may be related to hepatic necrosis or inflammation and to altered hepatic metabolism of steroids. Elevated levels of endotoxins and cytokines, for example, tumor necrosis factor-alpha (TNF-alpha), interleukin-1-beta (IL-1-beta), and interleukin-6 (IL-6), have also been demonstrated in patients with cirrhosis and may be involved in the pathogenesis of low-grade fever observed in cirrhosis (1).

The first formal definition of FUO to attain broad acceptance was one proposed by Petersdorf and Beeson four decades ago: "fever higher than 101°F (38.3°C) on several occasions, persisting without diagnosis for at least three weeks in spite of at least one week's investigation in hospital." (2).

FUO is currently classified into four distinct subclasses: classic FUO, nosocomial FUO, immune-deficient FUO, and human immunodeficiency virus (HIV)-associated FUO.

FUO in cirrhosis is classified under miscellaneous causes of fever.

The initial evaluation of the patient with FUO typically includes a comprehensive history, repeated physical examinations, and a host of laboratory investigations. The first step in evaluating, the patient is to verify the presence of fever. The importance of this step is self-evident and yet, all too often, overlooked.

Although fever patterns are rarely diagnostic, they may contain diagnostically useful information and should, therefore, be examined carefully. Cirrhosis associated with a liver abscess maybe associated with a double-quotidian spike (am and pm spike).

The prognosis of FUO is determined by both the cause of the fever and the underlying disease or diseases on which the disorder is superimposed. The time required to make the diagnosis is less important. Patients in whom FUO remains undiagnosed after extensive evaluation generally have a favorable outcome, characteristically with resolution of their fever in four or more weeks without sequelae.

CIRRHOSIS-CAUSING FEVER—NONINFECTIOUS

Fifty consecutive patients with fever and cirrhosis were prospectively studied to assess if cirrhotic fever was a true clinical entity and to determine its characteristics and outcome (1).

In 20% (10) of the 50 patients, an identifiable source of fever or infection was not documented (these patients were defined as having cirrhotic fever). The patients with cirrhotic fever were significantly less toxic, as indicated by lower temperature, tachycardia, and tachypnea, but had a fever of longer duration than did patients with infectious fever. Patients with cirrhotic fever were significantly less likely to have focal signs or symptoms or a portal of infection confirmed by culture as compared with patients with infectious fever. Outcome (at 30 days or long term) was not different for patients with cirrhotic fever versus patients with infectious fever or matched controls that did not have fever. Eight (80%) of the 10 patients with cirrhotic fever underwent transplantation: Fever did not recur after transplantation in any of these patients.

Thus, fever in up to 20% of the febrile patients with cirrhosis may be attributable to cirrhosis itself; such patients may be spared the ongoing diagnostic maneuvers and unnecessary trials of antibiotics.

INFECTIONS IN CIRRHOTICS

Infectious complications in cirrhotic patients can cause severe morbidity and mortality. Bacterial infections are estimated to cause up to 25% of deaths in cirrhotic patients (2). The most frequent are urinary tract infection, spontaneous bacterial peritonitis, respiratory tract infection, and bacteremia. It has been said that cirrhosis is the most common form of acquired immunodeficiency, exceeding even AIDS. The specific risk factors for infection in cirrhotic patients are low serum albumin, gastrointestinal bleeding, intensive care unit admission for any cause, and therapeutic endoscopy. Certain infectious agents are more virulent and more common in patients with liver disease. These include *Vibrio, Campylobacter, Yersinia, Plesiomonas, Enterococcus, Aeromonas, Capnocytophaga,* and *Listeria* species, as well as organisms from other species (Table 1) (spontaneous bacterial peritonitis is a frequent, severe, life-threatening complication in patients with ascites).

PERITONITIS IN CIRRHOTICS

Other entities that cause fever in cirrhosis include the following.

In adults, primary peritonitis has usually been reported in patients with cirrhosis and ascites (2). The prevalence of primary peritonitis in hospitalized patients with cirrhosis and ascites has been estimated at 10% to 30%. In cirrhotic patients, micro-organisms presumably of enteric origin account for 69% of the pathogens. *Escherichia coli* is the most frequently recovered pathogen, followed by *Klebsiella pneumoniae, Streptococcus pneumonae* and other streptococcal species, including enterococci. In a review of 126 cases of primary peritonitis in cirrhotic patients recorded in the literature, only eight patients (6%) had diseases caused by anaerobic or microaerophilic bacteria, including *Bacteriodes* spp., *Bacteriodes fragilis,*

TABLE 1   Causes of Fever in Cirrhotics

Cirrhosis
Pathogens (systemic)
Cryptococcus especially
meningitis
Tuberculosis
Listeria sp.
Streptococcus pneumoniae
Escherichia coli—especially
cholangitis
Spontaneous peritonitis
Gramnegative bacteria
Listeria sp.
S. Pneumonae
Cryptococcus sp.,
Chlamydia
Mycobacterium sp.
Anaerobes sp.
Polymycrobial
With iron overload
Salmonella sp.
Yersinia sp.
Vibrio sp.
With hyposplenic function
S. pneumoniae
Hemophilus influenzae
Type B
Babesia
Varicella-Zoster
Neisseria sp.
E. coli
Capnocytophagia (DF2)
With portal hypertension
Esophageal lesions
Candida sp.
Herpes Simplex

Clostridium perfringes, Peptostreptococcus spp., *Peptococcus* spp., and *Campylobacter fetus*. Polymicrobial infection was present in four of these eight cirrhotic patients with peritonitis caused by anaerobes, in contrast to the relatively low frequency of polymicrobial infection (only 10 of 118 cases of peritonitis) when aerobes were involved. Occasionally, peritonitis may result from infection with *Mycobacterium tuberculosis, Neisseriae gonorrhoeae, Chlamydia trachomatis,* or *Coccidioides immitis,* but this is usually the result of disseminated infection or sometimes spreads from adjacent foci of infection.

Cryptococcal peritonitis can present in two distinct patient groups:

1. Those receiving chronic ambulatory peritoneal dialysis, and
2. those with underlying liver disease and cirrhosis.

Fever in cirrhotics is also noted with hyposplenic function due to the following organisms.

Streptococcus pneumoniae—Pneumococcus is singularly the most important organism implicated in postsplenectomy sepsis (PSS), involved in 50% to 90% of cases. Although common in all age groups, the percentage of pnemococcal PSS cases increases with age. Antimicrobial drug generally tetracycline, and macrobial resistance in *S.pneumoniae* is increasingly prevalent (3).

Hemophilus influenzae—Type b *H.influenzae* (Hib) is the second most common organism related to PSS. Most Hib-associated PSS cases have occurred in children less than 15 years old. Use of the conjugated Hib vaccine has dramatically decreased the incidence of invasive Hib disease. Importantly, β-lactamase production by many *H. influenzae* strains needs accounting for choosing empirical therapy (3).

Neisseria meningitides, the meningococus, is often cited as the third most common cause of PSS. Meningococcemia does occur in the aspenic host. It is neither more frequent nor more severe in splenic or hyposplenic patients than in healthy individuals. Certainly, fulminant meningeal infection occurs in the normal host (3).

Capnocytophagia canimorsus, a fastidious gram-negative rod, formerly classified as CDC group DF-2, is part of canine and feline oral flora. It is typically transmitted to humans from dog contact, usually a bite. *C. canimorsus* infection does occur in healthy immunocompetent persons but usually is relatively mild. Asplenia and hyposplenic states seem to be predisposing factors in 80% of the reported cases. Finding gram-negative bacilli in the buffy coat or peripheral blood smear or observing an eschar at the bite site, manifesting one to seven days after the bite, suggests *C. canimorsus* as the cause of PSS (3).

Salmonella species have been associated with PSS. Severe salmonellosis is associated with the hyposplenism of chronic reticuloendothelial blockage in bartonellosis, and the infection is prominent in children with sickle-cell anemia associated with splenic dysfunction; despite these observations, the organism does not play a large role in PSS (3).

Babesiosis—Most cases of morbidity and mortality occur in the asplenic host. It is these splenectomized individuals who have a higher grade parasitemias, have significant hemolysis, and require specific treatment for the infection. Babesiosis in eusplenic persons is by and large mild or subclinical, not requiring therapy.

Ehrlichiosis—Human granulocytic ehrlichiosis, a tick-borne infection, has been reported to be recurrent, prolonged, and/or more severe in asplenic persons.

IRON OVERLOAD ASSOCIATED WITH CIRRHOSIS

In cirrhotic patients, iron overload is fairly common. Of course hemochromatosis, which produces cirrhosis, has severely elevated iron levels. There are three organisms that thrive when the iron levels are elevated, namely, *Salmonella*, *Yersinia*, and *Vibrio* species (2). These organisms can cause fever and remain hidden in foci such as prostate, spleen, bone aneurysm, bowel, and other remote areas. Finding their foci can be difficult, even with detailed modern screening.

PORTAL HYPERTENSION

Cirrhotic patients with portal hypertension and varice which can also be accompanied by herpes simplex, often have severe esophagus lesions, which can contain *Candida* species, herpex simplex. However it is extremely rare to have fever from this source unless there is an erosive lesion present.

MENINGITIS IN CIRRHOTIC PATIENTS

Cryptococcal meningitis in cirrhotic patients presents with and without fever and no stiff neck. The diagnosis is difficult. Tuberculosis meningitis can produce the same findings. In cirrhotics with FUO a spinal fluid examination is extremely important. The serum and spinal fluid cryptococcal antigen is usually positive. Listeria meningitis can also occur in cirrhosis.

CIRRHOSIS WITH CHOLANGITIS—CHARCOT'S FEVER

This is a rare event. Charcot's fever with shaking chills is the most common presentation. The common duct may be partially obstructed or dilated. Gallstones are often present. *E. coli* bacteremia is the most common pathogen and process.

Vibrio vulnificus (2) is part of the normal marine flora and, in the temperate zones, reaches sufficient concentration to cause clinical illness only in the warmer months of the year. Nearly all oysters harvested in the summer from the Chesapeake Bay contain this pathogen, as do 10% of crabs. It is primarily associated with a severe, distinctive soft-tissue infection and/or septicemia rather than a diarrheal disease. It may produce purpura fulminans.

Yersinia enterocolitica (2) is a gram-negative bacillus that thrives in conditions associated with iron overload, and leads to the formation of multiple liver and spleen abscesses. Liver biopsy reveals moderate fibrosis and early cirrhosis, with large amounts of hemosiderin granules deposited in hepatocytes and bile duct epithelium.

SUMMARY

Patients with cirrhosis who have fever present a challenge to the physician. The literature is sparse about the differential diagnosis of fever in such patients. This article has compiled accumulated data and clinical experience on the subject.

REFERENCES

1. Singh N, Yu VL, Wagener MM, et al. Cirrhotic fever in the 1990s: a prospective study with clinical implications. Clin Infect Dis 1997; 24(6):1135–1138.
2. Mandell GL, Bennett JE, Dolin R. Principles and Practice of Infectious Diseases. 5th ed, ch. 44. 622–631, 2000.
3. Sumaraju V, Smith LG, Smith SM. Infectious complications in asplenic hosts. Infect Dis Clin North Am 2001; 15(2):551–565 x review, 1989.

5 Fever of Unknown Origin in Malignancies

Burke A. Cunha

Infectious Disease Division, Winthrop-University Hospital, Mineola, New York, U.S.A.

OVERVIEW

Malignancies have superseded infections as the most common cause of fever of unknown origin (FUO). In Petersdorf's classic paper on FUO, published in 1961, infectious diseases were the most common etiology of FUO, and neoplasms constituted the second most frequent category. This shift from infectious to malignant etiology as the most frequent cause of FUO is related to several factors. Firstly, due to the widespread introduction of computed tomography (CT) and magnetic resonance imaging (MRI), many intra-abdominal causes of infection are diagnosed early and therefore do not meet the definition of prolonged fever required to make the diagnosis of FUO. Secondly, radionucleotide imaging studies, that is, indium scans, gallium scans, and bone scans, have been useful in identifying occult malignancies undetectable by other means. Thirdly, transthoracic echocardiography (TTE) and transesophageal echocardiography (TEE) have helped to identify those cases of atrial myxoma presenting as FUO. Lastly, the population is aging, and malignancies are more common in the elderly population. The combination of these factors has resulted in malignancies becoming the most frequent overall cause of FUO in adults (1–12).

PATHOPHYSIOLOGY OF FEVER WITH NEOPLASTIC FUOs

Most malignancies are not associated with fever: A few malignancies are associated with acute or subacute fevers, and fewer yet are associated with prolonged fevers that may present as FUOs. Malignancies may cause fever directly or indirectly. Malignancies may cause fever indirectly by compression/obstruction of a hollow viscus, with subsequent infection and an increase in temperature due to the infectious component. Another way neoplasms cause fever indirectly is perforation of a hollow viscus. Perforation of an intra-abdominal viscus results in peritonitis, the severity of which is related to the size of the perforation and location in the gastrointestinal tract or pelvis.

Malignancies may cause fever directly via cytokine production. Infections elicit a different cytokine response than do neoplasms, that is, interleukins are released in infection, whereas tumor necrosis factor is the usual mechanism of fever from neoplasms. Fever may also be multifactorial and due to the neoplasm itself and/or indirect mechanisms. In the patients with FUO due to malignancies, the innate ability of the neoplasm to produce cytokines is the most common etiology. The fever generated by malignancies presenting as FUOs is either of the prolonged, low-grade variety or it may be a high-grade spiking fever that mimics infection (10–12) (Table 1).

TABLE 1 Fevers in Neoplastic Disorders

Commonly associated with fever	Rarely associated with fever
High-grade fevers (>102°F)	CML
Hodgkin's lymphoma	CLL
Non-Hodgkin's lymphoma	Multiple myeloma
Hypernephromas (renal cell carcinomas)	Malignant melanoma
	Gastrointestinal malignancies
	Pancreatic carcinomas
Low-grade fevers (<102°F)	Breast carcinomas
Hepatomas	Adrenal tumors
Liver metastases (involving hypothalamus)	Sarcomas
Inflammatory breast carcinoma	CNS tumors
AML	(mostly involving the hypothalamus)
ALL	CNS metastases
Hairy cell leukemia	Testicular tumors
Preleukemias	Ovarian carcinoma
Myeloproliferative disorders	Cervical carcinoma
Castleman's disease	Skin cancers

Abbreviations: ALL, acute lymphocytic leukemia; AML, acute myelogenous leukemia; CLL, chronic lymphatic leukemia; CML, chronic myelogenous leukemia; CNS, central nervous system.
Source: From Ref. 12.

TYPES OF MALIGNANCIES PRESENTING AS FUO
Solid Tumors
FUOs due to malignancies that present as high-spiking fevers, resembling an infectious process, have been classically associated with lymphomas. Fevers of the high-spiking variety, that is, so-called "Pell-Epstein" fevers, were initially described in lymphoma patients. Either B-cell or T-cell lymphomas may present as FUOs with high-spiking fevers or low-grade, continuous fevers. Aside from lymphomas, which may present with continuous low-grade fevers, selected lymphoreticular malignancies or solid tumors are the neoplasms most likely to present as FUOs. Of the nonlymphoreticular malignancies causing FUOs, the most common neoplasms are hepatomas and hypernephromas (renal cell carcinomas). Metastatic disease of the liver or central nervous system (CNS) may also cause fever. Any involvement of the preoptic nucleus, the intrahypothalamus by a primary or secondary neoplasm will result in fever because the anterior hypothalamus mediates the febrile response. The primary hepatic tumors or metastases to the liver are also frequently associated with fever. The liver is part of the reticuloendothelial system and contains Küffer cells, which are capable of elaborating fever-producing cytokines. Splenic malignancies presenting as FUOs should properly be considered as lymphomas rather than as an histologically distinctive type of splenic malignancy. Although other solid malignancies, such as inflammatory breast carcinoma, may be associated with fevers, they do not present as FUOs because they are readily diagnosable and do not meet FUO criteria (10,11).

Pancreatic carcinomas are a rare case of solid tumors presenting as FUOs. Most patients with pancreatic carcinoma present with painless jaundice because most pancreatic carcinomas involve the head of the pancreas. In patients presenting with pancreatic carcinoma and FUO, the tumor usually involves the tail of the pancreas; in such patients, there is no jaundice to suggest the potential etiology. Furthermore, unless patients with pancreatic carcinoma are complicated with obstruction, that is, cholangitis, prolonged fevers are not a usual component of pancreatic carcinomas involving the head of the pancreas. Pancreatic carcinomas involving the tail or middle portion of the pancreas are those that may rarely present with fever as the only sign of the malignancy and present as an FUO (10,13–16).

Another solid malignancy that rarely presents as FUO is atrial myxoma. Atrial myxomas are more common in the left atrium than in the right atrium and are often confused with subacute bacterial endocarditis (SBE) in patients with a heart murmur and prolonged fever. Patients with atrial myxoma usually present with symptoms similar to SBE or malignancy, that is, fever, weight loss, night sweats, and fatigue. Laboratory abnormalities, for example, thrombocytosis, highly elevated erythrocyte sedimentation rate (ESR) ≥100 mm/hr, also may mimic SBE or another malignancy. As with SBE, atrial myxomas may present with embolic phenomena. Atrial myxomas are rarely infected, therefore the possibility of atrial myxoma and SBE is exceedingly rare. Metastatic disease of the heart usually presents with cardiac arrhythmia rather than as prolonged, unexplained fever (17–20).

Lymphoreticular Malignancies

The group of lymphoreticular disorders most likely to present as FUO include preleukemias secondary to acute myelogenous leukemia (AML) or preleukemia as part of a myeloproliferative disorder (MPD). During blast crises, acute leukemias are often associated with fever in the absence of infection. Because patients with acute leukemias have systemic symptoms, they usually seek medical attention early, and the diagnosis is made on the basis of abnormal blast cells in the peripheral smear or bone marrow aspirate. Such patients do not remain undiagnosed for sufficient time to present as FUOs. In contrast, patients with preleukemia may present with fever as the sole manifestation of their underlying preleukemic state. By definition, patients with preleukemia do not have blasts in the peripheral smear, but, in some cases, immature cells, that is, nucleated red cells or myelocytes/metamyelocytes may be present and are a clue to an underlying myelocystic problem. A blast crisis is often the final common pathway for many malignancies that have been previously treated with radiation therapy or chemotherapy.

An AML blast crisis is a not an uncommon complication of malignancies previously treated. Preleukemia preceding AML or MPD, are the most common clinical scenarios in this population of patients presenting as FUOs. MPD itself may also present as FUO. However, in patients with MPD presenting with fevers, the diagnosis of AML preleukemia should be considered as a diagnostic possibility (10,11,21–25).

Chronic leukemias, that is, chronic myelogenous leukemia (CML) or chronic lymphatic leukemia (CLL), are not ordinarily accompanied by sustained fevers. Patients with CLL or CML and fever should be suspected of having an infection until proven otherwise. Patients with CLL in particular are predisposed to infection due to impaired B- and T-lymphocyte dysfunction. Infections due to encapsulated and intracellular pathogens frequently complicate CLL. In patients who have CLL and without infection, the possibility of a lymphoma should be suspected. The Richter's syndrome or transformation refers to the malignant transformation in CLL patients into a lymphoma. It is the lymphoma in Richter's transformation that produces the fever in CLL. Patients with CLL and Richter's transformation may present as FUO. Although Richter's transformation is a rare complication of

TABLE 2   FUO: Neoplastic Disorders

Common causes	Uncommon causes
Hodgkin's lymphomas	CLL (Richter's transformation)
Non-Hodgkin's lymphomas	Myelodysplastic syndrome
Hepatomas	AML (preleukemia)
Hypernephromas	Rare causes
(renal cell carcinomas)	Pancreatic carcinomas
CNS/hepatic metastases	Multiple myelomas
	Arial myxomas

Abbreviations: AML, acute myelogenous leukemia; CLL, chronic lymphatic leukemia; CNS, central nervous system.

CLL, fever is a common accompaniment of CLL patients with Richter's transformation and lymphoma (26–30).

Multiple myeloma is a common lymphoreticular malignancy. Patients with multiple myeloma are predisposed to intracellular pathogens because of impaired B-lymphocyte function. Ordinarily, multiple myeloma is not accompanied by fever and therefore is a rare cause of FUO. Patients with multiple myeloma presenting with fever should be suspected as having an infection until proven otherwise. In a myeloma patient, where infection has been eliminated as a consideration and the patient presents with otherwise unexplained fevers, FUO should be considered a diagnostic possibility. In such patients, plasma-cell leukemia should be ruled out as a cause of fever. In patients with multiple myeloma who have not undergone a malignant transformation to plasma-cell leukemia, or have a neoplasm secondary to chemotherapy or radiation therapy, that is, lymphoma, FUO should be considered as a definite diagnostic possibility (11,22,23) (Table 2).

DIAGNOSTIC TESTS FOR PATIENTS WITH NEOPLASTIC FUO

In patients presenting with prolonged unexplained fevers, routine laboratory tests and selected radiologic imaging studies can be helpful in suggesting a neoplastic etiology or ruling out an infectious etiology. In FUO diagnosis, tests helpful in suggesting a neoplastic etiology include a complete blood count (CBC) with a manual differential count, ESR, serum ferritin level, serum protein electrophoresis (SPEP), and imaging tests. Patients presenting with FUOs usually have had routine radiologic tests including chest X-rays and abdominal films. A CT/MRI scan of the abdomen and pelvis is an essential part of the FUO workup. A CT/MRI scan of the head or chest or extremities is indicated if there are symptoms referable to these areas. In FUO patients with no localizing signs, gallium or indium scanning may be useful in localizing the pathological process responsible for the prolonged fever. Abnormalities detected on gallium or indium scans should be further studied using CT/MRI scanning of these areas. CT/MRI scanning of areas of indium or gallium pickup will provide further anatomical definition and may provide a clue to the nature of the underlying process. Bone scans are useful to detect otherwise unsuspected osteomyelitis or neoplastic bone involvement. Gallium scans are as sensitive and specific as bone scan, but indium scans have a high incidence of false-negatives in osteomyelitis. Patients with FUO and heart murmur should have blood cultures obtained for SBE and to rule out atrial myxoma. TTE or TEE should be obtained in such patients to detect vegetations in the case of SBE and to detect cardiac neoplasms, particularly atrial myxomas. Other diagnostic tests are also helpful (10,11,31).

In FUO patients, the Naprosyn test is particularly useful in differentiating infectious from neoplastic disorders. If, during the Naprosyn test, the patient experiences a rapid drop in temperature, then the origin of the fever is neoplastic, whereas a slight or no change in temperature suggests an infectious etiology of the fever. The Naprosyn test is especially useful in patients who have an underlying malignancy that predisposes into an infection, for example, multiple myeloma or CLL, where the etiology of the fever may be due to the underlying neoplasm or superimposed infection. The Naprosyn test helps in making this distinction and is a noninvasive, simple, and reliable way to distinguish neoplastic from infectious causes of FUO (32–35).

DIAGNOSTIC APPROACH

The diagnostic approach involves utilizing clues from the history and physical examination or routine laboratory tests to narrow diagnostic possibilities that will lead to a definitive diagnosis. Important clues are often overlooked with routine laboratory tests. In the CBC, for example, a manual differential count should be ordered and reliance not placed on an automated differential count. An automated CBC is helpful in detecting leukopenia, monocytosis, anemia, thrombocytosis, thrombocytopenia, relative lymphopenia, eosinophilia, and basophilia, all of which are potentially indicative of an underlying neoplastic disorder in a patient with FUO. None of these abnormalities, of themselves, are specific, but in concert with other tests can point to a neoplastic etiology. For example, if the CBC reveals a normal white blood cell count (WBC) with otherwise unexplained mono-cytosis and thrombocytosis, differential diagnostic possibilities are quickly limited to a chronic infectious disorder, such as osteomyelitis or SBE versus an occult neo-plasm. Otherwise unexplained eosinophilia or basophilia should at least suggest the possibility of malignancy in an FUO patient. If an infectious etiology can be ruled out as a cause of the patient's eosinophilia, that is, fungal disorders, particu-larly coccidioidomycosis or histoplasmosis, then eosinophilia might suggest vascu-litis, particularly periarteritis nodosum (PAN) or a neoplastic process. Allergic reactions are not in the differential diagnosis because the presence of a rash with a detailed drug history is usually readily diagnosed, and they do not present as pro-longed, otherwise unexplained fevers. Basophilia in a peripheral smear should immediately suggest a myeloproliferative disorder or a malignancy. Relative lym-phopenia plus eosinophilia or basophilia further increases the probability that the patient's fevers are of a neoplastic basis. A manual CBC offers advantages over an automated CBC in the detection of atypical lymphocytes and eosinophils. Atypical lymphocytes rule out the presence of a malignancy, but are not to be confused with abnormal lymphocytes, which indicate a malignancy. Atypical lymphocytes, for example, Epstein-Barr virus (EBV), cytomegalovirus (CMV), and human herpes virus-6 (HHV-6) are most often present due to a viral infection, but they are not present in all viral infections. The atypical lymphocytes associated with viral infections each have a different morphology, that is, no two lymphocytes look the same. Atypical lymphocytes are "reactive viral" lymphocytes, and do not resemble each other in their shape/morphology. In contrast, "abnormal lympho-cytes" are exactly the same and have a monotonous morphological appearance. Abnormal lymphocytes are always indicative of a lymphatic malignancy, for example, ALL or CLL. The presence of myelocytes/metamyelocytes or nucleated RBCs in the peripheral smear immediately suggests a bone marrow problem and a myelocystic process. A bone marrow biopsy should be obtained in these cases, which will be diagnostic of the neoplastic process in the bone marrow in patients with FUO. The ESR test is highly sensitive without being very specific. The diagnostic usefulness of the ESR, as with other laboratory tests, depends upon its association with other laboratory abnormalities, as well as the degree of ESR elevation. The degree of any abnormality limits diagnostic possibilities. Although many disorders are associated with an increased sedimentation rate, only six disorders are associated with a very highly elevated sedimentation rate (≥ 100 mm/hr), that is, SBE, osteomyelitis, abscess, drug fevers, collagen vascular diseases, and malignancies. It is usually relatively straightforward in an FUO patient to eliminate most of these diagnoses with simple blood and radiologic tests.

Liver function tests are also useful in limiting diagnostic possibilities. In the approach to the patient with FUO, if the clinician can localize the disorder to a particular organ/organ system, then diagnostic possibilities are limited. The pattern of organ involvement determines the differential diagnosis. Liver function tests are helpful in indicating infiltrative liver diseases characterized by moderate to high elevations of the alkaline phosphatase and γ-glutamyltransferase (GGTP) associated with normal/near normal serum transaminases. Elevations of the alkaline phosphatase/GGTP should suggest primary or metastatic liver disease, as well as non-neoplastic infiltrative liver disease, for example, fatty liver, hepatic abscesses, temporal arteritis, or biliary tract obstruction due to any cause.

Other blood tests are helpful for the FUO patient suspected of having a malignancy. SPEP abnormalities include a polyclonal gammopathy or a monoclonal spike. A monoclonal spike on the SPEP suggests multiple myeloma or Waldenström's maculoglobulinemia as the most likely diagnostic possibilities. A slight monoclonal increase may be indicative of benign gammopathy of the elderly and must be differentiated from multiple myeloma by the presence or absence of skeletal involvement, skeletal/renal involvement, and bone marrow analysis. Polyclonal gammopathy suggests impaired T-lymphocyte function and secondary reactive B-lymphocytes over reactivity manifested by excessive polyclonal gamma globulin production. Polyclonal gammopathy in an FUO patient with a murmur should suggest atrial myxoma and argues against endocarditis because SPEP abnormalities are not a feature of SBE. There are other abnormalities in the SPEP that may be useful in suggesting a malignancy. Increases in alpha I/alpha II (or α_1/α_2) in the SPEP may indicate a collagen vascular disease, or, not uncommonly, are present in patients with lymphomas. Increase in α_1/α_2 are often dismissed as acute phase reactants, but it should be recalled that acute phase reactants have long since disappeared in patients presenting with FUO, and, in this setting, elevations of the α/β globulins have a different diagnostic significance. The serum ferritin test is another extremely useful screening test for malignancy. Serum ferritin is an acute phase reactant and minimal transient elevations of the serum ferritin in an acute process are expected. However, highly elevated, persistent, ferritin levels found in FUO patients are not on the basis of acute phase reactivity. Highly elevated ferritin levels should suggest a collagen vascular disease, particularly juvenile rheumatoid arthritis (JRA). If adult JRA can be ruled out, then an otherwise highly elevated, unexplained, ferritin level should suggest malignancy until proven otherwise. Once again, it is the combination of several nonspecific tests, which, when taken together, have increased diagnostic specificity. For example, highly elevated serum ferritin level with no other findings is not as diagnostically specific as an elevated ferritin level with relative lymphopenia, myelocytes/metamyelocytes in the peripheral smear and a highly elevated ESR (10,11). Urinalysis is helpful primarily in detecting microscopic hematuria. In a patient with FUO with otherwise unexplained microscopic hematuria, the possibility of a renal cell carcinoma should be considered if benign prostatic hypertrophy and bladder tumors can be excluded.

Gallium or indium scans should be ordered early in the diagnostic workup to localize the focus of the febrile disorder. If a focal abnormality is detected by gallium or indium scanning, then a CT or MRI scan should be obtained to define the possible pathology at the site of the increased uptake. The indium and gallium scanning focus where the CT/MRI scans may be of benefit. Abdominal/pelvic CT/MRI scans should be obtained in all patients with an FUO, because there are so many processes in the abdomen/pelvis that are potentially responsible for most noninfectious and infectious disorders presenting as an FUO. The differential diagnostic possibilities can be limited if radiologic tests can localize the process to a particular organ, which in turn limits diagnostic possibilities. The Naprosyn test is another test that can direct the diagnostic workup by suggesting an infectious or neoplastic etiology in the FUO patient. The Naprosyn test should not be applied to patients with acute fevers but has proven as a useful way to determine neoplastic versus infectious fevers in the FUO population. A positive Naprosyn test, that is, a rapid fall in temperature during the three days of Naprosyn, should prompt the clinician to order a gallium or indium scan as well as an abdominal/pelvic CT/MRI scan, if not already ordered. Once the organ system is identified in the FUO process, definitive diagnostic testing is relatively straightforward. Biopsy of the liver is indicated if other laboratory tests indicate an infiltrative liver process. Renal biopsy is indicated if hypernephroma is suspected. Bone marrow biopsy is needed when a myelocystic process is identified or is suggested by immature cells in the peripheral smear. Monoclonal abnormalities on the SPEP should be followed up with a bone marrow aspirate in FUO patients. Biopsy of an atrial myxoma may be necessary for a definitive diagnosis, and certainly any lymph nodes or masses should be biopsied to confirm a pathological explanation for the FUO (10,11,36).

REFERENCES

1. Petersdorf RG, Beeson PB. Fever of unexplained origin: report on 100 cases. Medicine (Baltimore) 1961; 40:1–30.
2. Petersdorf RG. Fever of unknown origin: an old friend revisited. Arch Intern Med 1992; 152:21–22.
3. Arnow PM, Flaherty JP. Fever of unknown origin. Lancet 1997; 350:575–580.
4. Brusch JL, Weinstein L. Fever of unknown origin. Med Clin North Am 1988; 72: 1247–1261.
5. Larson EB, Featherstone HJ, Petersdorf RG. Fever of undetermined origin: diagnosis and followup of 105 cases 1970-1980. Medicine (Baltimore) 1982; 61:269–292.
6. Kazanjian PH. Fever of unkown origin: review of 86 patients treated in community hospitals. Clin Infect Dis 1992; 15:968–973.
7. Knockaert DC, Vanneste LJ, Vanneste SB, et al. Fever of unkown origin in the 1980s. An update of the diagnostic spectrum. Arch Intern Med 1992; 152:51–55.
8. Gleckman R, Crowly M, Esposito A. Fever of unknown origin: a view from the community hospital. Am J Med Sci 1977; 274:21–25.

9. de Kleijn EM, Vandenbroucke JP, van der Meer JW, for the Netherlands FUO Study Group. Fever of unknown origin (FUO), I: a prospective multicenter study of 167 patients with FUO, using fixed epidemiologic entry criteria. Medicine (Baltimore) 1997; 76:392–400.

10. Cunha BA. Fever of unknown origin (FUO). In: Gorbach SL, Bartlett JB, Blacklow NR, eds. Infectious Diseases. 3rd ed. Philadelphia: Elsevier 2004:1568–1577.

11. Cunha BA. Fever of unknown origin. Infect Dis Clin North Am 1996; 10:111–127.

12. Cunha BA. Fever in malignant disorders. Infect Dis Pract 2004; 26:335–336.

13. Strollo S, Eisenstein L, Cunha BA. Fever of unknown origin (FUO): pancreatic carcinoma. Infect Dis Pract 2006; 30:497–498.

14. Luft FC, Rissing JP, White A, et al. Infections or neoplasm as causes of prolonged fever in cancer patients. Am J Med Sci 1969; 272:65–72.

15. Meytes D, Ballin A. Unexplained fever in hematologic disorders. Sec 2: Malignant hematologic disorders. In: Isaac B, Kernbaum S, Burke M, eds. Unexplained Fever. Boca Raton, Florida: CRC Press, 1991:209–224.

16. Klastersky J, Weerts D, Hensgens C, et al. Fever of unexplained origin in patients with cancer. Eur J Cancer 1973; 9:649–656.

17. Pinede L, Duhaut P, Loire R. Clinical presentation of left atrial cardiac myxoma. A series of 112 consecutive cases. Medicine (Baltimore) 2001; 80:159–172.

18. Revankar SG, Clark RA. Infected cardiac myxoma case report and literature review. Medicine 1998; 77:337–344.

19. Reynen K. Cardiac myxomas. N Engl J Med 1995; 333:1610–1617.

20. Savas L, Onlen Y, Kiziltan T, et al. Fever of unknown origin due to left atrial myxoma. Infect Dis Clin Pract 2006; 14:170–172.

21. Mueller PS, Terrel CL, Gertz MA. Fever of unknown origin caused by multiple myeloma: report of 9 cases. Arch Intern Med 2002; 1262:1305–1309.

22. Lambotte O, Royer B, Genet P, et al. Multiple myeloma presenting as fever of unknown origin. Eur J Intern Med 2003; 14:94–97.

23. Cunha BA, Goldstein D. Fever of unknown origin (FUO): preleukemia due to AML. Infect Dis Pract 2006; 30:540–541.

24. Oguma S, Yoshida Y, Uchino H, et al. Infection in myelodysplastic syndromes before evolution into acute nonlymphoblastic leukemia. Int J Hematol 1994; 60:129–136.

25. Cunha BA, Hamid N, Krol V, et al. FUO due to preleukemia/myelodysplastic syndrome: the diagnostic importance of monocytosis with elevated serum ferritin levels. Heart Lung 2006; 35:277–282.

26. Robertson LE, Pugh W, O'Brien S, et al. Richter's syndrome: a report on 39 patients. J Clin Oncol 1993; 11:1985–1989.

27. Armitage JO, Dick FR, Corder MP. Diffuse histocytic lymphoma complicating chronic lymphocytic leukemia. Cancer 1978; 41:422–427.

28. Foucar K, Rydell RE. Richter's syndrome in chronic lymphocytic leukemia. Cancer 1980; 46:118–34.

29. Giles FJ, O'Brien S, Keating M. Chronic lymphocytic leukemia in (Richter's) transformation. Semin Oncol 1998; 25:117–125.

30. Cunha BA, Mohan S, Parachuri S. FUO: CLL vs. lymphoma (Richter's transformation). Heart Lung 2005; 34:437–441.

31. Krol V, Cunha BA. Diagnostic significance of serum ferritin levels in infectious and noninfectious diseases. Infect Dis Pract 2003; 27:196–197.

32. Chang JC, Gross HM. Utility of naproxen in the differential diagnosis of fever of undetermined origin in patients with cancer. Am J Med 1984; 76:597–603.

33. Chang JC, Gross HM. Neoplastic fever responds to the treatment of an adequate dose of naproxen. J Clin Oncol 1985; 3:551–558.

34. Chang JC. How to differentiate neoplastic fever from infectious fever in patients with cancer: usefulness of the naproxen test. Heart Lung 1987; 16:122–127.

35. Remé P, Cunha BA. NSAIDS and the Naprosyn test in FUOs. Infect Dis Pract 2000; 24:32.

36. Cunha BA. Diagnostic significance of nonspecific laboratory tests in infectious diseases. In: Bartlett JG, Blacklow NR, eds. Infectious Diseases. 3rd ed. Baltimore: Lippincott Williams 2004:158–166.

6

Fever of Unknown Origin in Febrile Leukopenia

Anastasia Antoniadou and Helen Giamarellou

Fourth Department of Internal Medicine of Athens University Medical School, University General Hospital ATTIKON, Athens, Greece

OVERVIEW

Definitions, Epidemiological Features, Risk Factors

As the first cellular component of the inflammatory response and a key component of innate immunity, neutrophils are the first line of defense against infection (1). Nearly 40 years ago, Bodey et al. reported that the risk of infection increases significantly when the absolute neutrophil count is reduced to <500 cells/mm^3 (2). Neutropenia defined as neutrophils of <500/mm^3 remains the best characterized and most prominent form of immunocompromise in patients undergoing treatment for cancer, either solid tumors or hematological malignancies. It is the leading cause of infectious complications in patients receiving antineoplastic chemotherapy, accounting for the majority of chemotherapy-associated mortalities and compromising treatment outcomes by causing dose reductions and treatment delays.

Neutropenia blunts the inflammatory response to nascent infections, allowing bacterial multiplication and invasion and compromising the mounting of clinically apparent inflammatory responses, except from the presentation of fever (1). Sickle et al. demonstrated early the lack of typical manifestations of infections in neutropenic patients. In their study, 84% of patients with pneumonia and an adequate neutrophil count (>1000/mm^3) produced purulent sputum, compared to only 8% of those with pneumonia and severe neutropenia (<100/mm^3) (3). In a prospective study of 1001 cancer patients with febrile neutropenia, Pizzo et al. reported that only 45% of those with documented bacteremia had signs of infection other than fever (4). When neutrophils were <100/mm^3, purulent exudates in patients with pharyngitis were present in 22%; dysuria, frequency, and pyuria were present in 44%, 33%, and 11%, respectively, of patients with urinary tract infections, while clinical signs of meningeal inflammation were absent in meningitis and fluctulence from perineal abscesses (3,4). Fever can be the only sign of infection, and 60% of febrile episodes in neutropenic patients are initially considered as FUOs. Since 70% of these FUOs respond to empirical antimicrobial treatment, it is likely that many of these episodes represent undetected infections, which, if left untreated, share a considerable mortality, especially if they represent an occult gram-negative bacteremia (5).

Febrile leukopenia and, most precisely, febrile neutropenia represent a syndrome comprising two components, as defined by the Infectious Diseases Society of America (IDSA) (6) and the Immunocompromised Host Society (IHS) (7). Fever is defined as an oral temperature of 101°F (38.3°C) in a single measurement or a temperature of 100°F (38.0°C) lasting for ≥ 1 hour. IHS and other scientific societies (8) add also as a criterion of fever the presence of an oral temperature of 38.3°C=101°F measured twice in 12 hours. Fever as a manifestation of infection or inflammation is not blunted in neutropenic patients, because the proinflammatory cytokines necessary for its production are released from many types of cells (macrophages, lymphocytes, fibroblasts, epithelial, and endothelial cells) (9). In the context of febrile neutropenia, every effort should be made to exclude fever related to uninfectious causes (drug fever, disease fever, transfusion related, etc.). Rectal measurement of temperature should be avoided (along with other rectal-related procedures, such as rectal examination, enema, or endoscopy), because it may serve as a portal of entry for micro-organisms, especially in patients with mucositis (diarrhea is the common presentation), hemorrhoids, or other topical lesions. Occasionally, the presence of fever can be blunted by immunosuppressive therapies (e.g., corticosteroids) or in very old, or in patients in shock (10).

Neutropenia is defined as an absolute neutrophil count of either ≤ 500 cells/ mm^3, or ≤ 1000 cells/mm^3 initially, predicted to decline to ≤ 500 cells/mm^3 in 24 to 48 hours.

The incidence, severity, and recovery of infection are inversely proportional to the degree or depth of neutropenia (11,12). The Common Toxicity Criteria of the National Cancer Institute delineates four grades of anticancer chemotherapy-related neutropenia: grade 0 is within normal limits (≥ 2000 cells/mm^3) and grades 1, 2, 3, and 4 are defined when the absolute neutrophil count is within the ranges of ≥ 1500 to < 2000 cells/mm^3, ≥ 1000 to < 1500 cells/mm^3, ≥ 500 to < 1000 cells/mm^3, and < 500 cells/mm^3, respectively (13).

Duration of neutropenia is another variable that bears a direct relationship to the risk of infection (14). It has been estimated (12) that all patients with grade 4 neutropenia that is prolonged for three weeks will develop an infection. Duration of neutropenia after the onset of a febrile episode also affects response to antimicrobial treatment and the incidence of complications. Neutropenia lasting seven days or less leads to 95% response rates compared to 32% in patients with neutropenia lasting more than 15 days (15).

The frequency of neutropenia is greatly influenced by the type and intensity of the chemotherapy regimen used, the type and stage of the underlying disease [high-dose chemotherapy, peripheral blood stem cells transplantation, and bone marrow transplantation (BMT) procedures, induction chemotherapy for acute myelogenous leukemia (AML)], the use of concomitant radiation therapy, the phase of therapy (greater risk in the earlier cycles), the degree of bone marrow involvement, and patient-specific factors such as age, performance status, and comorbid conditions (16). The risk of febrile episodes is increased if the neutrophil nadir at day 10 after cycle 1 of chemotherapy is < 500 cells/mm^3 (Silber's model of prediction) (17).

Febrile episodes during neutropenic periods after antineoplastic chemotherapy, either FUO or documented infections, affect overall survival, probably due to substantial delays in treatment delivery or the need for dose reductions. A study linking data from the National Cancer Institute with data from a survey in patients with aggressive nonhodgtin lymphoma found a significant association between the occurrence of febrile neutropenia, reduction in the number of cycles of cyclophosphamide + Adreamycin (hydroxydoxocubicin) + Vincristine (Oncovin) + Predrizone delivered, and lower five-year overall survival (18).

Neutropenic patients may present with other factors that further increase the risk and spectrum of potential complications, such as: (*i*) the damage of mechanical barriers by chemotherapy-induced mucositis, bleeding disorders (low platelet count) or due to the presence of invasive devices such as central venous catheters

(CVC) (implanted or not), (*ii*) the alteration of patients' own flora by multiple hospitalizations and extensive use of antimicrobials and antifungals, (*iii*) organ function alterations caused by the underlying disease (e.g., kidney or liver failure), and (*iii*) medications that affect other arms of the immune defense such as the phagocytic function or the humoral response (monoclonal antibodies, fludarabine, corticosteroids) (16,19,20–23). Recent studies point also at genetic factors that might influence the risk of infection and response to treatment in patients with neutropenia (24).

Patients with neutropenia not related to cancer, such as after a viral disease or due to drug toxicity, do not have the same risk of acute infection, probably because they retain mucosal integrity (25). Lower risk also characterizes patients with congenital neutropenia or aplastic anemia. HIV-positive patients with febrile neutropenia have a possible infectious complication but with a lower relative risk compared to those who are neutropenic after cytotoxic chemotherapy (25).

Febrile neutropenia for patients at high risk of infectious complications represents a medical emergency. In 50% of patients presenting with fever and neutropenia, an occult infection may be present, while in 20% of those with grade 4 neutropenia, bacteremia is present (26). Pseudomonal bacteremia, if untreated, bears a grave prognosis, with a 33% to 75% mortality rate within the first 24 to 48 hours (27–29). This is the reason why, since 1971, empiric use of intravenous broad-spectrum antibiotics has been introduced (30) and their initiation is immediately recommended (within the first hour after fever) in patients presenting with the syndrome of febrile neutropenia (6). Schimppff et al. showed that using this strategy, mortality from febrile neutropenia could be dramatically decreased from 60% to 70% in the 1970s to 4% to 6% in adults and 0.4% to 1% in children today (31–33). During recent years, and with the introduction of growth factors, it was realized that all febrile neutropenic patients were not the same. Patients with febrile neutropenia and a low risk for life-threatening infectious complications had a 70% chance to be treated as outpatients, with reduced costs and increased patient comfort, by orally administered broad-spectrum antimicrobial agents (16,34). Validated prediction models have been developed to distinguish patients falling into different risk categories, and they should be applied during the initial evaluation of the patient with febrile neutropenia and FUO.

Patient Risk-Assessment Stratification

Talcott et al. were the first to develop a prospectively validated risk-assessment tool (35,36). Before that only a variety of exclusion criteria for the prediction of patients at low risk for serious infectious complications had been used in studies, such as the presence of renal failure, shock, respiratory failure, HIV status, receipt of intravenous supportive therapy, allogeneic BMT, catheter-related infection, coagulase-negative *Staphylococcus* (CNS) infection or risk of death within 48 hours, postulated by Kern et al. (37), or the following factors proposed by Freifeld et al: hemodynamic instability, abdominal pain, nausea and/or vomiting, diarrhea, neurological or mental changes, new pulmonary infiltrates, catheter-related infection, and kidney or liver insufficiency (38). The clinical model by Talcott consisted of clinical factors assessable within 24 hours of admission and involved four categories of patients. Categories I, II, and III included patients at high risk: those being hospitalized at presentation of febrile neutropenia (I), outpatients who presented with serious acute comorbidity, which could have been the reason for hospitalization, independent of fever and leukopenia (II), and patients without acute comorbidity but with uncontrolled cancer (leukemia not in complete remission and other cancers, which progressed during the last assessable chemotherapy regimen (III). Complications in Groups I to III were >30% compared to 2% in Group IV, which included patients not possessing risk factors present in the other groups (35,36). Later, Klastersky et al. postulated a scoring system based on the Multinational Association for Supportive Care in Cancer (MASCC) predictive model, which consists of seven variables with a maximum score of 26 (39): (*i*) burden of illness with moderate (score 3) or mild (5) or absent symptoms (score 5), (*ii*) absence of hypotension (scores 5), (*iii*) absence of chronic obstructive pulmonary disease (4), (*iv*) presence of solid tumor (4) or no history of previous fungal infection in case of hematological malignancy (4), (*v*) outpatient status (3), (*vi*) absence of dehydration (3), and (*vii*) age less than 60 years for adults (score 2). A score of ≥21 predicts a <5% risk for severe complications. Compared to the Talcott model, it offers increased sensitivity (71% vs. 30%) and fewer miscalculations in the identification of low-risk patients at a cost of lower specificity (68% vs. 90%) (39). A prospective survey is now validating the MASCC index in a mixed population of patients with solid tumors or leukemia who present with febrile neutropenia (40,41). It seems that patients should be followed for 24 hours and considered low-risk if the index continues to have a value of ≥ 21. FUO seems to be a benign presentation, most commonly present in low-risk patients (49% vs. 35% in high-risk patients). High-risk patients are more often bacteremic with gram negatives (59% vs. 31%), and less often with gram positives (38% vs. 62%). Bacteremic high-risk patients bear a higher complication (68% vs. 24%) and mortality rate (28% vs. 2%). A 45% mortality rate accompanies high-risk patients compared to no deaths in the low-risk group (40). Differences are less impressive between high- and low-risk groups in the subpopulation of patients with gram-positive bacteremia. High-risk febrile neutropenic patients have a significantly longer duration of neutropenia and an increased incidence of complications among patients not responding to the initial empiric therapy, with no differences in complications or mortality between patients with solid tumors and those with hematological malignancies. Patients in the high-risk category (score ≤21) may not be identical: a score of 7 to 14 bears twice the mortality of a score of 19 to 20. Efforts continue for the precise identification of patients at high risk who would benefit from an aggressive therapeutic approach (40).

INITIAL PATIENT CLINICAL EVALUATION

Despite the fact that FUO, as a term, entails the absence of signs of a localized infection, clinical evaluation of the febrile neutropenic patient should be thorough and repeated daily for the duration of the febrile episode. Although signs can be minimal, it should be mentioned that the commonest sites of infection noted in patients with febrile neutropenia, observed during the first consecutive European Organization for the Research and Treatment of Cancer (EORTC) trials, are the lungs (25%), mouth and pharynx (25%), soft tissue, skin and CVC sites (15%), the perineum (10%), and, less often, the gastrointestinal and urinary tracts (5%) and the nose sinuses (5%). The sites mentioned earlier serve also as portals of entry for the offending pathogens (42).

During initial evaluation, any piece of information leading to the probable occult infection must be gathered. From a patient's history, bits include the type and timing of antineoplastic chemotherapy, environmental exposures, contact with persons with viral diseases (common cold, chickenpox, measles, etc.), administration of antibiotics or antifungals, either as prophylaxis or treatment of previous infections, known allergies and drug interactions, and recent transfusion of blood or blood products.

Physical examination should include careful search for potential sites of infection such as the oropharynx, skin and skin folds, the axilla, perineum, nails, eyes, sinuses, vascular access sites, and the lungs. If febrile neutropenia presents as FUO, physical examination initially is unrevealing, but it must be repeated daily, searching for skin nodules, ulcers, ecthyma gangrenosum, black eschars, pain in the perineum, facial or sinus pain, and swelling or eye redness, documenting clinical infection of microbial or fungal etiology. Vital signs, urine output, respiratory function parameters, and mental state should be evaluated and monitored, as hemodynamic instability, hypoxemia, and confusion are signs of clinical deterioration and life-threatening infectious complications (43).

LABORATORY EVALUATION

Laboratory evaluation of all patients with febrile neutropenia should include complete blood count and biochemical tests and two sets of blood cultures. If a CVC is present, a set of cultures drawn, one from a peripheral vein, and the others from each CVC lumen, is obligatory to serve as a diagnostic criterion of catheter-related blood stream infection, especially if differential time to positivity is used as a diagnostic method (i.e., centrally drawn blood culture becomes positive $\geq$120 minutes earlier compared to the peripherally drawn sample) (44); urine cultures are recommended even if pyuria and dysuria are absent because neutropenia blunts these signs of urinary tract infection. Expectorated sputum samples are processed and cultured even in the absence of neutrophils in a Gram stain, for the reason mentioned earlier. Cultures from other sites are sent if clinical suspicion of infection is present. Screening of normal flora is not indicated because it has not proved useful and cost effective in identifying early the causal pathogen.[0] Screening for multidrug-resistant (MDR) pathogens such as methicillin-resistant *Staphylococcus Aureus* (MRSA), vancomycin-resistant *enterococcus* (VRE), or MDR gram-negative pathogens is recommended only for infection control purposes (6).

A chest radiogram, though not expected to be abnormal even in the presence of pneumonia, should be done initially for later comparison (45). It should be repeated if FUO persists and should be accompanied by a high-resolution computed tomography (CT) of the thorax, which can reveal early signs of fungal pneumonia (the "halo sign" in lung hyphomycoses) (46–48). Right-sided abdominal pain and distention should prompt for a CT of the abdomen, which might reveal bowel wall thickening (>4 mm), indicative of typhlitis or neutropenic enterocolitis (49). An ultrasound or CT examination of the abdomen can be also useful in the case of persisting FUO after neutrophil-count recovery to normal levels, where multiple, hypodense lesions of liver and spleen are suggestive of chronic, disseminated candidiasis in the form of hepatosplenic candidiasis (a condition with no other symptoms and signs except fever, increased serum alkaline phosphatase, and negative blood cultures, that necessitates administration of antifungal treatment for the duration of the chemotherapy cycles and for $\geq$6 months afterwards) (50).

Considering that acute bacterial infections, especially bacteremic infections, have an increased rate of complication and mortality compared to FUO not representing an occult infection, it would be useful for the successful management of the febrile episode in the neutropenic patient to have markers indicative, in the case of FUO, of the infectious and bacterial origin of fever. Serum concentrations of several acute-phase proteins (C-reactive protein, serum amyloid A), proinflammatory cytokines [tumor necrosis factor-alpha (TNF-alpha), interleukin-1 (IL-1), Interferon-gamma (IFN), interleukin-6 (IL-6), interleukin-8 (IL-8)], and soluble adhesion molecules (soluble E-selectin, vascular cell adhesion molecule 1, intercellular adhesion molecule 1) have been investigated as to whether these may contribute to identifying infections as the cause of neutropenic fever. Unfortunately, at present, the predictive values of all these parameters, based on the small and inconsistent amount of data available, are too low to influence the clinically based initial treatment decisions in patients with neutropenic fever (51,52). More recently, procalcitonin (PCT), a precursor of calcitonin, has been shown to increase in systemic bacterial infection, especially if severe sepsis is present (53,54). In healthy humans, PCT levels are almost undetectable (<0.1 ng/mL) (55). PCT was measured daily for the whole duration of the febrile episode in patients with neutropenia and cancer in several studies, and it was found that it increases in serious systemic infections (values >5 ng/mL), with levels particularly elevated in patients with bacteremia and severe sepsis, while in viral or localized infections its levels remain much lower (≤0.1 ng/mL) (56–59). In one of the studies (56), blood samples were obtained from 115 patients with febrile neutropenia for determination of PCT levels before onset of fever and daily until the resolution of fever. The rise in PCT levels appeared early, with median values on the first day of fever of 8.23 ng/mL in patients with bacteremia, compared to 0.86 ng/mL in patients with localized bacterial infections ($p < 0.017$), 2.62 ng/mL in patients with severe sepsis, and 0.57 ng/mL in patients with clinically localized infections ($p < 0.001$). A dramatic decrease in PCT levels was documented after resolution of the infection, while elevations were noted when infections worsened, indicating that PCT may also serve as a marker useful for the follow-up of patients during the febrile episode. Pronounced PCT levels were also found in patients with fever of unknown origin who were responding to antimicrobial chemotherapy (indicative of occult infection), compared with those not responding to treatment with antibiotics (60). In other studies, PCT levels were not found to rise during CNS bacteremia (60), while in only one study, levels >3 ng/μL were reported in BMT patients with invasive aspergillosis (IA) (61). For the moment, due to low sensitivity and specificity, PCT adds little or no help to the diagnosis of invasive fungal infection (IFI) (62). Accumulated data offer PCT a sensitivity range of 44% to 83% and a specificity range of 64% to 100% depending on the severity of the underlying infection and the cutoff value used. Most powerful is its negative prognostic value (NPV) for the presence of bacterial infection when levels are <0.5 ng/mL, which is >85% (55). If PCT evaluation is to be used, serial measurements are more helpful than an isolated determination. A relevant issue studied recently is the prospective evaluation of PCT in the context of febrile neutropenia and the challenge of being able to discriminate early between patients at low or high risk of complications, and how this would be compared and combined with the Talcott and MASCC criteria. Of particular interest would be the ability to identify low-risk patients efficaciously, without falsely including high-risk patients, and to offer outpatient management confidently to this patient population. The addition of PCT to clinical risk assessment scales, although not in a statistically significant way, appeared to augment sensitivity but, more important, incremented the NPV for the detection of bacteremia or treatment failure up to 98%, a determinant factor in deciding whether a patient can be discharged safely and treated on an outpatient basis (55).

C-Reactive Protein (CRP) is an acute phase protein that has proved less useful in discriminating occult bacteria infection during an episode of FUO in febrile neutropenic patients, correlating more with the course of fever than with that of infection (63), and its value can be affected by the underlying disease or the presence of graft versus host disease (GVHD). It increases late in the course of infection (≥ 3 days after the onset of fever) (64) and its normalization is also prolonged due to a long half-life. It is reported that serial measurements of CRP can be of help (64,65), with two consecutively low measurements bearing a good NPV for the presence of bacterial infection and stable, consecutively increasing values (levels >200 mg/mL) in patients still febrile the fifth day of the febrile episode to be strongly predictive of mortality (66). In a recent study, levels of PCT and IL-6 varied significantly between bacteremic and not bacteremic episodes of FUO and neutropenia, while no differences were found in CRP concentrations, indicating that PCT and IL-6 are more reliable markers than CRP for predicting bacteremia in patients with febrile neutropenia (67).

IFIs, especially those caused by molds, have minimal signs and cultures are often negative (except for a 60% probability of positive blood cultures in fusariosis). The detection of specific antibodies or circulating fungal antigens or fungal metabolites is being investigated in order to lead to early or pre-emptive diagnosis of IFI. Among the most promising are the Candida antigens and antibodies in combination, the Aspergillus galactomannan [a major constituent of Aspergillus cell wall detected in bronchoalveolar lavage (BAL) and blood and recently in Cereprospinal Fluid (CSF)], and the polymerase chain reaction (PCR) for Aspergillus.

The recent advent of an improved, commercial-serum, enzyme-linked immunosorbent assay (ELISA) for the detection of circulating galactomannan (GM) has contributed to the diagnosis of invasive aspergillosis (IA) in many haematology and transplant centres (68,69). The optimal threshold for positivity remains a matter of debate, and measurements must be repeated consecutively on a twice or thrice-a-week basis in patients with neutropenia. Decreasing the index cutoff for positivity to 0.5 increases its sensitivity (with minimal loss of specificity) and the duration of test positivity before diagnosis by clinical means (70). Sensitivity is highest in patients who did not receive antifungal prophylaxis with mold-active agents (87.5%) (71). A rabbit model demonstrated that the level of circulating antigen correlated with the tissue fungus burden and a quantifiable response to antifungal therapy (72).

A series of allogeneic stem-cell transplant recipients were monitored prospectively, and the relationship between antigenemia and other diagnostic triggers for initiation of antifungal therapy was analyzed. Antigenemia preceded diagnosis on the basis of radiologic examination or Aspergillus isolation by eight and nine days in 80% and 88.8% of patients, respectively, and initiation of therapy in 83.3% of patients. Detection of GM was especially useful when patients were receiving steroid treatment or when coexisting conditions masked the diagnosis of IA. Prospective screening for GM allows earlier diagnosis of aspergillosis than do conventional diagnostic criteria (68). Studies have shown a sensitivity range of 75% to 100%, a specificity of 80% to 98%, and a high NPV of about 95% (with a sensitivity of 81% and a specificity of 89% in the studies leading to its FDA clearance) (73). Physicians still must be aware of the potential for false-positive and false-negative results; the test does not replace careful microbiological and clinical evaluation.

The following have been identified as causes related to false-positive results (false-positive reactivity has been reported from 5% in adults to 83% in neonates) (72): treatment with amoxicillin/clavulanate or piperacillin/tazompactam (74), early after lung transplantation (first week) (75) or BMT (first 15–30 days) (76), in neonates (because of the heavy colonization of the neonatal gut by the cross-reacting *Bifidobacterium* spp.) (77), several cross-reacting food components such as milk, rice, pasta, sogia, canned vegetables, food supplements rich in proteins (78), and technical factors, such as specimen transportation or airborne contamination with cross-reacting fungi (*Penicillium* sp., *Paecilomyces variotii, Alternaria* spp., etc.) (79).

In a prospective study including 205 treatment episodes in 165 patients, PCR for Aspergillus was validated in comparison to GM and was found superior to GM with respect to sensitivity rates. In patients at high risk for IA, positive results for Aspergillus by PCR of blood samples are highly suggestive for IA and contribute to the diagnosis (80).

Detection of Candida antigens and antibodies is still under study in the evaluation of the febrile neutropenic patient at risk of candidiasis. In one study, circulating candidal antigens [mannan and (1–3) glucan] and immunoglobulin G subclass antibodies to these cell wall antigens were analyzed in a limited number (14) of intensive care unit (ICU) or surgical patients with systemic candidiasis and cancer or diabetes. The (1–3) glucan antigen and the two subclass antibodies appeared to be early, specific markers for the laboratory diagnosis of candidiasis, while the kinetics of (1–3) glucan appearance in serum were found to assist in evaluating the therapeutic efficacy of antifungal treatment. Combined, they offered a 92% sensitivity and a 100% specificity and positive peredicitive value (81). In another study, the Platelia Candida-specific antigen and antibody assays were used to test serial serum samples from seven neutropenic adult patients with hematological malignancies who had developed systemic *Candida tropicalis* infections. High and persistent mannanemias were detected in all patients during the neutropenic period, confirming the value of the combined detection of mannanemia and antimannan antibodies in individuals at risk of candidemia (82). Further studies are needed to confirm these preliminary results.

In vitro fungal-susceptibility testing still needs to be clinically interpreted and in vivo correlated with clinical outcomes. More solid and meaningful data exist about the in vitro sensitivity of *Candida* sp. against fluconazole, itraconazole, and flucytosine, using the standardized and clinically relevant methodology developed by the National Committee for Clinical Laboratory Standards (recently Clinical and Laboratorcy Standards). Breakpoints were developed from data derived from patients with oropharyngeal or esophageal candidiasis (for fluconazole and itraconazole) and from non-neutropenic patients with candidemia (for fluconazole only) (83). Application and clinical relevancy of data in the setting of febrile neutropenic patients with cancer is still under study, and indications exist that in vitro susceptibility is a factor affecting outcome (84). Reliable and convincing interpretative breakpoints are not available for amphotericin B, and meaningful data do not exist yet for other compounds (echinocandins, newer azoles), although minimal inhibitory concentration (MIC) data are available (85). Epidemiological studies have shown that Candida species such as *C. albicans, C. tropicalis, C. parapsilosis* should be considered susceptible to fluconazole[0]. Concern exists about the sensitivity of *C. glabrata* for which resistance rates of 15% against fluconazole are reported (86). Identification of Candida to species level is thus of paramount importance, for antifungal-treatment selection and sensitivity testing is indicated in case of lack of clinical response after treatment initiation or when a change from a parenteral agent to oral fluconazole is considered.

THERAPEUTIC CONSIDERATIONS
The Empirical Approach

Prompt administration of empirical antibiotic therapy is essential for patients with febrile neutropenia and FUO, because underlying infections may progress rapidly. Selection of proper empiric antimicrobial therapy should primarily be influenced by the local epidemiology, drug-susceptibility patterns of bacterial pathogens at a certain institution and exposure of the patient to previous antimicrobial therapy (6). Initial empiric therapy is primarily directed against bacterial pathogens, since fungal, viral, or protozoan etiology is rarely the initial cause of infection (87). The local epidemiological data are subject to dynamic changes and are influenced by: (*i*) Resistance patterns in the community and the use of chemoprophylaxis. In environments where prophylaxis is not widely used, gram-negative pathogens tend to predominate (88). If prophylaxis is extensively used with agents active against gram-negatives, gram-positives consist of >65% of pathogens (89). In two large trials including more than 1000 patients, prophylaxis was given to <25% of patients and gram-negatives remained the majority of isolates (89,90). In two recent studies, the one using chemoprophylaxis in >90% of patients and the second using nonabsorbable colistin for gut decontamination, gram-positives consisted of 66% and 67% of isolates, respectively, with CNS predominating in the first and *Streptococci* sp. in the latter (91,92). (*ii*) The type of chemotherapy. Intensively cytotoxic and damaging-to-the-mucosa regimens increase the presence of *Viridans streptococci*, *Enterococci*, and gram-negative pathogens (87). The type of pathogens that prevail during certain periods must not rely on data extracted only from blood isolates (93). Bacteremias are documented only in 25% of patients with FUO and neutropenia (93). Infections at other sites are commonly due to gram-negative pathogens or are polymicrobial, a pattern that is currently emerging in 23% and 31% of documented bacterial infections in patients with hematological malignancies or solid tumors, respectively. In these polymicrobial infections, 80% of pathogens are gram-negatives, and in 33% of cases, pathogens include only gram-negatives (94). If data from all sites of infection are pooled together, gram-positives, which, for the last 15 years, are mentioned to predominate in bacteremias of febrile neutropenic patients, prove to have a prevalence of <50% (93). *Pseudomonas aeruginosa* rates are stable, being the second most common gram-negative pathogen, at least at M.D. Anderson Cancer Center (18%), following *Escherichia coli* (29%), and followed by *Klebsiella* sp. (16%) (95). It appears to be more prevalent in warmer climates (96). Thus, the initial empiric antimicrobial regimen should include coverage against negativegram-negatives, including *P. aeruginosa*, as traditionally is practiced since 1971, taking into consideration local resistance patterns at each institution.

Today, a challenging issue is the emergence of drug resistance among nosocomial pathogens, compromising the efficacy of the initial empiric antimicrobial regimen. Resistance to methcillin among CNS is 70% to 90% and among *S. aureus* is >50%. Rates of VRE are ≥30%, whereas 50% to 60% of *S. viridans* and *S. pneumoniae* are resistant to penicillin (93,97). *S. viridans* can be the cause of fulminant bacteremia associated with adult respiratory distrese syndrome, renal failure, and rapid death (98). vancomycin resistant enterococci (VRE) is reported as the cause of outbreaks of bacteremias in leukemic patients, associated with high mortality (88). Unusual gram-positive pathogens, intrinsically resistant to vancomycin are emerging as pathogens causing catheter-related blood stream infections or other systemic infections (*Leuconostoc* sp., *Pediococcus* sp., *Lactobacillus* sp., *Corynebacterium jeikeium*). *P. aeruginosa* resistant to ciprofloxacin is a fact in many institutions, and nonfermenting, intrinsically drug-resistant bacteria are rising in incidence (*Acinetobacter* sp., *S. maltophilia*, *Alcaligenes* sp., *P. non-aeruginosa*). Extended Specture β-lactamases (ESBL) producing *E. coli* and *Klebsiella pneumoniae*, along with *Enterobacter* sp., renders problematic the use of cephalosporins. Extensive use of carbapenems led to 15% to 30% rates of MDR *P. aeruginosa* reported from different parts of the world, sensitive only to colistin, which, because of suboptimal efficacy cannot be used as a single agent (99,100). Anaerobes are rarely isolated in blood cultures of patients with febrile neutropenia (<5%) for reasons that are not clearly defined (97,101), although their presence should be suspected in perineal abscesses, periodontal infections, or neutropenic enterocolitis.

Empiric antimicrobial therapy must be adapted to local epidemiology data, according to the mentioned factors. Usually it consists of an antipseudomonal cephalosporin (ceftazidime if ESBL do not prevail), piperacillin/tazobactam, cefepime, or an antipseudomonal carbapenem (imipenem, meropenem), combined with an aminoglycoside (6). The combination is used for spectrum extension and rapid pathogen killing and not for synergy purposes, which could not be proved in meta-analysis studies (102). Aminoglycosides, as drugs exhibiting a dose-dependent pattern of Pharmacokinetics/Pharmacodynamics (PK/PD), can be safely and effectively used in a once-daily dose regimen (103). It is essential that if bacteremia or pseudomonas infection is not proved, the aminoglycoside is discontinued early (at 72–96 hours) (6). Otherwise, monitoring of kidney function and drug levels is recommended.

Monotherapy with ceftazidime, cefepime, meropenem, and imipenem or piperacillin/tazobactam was found in several studies to be equally effective with the conventional combination of a β-lactam and an aminoglycoside (104–107). When ESBL-producing pathogens prevail, cephalosporins may be problematic as empiric treatment, and antipseudomonal carbapenems remain the first choice, probably followed by piperacillin/tazobactam as an alternative. Aminoglycosides clearly are not suitable as monotherapy (108), and the use of quinolones is discouraged in institutions where they are used as prophylaxis, although data are scarce and contradictory (109). No universal guidelines can be applied. Clinicians should be alert about the pathogen predominating in their institution.

Patients with intermediate or high risk must be hospitalized and receive Intravenous or Parenteral (IV) antibiotics. Patients falling in the low-risk category, after 24-hour evaluation at the hospital, can be either sent home on oral regimen or be hospitalized until defervescence and sent home to complete therapy with an oral regimen. An extensively used oral regimen is the combination of ciprofloxacin plus amoxicillin/clavulanate. The newer quinolones (moxifloxacin) are under study, with data limited stin about their potential use as monotherapy in low-risk patients treated as outpatients (110). The decision to treat a low-risk patient on an outpatient basis should rely or prerequisites like the patient's ability to understand the risk, to receive oral medication, to have a telephone, to reach a hospital within one hour, to have help at home, and the ability to offer a 24-hour service seven days a week (111).

Addition of Vancomycin to the Initial Empirical Regimen

The increased predominance of gram-positive micro-organisms in bacteremias of patients with febrile neutropenia has led during the last 15 years to the increased use of vancomycin as part of the initial empiric antimicrobial regimen. Study V of the EORTC in 1990 showed that the nonincorporation of vancomycin in the initial regimen and its use only when indicated by the isolation of a gram-positive micro-organism did not lead to increased morbidity and mortality rates, except in patients with *S. viridans* bacteremia not receiving a carbapenem, pip/tazo, or cefepime (112). In another study, the addition of vancomycin to imipenem did not affect efficacy (113). A study by National Cancer Institute (NCI) confirmed that the gram-positive pathogens are not quickly lethal (114). A recent meta-anlaysis of randomized controlled trials comparing antibiotics with antigram-positive spectrum to control or placebo, in addition to the same baseline antibiotic regimen in both arms (which included 13 studies with 2392 participants in total), concluded that the use of glycopeptides can be safely deferred until the documentation of a resistant gram-positive infection. Empirical antigram-positive antibiotics were assessed for the initial treatment in 11 studies, and for persistent fever in two. Glycopeptides were assessed in nine trials. No significant difference in all-cause mortality and overall failure was observed, whereas adverse events were significantly more common with the additional antibiotic, and nephrotoxicity was significantly more common with additional glycopeptides (115,116). The IDSA, in its latest guidelines and taking into consideration the emergence of VRE under the selective pressure of vancomycin, recommends the addition of vancomycin to the initial regimen: (*i*) in patients with hemodynamic instability (threat of septic shock), (*ii*) when signs of or a documented gram-positive infection are present (tunnel infection, soft tissue infection), and (*iii*) when high rates of *S. viridans* or MRSA infections are prevalent in the institution, especially if the patient is known to be colonized with MRSA (6). Considerations exist in some physicians for patients with chemotherapy-related, substantial mucosal damage and history of quinolone prophylaxis during the period of a febrile neutropenia. Sudden spikes of temperature $>40°C$ may be predicted of streptococcal sepsis (6). Ceftazidime in this case should be avoided as empiric treatment because it lacks streptococcal activity.

Vancomycin remains the most widely used glycopeptide. Teicoplanin, widely used in Europe, is not approved in the United States. It is administrated once daily, rarely causes red-man syndrome, and is less nephrotoxic. However, drug fever and thrombocytopenia should be a consideration. In vitro studies have shown strains of *Stapylococcus hemolyticus* to be resistant to teicoplanin, whereas vancomycin retains its activity against them. The activity of teicoplanin in cancer patients has been proved in several open, comparative trials (117,118).

Linezolid, an oxazolidinone active against MDR gram-positive pathogens (MRSA, VRE), has not been evaluated as empiric therapy in febrile neutropenia. Hematological toxicity of the drug could be problematic (6). Quinopristine—dalfopristin, also active against VRE, awaits further studies for evaluation in neutropenic patients (6).

Empiric Antifungal Therapy

During the first week of neutropenia, efforts to evaluate fever primarily focus on the search for a bacterial pathogen because, at point, bacteria account for the majority of infections during febrile neutropenia. With the administration of antibiotics and the prolongation of neutropenia, the risk of fungal infection emerges. *Candida* spp. and *Aspergillus* spp. are the most common fungal pathogens encountered. Candida infections occur during the second or subsequent week of neutropenia and Aspergillus infection later, during the third and subsequent weeks of neutropenia (119). Therapies that cause short-term neutropenia, lasting less than a week, do not meet the risk of fungal infection. BMT patients are the patients at highest risk due to prolonged and deep neutropenia and the presence of other factors compromising immunity as well (GVHD corticosteroids) (119).

Candida may be the cause of fungemia, acute- or chronic-, disseminated or single-organ disease. Non-ablicans strains are emerging. Aspergillosis initially is a lung or sinuses disease, to disseminate in 30% of patients, causing primarily CNS disease with 90% mortality rate. *Aspergillus* resistant to amphotericin B, such as *A. terreus* and *A. flavus*, have also emerged as pathogens. Numerous other fungi are emerging as opportunistic pathogens: *Fusarium* spp. (sinopulmonary infection, skin lesions, fungemia), *Muror* spp. (sinopulmonary or disseminate disease), *Scedosporuim* spp., *Acremonium spp.*, *Trichosporon spp.*, and *Alternarnia spp.*, among others. They tend to present as breakthrough infections due to resistance to many antifungals (120).

Reasons necessitating the administration of empirical antifungal therapy include the high rates of morbidity and mortality associated with fungal infections, the difficulty of diagnosing IFI early during the course of infection, and the ineffectiveness of treatment when it is delayed.

Empiric antifungal therapy has been shown quite early (121,122) to improve patient's outcome. In the recent IDSA guidelines, the introduction of antifungal therapy is recommended in neutropenic patients with FUO not responding to ≥5 days of appropriate antimicrobial treatment. Decisions could be individualized. For example, the appearance of lung infiltrates on chest X-ray, suspicious mucosal skin lesions or eye/sinuses inflammation, should prompt at any time point the initiation of antifungal treatment. History of a documented IFI is an indication for the administration of antifungal therapy as secondary prophylaxis, as soon as the patient is rendered neutropenic (and for the whole duration of neutropenia) (119). Amphotericin B, its lipid formulations, and caspofungin have been shown equally effective as empiric antifungal therapy in the management of neutropenic FUO (123–125). Voriconazole has proved to cause less breakthrough fungal infections, but failed to reach the noninferiority end point compared to liposomal amphotericin B in the empiric antifungal treatment of neutropenic FUO (125). Its extensive use nowadays as treatment or prophylaxis in patients with cancer is accompanied by reports of an increase in invasive zygomycosis incidence at the same centers (126,127).

The optimal duration of empirical antifungal treatment has not been clearly established. If the patient is afebrile and the neutropil count has recovered ($>500/cells/mm^3$), treatment can be discontinued. If the patient is afebrile and stable but neutropenia persists, treatment can be stopped after two weeks of administration. In an unstable, febrile, neutropenic patient, treatment should continue until fever and neutropenia resolves (120).

In the future, empiric antifungal therapy may be transformed to pre-emptive antifungal therapy, based on nonculture methods (GM, PCR) and risk stratification efforts (119).

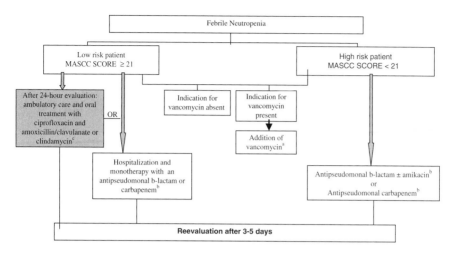

^ahemodynamic instability, MRSA carriage, clinical signs of gram-positive infection
^baccording to local epidemiology of resistance and previous antibiotic exposure
^cadequate home care is necessary and ability of rapid access to the hospital

FIGURE 1   Febrile neutropenia and initial empiric treatment. *Abbreviations*: MASCC, Multinational Association for Supportive Care in Cancer; MRSA, methicillin-resistant *Staphylococcus aureus*.

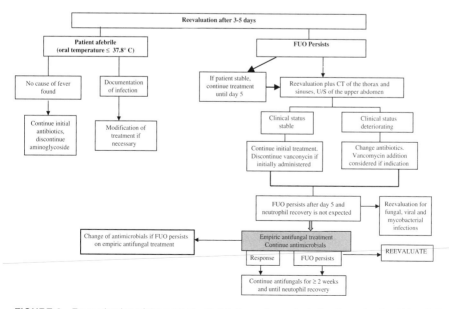

FIGURE 2   Re-evaluation of the patient with febrile neutropenia during the episode. *Abbreviations*: CT, computed tomography; U/S, Ultrasound.

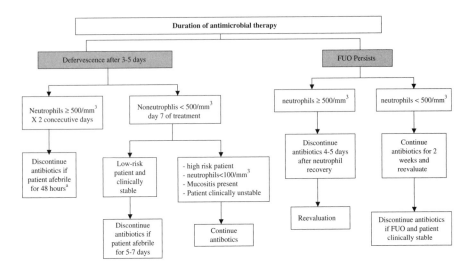

FIGURE 3   Duration of antimicrobial treatment.

Strategy of Treatment During the Febrile Episode

The first time point for the evaluation of the initial, empiric antimicrobial treatment is after 72 hours of treatment have been completed (Figs. 1–3). Elting et al. found that the median time to clinical response in hospitalized patients with cancer is five to seven days, while in low-risk patients, defervescence may be achieved in only two days (128,129). If the patient is afebrile after 72 hours and the episode was an FUO, in a low-risk stable patient without mucositis, treatment will continue until at least seven days of treatment have been completed, or it could also be stepped down to an oral regimen and the patient could be sent home. For some clinicians, resolution of neutropenia before treatment discontinuation may be preferable (6). If a pathogen has been identified, treatment can be modified, but change of a broad to a narrow, spectrum therapy is not recommended because of the risk of breakthrough infections (130). For unstable patients with mucositis and profound neutropenia, treatment should be continued for at least two weeks and for as long the patient is unstable or neutropenia profound ($<100/$ cells/mm^3) (6).

If fever as FUO persists after five days, the patient needs to be reassessed for occult fungal infection, a bacterial site of infection, for atypical opportunistic infections (viruses, mycobacteria), resistant organisms, suboptimal dosing of antibiotics, or noninfectious causes of fever (drug fever, underlying disease, GVHD, phlebitis, transfusions, etc.). Removal of CVCs without clear-cut evidence in case of FUO is not helpful (129). If no other causes of persisting fever are revealed, the next step is the addition of empiric antifungal therapy, with or without modification of the initial antimicrobial regimen (119). Simultaneous continuation of the same antimicrobial regimen may be preferable for stable patients who are expected to have a rapid recovery of neutrophils. Modifying by changing from one broad-spectrum antibiotic to another (e.g., from piperacillin/tazobactam to a carbapenem) may be done, epidemiology of resistance permitting, though is not supported by published evidence. Discontinuation of antimicrobials is not recommended (119). Empirical addition of vancomycin is also not recommended, because recent studies (116) have shown that the addition of a glycopeptide to persistently febrile neutropenic patients without evidence of a gram-positive infection is of no benefit. If a glycopeptide was a part of the initial regimen, it should be discontinued in patients with persistent FUO or no isolation of a gram-positive pathogen (6). If neutropenia and FUO persist, antimicrobial treatment should continue for at least two weeks (6). If neutropenia resolves and FUO persists, the patient must be evaluated for chronic disseminated candidiasis or other fungal or viral diseases, and antimicrobial treatment may be discontinued five days after neutrophil's recovery (6).

Empirical antiviral therapy is not recommended at any time point (6). It could be added in patients with oral lesions suggestive of herpes simple virus (HSV) infection (acyclovir), in patients with esophagitis (acyclovir or gancyclovir), or in patients with viral respiratory disease indicative of RSV (ribavirin), influenza, or parainfluenza infections (amantadine). HSV can cause serious morbidity in neutropenic patients after BMT, during the first month after transplantation, through systemic or CNS infection (131), while respiratory viruses can be the cause of serious pneumonias or interstitial pneumonitis leading to respiratory failure.

OTHER CONSIDERATIONS INCLUDING PROPHYLAXIS

Colony-stimulating factors and granulocyte transfusions are not routinely recommended. They might be helpful in documented infections that are not responding to appropriate treatment, in severe uncontrolled fungal infections, and in specific life-threatening infections such as pneumonia. They may be used as prophylaxis in high-risk patients with expected long duration of neutropenia (≥ 10 days) and with a high risk of a febrile episode ($>40\%$). The use of colony-stimulating factors in patients with febrile neutropenia due to cancer chemotherapy does not affect overall mortality, but reduces the amount of time spent in the hospital and the neutrophil recovery period. It is not clear whether colony-stimulating factors have an effect on infection-related mortality (132–134).

Routine use of antibacterial and antifungal prophylaxis for all patients with afebrile neutropenia is not recommended in the latest versions of IDSA's guidelines (6). It may be beneficial in high-risk patients with expected prolonged neutropenia (such as BMT patients) but it should be given for the shortest duration possible (6). Two recent meta-analysis (135,136), published in 2005, come to doubt and reverse what, during previous years, was established as evidence-based knowledge by previous meta-analysis (137,138) on which guidelines are based: that although oral antimicrobial prophylaxis reduces Gram($-$) and documented infections, the incidence of febrile episodes and, subsequently, duration of hospitalization and days of antibiotic use, it does not decrease overall, infection-related mortality, contributing to the emergence of resistance and accelerated toxicity. The first meta-analysis (135) (95 trials of, 52 were quinolone based) showed that in patients with hematological malignancies, quinolone prophylaxis reduces overall and infection-related mortality, whereas the second (136) (22 trials) also confirmed a reduction in infection-related mortality due to bacterial causes in a mixed population of patients with solid tumors or hematological malignances receiving corimoxazole or a quinolone. How this will affect future guidelines is not yet known, considering that studies have also shown that oral antimicrobials do not alter the protecting effect exhibited by growth factors in patients with chemotherapy-induced neutropenia.

Prophylaxis against *Pneumocystis jirovecii* pneumonia (PCP) (cotrimoxazole) should be given to all patients at risk [BMT, lymphoma, or chronic lymphatic lymphoma (CLL) patients, or patients treated with corticosteroids] (6).

Studies have shown the effective role of antifungal prophylaxis in the reduction of superficial infections and in the need for empirical antifungal treatment, in reduction of invasive fungal disease and with a trend for reduced mortality (139). The effective role of fluconazole against prevention of superficial infections and systemic candidiasis was shown in patients with BMT and is recommended for this population until engraftment in the dose of 400 mg/day (140). Considerations exist today about the narrow spectrum of fluconazole and the increasing incidence of mold infections and infections due to fluconazole-resistant Candida strains (141). New data have been added by studies using IV itrazonazole and liposomal amphotericin B as antifungal prophylaxis. A reappraisal of this issue through new recommendations is pending. New antifungal agents, such as the echinocandins and the new azoles, are available and may have a potential role in antifungal prophylaxis. Future studies should evaluate which strategy is more useful: prophylaxis or pre-emptive therapy (142).

High-efficiency particulate air (HEPA) filtration seems to be effective in reducing mold infections. It is recommended in BMT patients along with positive pressure rooms with >12 air exchanges per hour, especially in facilities undergoing construction and renovation. Debate exists about the effectiveness of the laminal airflow systems, which are not generally recommended. All neutropenic patients require careful barrier nursing, including strict hygienic practices (gown, mask, sterile gloves), daily patient skin care and strict adherence to hand hygiene rules, avoidance of plants and flowers, and dietary restrictions that include raw vegetables and salads and everything that is not well cooked, or boiled, or pasteurized. Visitors must be limited and without exposure to viral diseases. Adherence to such procedures is the first step toward effective prophylaxis (142,143).

Patients with febrile neutropenia, especially after BMT, who present with respiratory failure or hemodynamic instability may need the support of a medical intensive care unit (MICU). Admission of cancer patients with serious medical complications to the ICU remains controversial primarily because of the high short-term mortality rates in these patients. A number of studies (144–148) have evaluated the risk factors for mortality and the differences between survivors and nonsurvivors among neutropenic patients admitted in the ICU. Admission to the ICU worsens the prognosis substantially, but only the number of organ system failures at admission (expressed as number, SOFA, or SAPS II score) and respiratory failure [requiring intubation and mechanical ventilation (19% survival rates in intubated patients vs. 66% in nonintubated)] remains predictive of ICU mortality, which is comparable to severely ill noncancer patients (>47%). Septic shock among cancer patients admitted to the ICU has a mortality rate similar to that reported for mixed populations (>50%) and is particularly increased when hepatic or respiratory dysfunction develops. Neutropenia and its duration and underlying disease progression is not associated with a worse prognosis in terms of mortality, and general reluctance to admit cancer patients to an ICU does not seem to be justified. In the ICU, CSF administration does not seem to alter the clinical outcome (149).

SUMMARY

Febrile neutropenia is a syndrome commonly anticipated in patients receiving treatment for cancer. In 60% of cases and due to a blunted inflammatory reaction, it presents as FUO and constitutes a medical emergency because of the high mortality of occult gram-negative bacteremia that may be present. For the last three decades, its management has included the prompt administration of empiric antibacterial therapy, a tactic that resulted in a subsequent reduction in mortality. Challenges remain the administration of the most appropriate empiric treatment regimen adapted to the evolving and changing epidemiology of infections in neutropenic patients, the development of markers of early diagnosis of severe bacterial or fungal infections, the risk stratification of patients, the establishment of targeted empiric (pre-emptive) antifungal therapy criteria, and the containment of the antimicrobial resistance that compromises effective treatment efforts through effective antibiotic policies and implementation of infection control measures, especially hand hygiene. The need for targeted antimicrobial or antifungal prophylaxis and supportive strategies, such as the use of growth factors, awaits to be further clarified.

REFERENCES

1. Crawford J, Dale DC, Lyman GH. Chemotherapy-induced neutropenia. Risks, consequences, and new directions for its management. Cancer 2004; 100(2):228–237.
2. Bodey Gp, Buckley M., Sathe YS, et al. Quantative relationships between circulating leukocytes and infection in patients with acute leukemia. Ann Intern Med 1966; 64(2):328–340.
3. Sickles EA, Greene WH, Wiernick PH. Clinical presentation of infection in granulocytopenic patients. Arch Intern Med 1975; 135(5):715–719.
4. Pizzo PA. Management of fever in patients with cancer and treatment induced neutropenia. N Engl J Med 1993; 328(18):1323–1332.
5. Bodey GP. Unusual presentations of infection in neutropenic patients. Int J Antimicrob Agents 2000; 16(2):93–95.
6. Hughes WT, Armstrong D, Bodey GP, et al. 2002 Guidelines for the use of antimicrobial agents in neutropenic patients with cancer. Clin Infect Dis 2002; 34(6):730–751.
7. From the Immunocompromized Host Society. The design, analysis and reporting of clinical trials on the empirical antibiotic management of the neutropenic patient. J Infect Dis 1990; 161(3):397–401.
8. Link H, Bohme A, Cornely OA, et al. Guidelines of the Infectious Diseases Working Party (AGIHO) of the German Society of Hematology and Oncology (DGHO) Study Group Interventional Therapy of Unexplained Fever. Antimicrobial therapy of unexplained fever in neutropenic patients. Ann Hematol 2003; 82(suppl 2):S105–S117.
9. Oude Nijhuis CS, Daenen SM, Vellenga E, et al. Fever and neutropenia in cancer patients: the diagnostic role of cytokines in risk assessment strategies. Crit Rev Oncol Hematol 2002; 44(2):163–174.
10. Rolston KV. The Infectious Diseases Society of America 2002 guidelines for the use of antimicrobial agents in patients with cancer and neutropenia: Salient features and comments. Clin Infect Dis 2004; 39(suppl 1):S44–S48.
11. Dompeling EC, Donnelly JP, Raemaekers JM, et al. Evolution of the clinical manifestations of infection during the course of febrile neutropenia in patients with malignancy. Infection 1998; 26(6):349–354.
12. Rolston KV. Prediction of neutropenia. Int J Antimicrob Agents 2000; 16(2):113–115.
13. National Cancer Institute. Common toxicity criteria, version 2.0. Available at URL: http://ctep.cancer.gov/forms/CTCv20_4-30-992.pdf
14. Dale DC, Guerry D 4th, Wewerka JR, et al. Chronic neutropenia. Medicine (Baltimore) 1979; 58(2):128–144.

15. Rubin M, Hathom JW, Pizzo PA. Controversies in the management of febrile neutropenic cancer parients. Cancer Invest 1988; 6(2):167–184.
16. Scott S. Identification of cancer patients at high risk of febrile neutropenia. Am J Health-Syst Pharm 2002; 59(Suppl 4):S16–S19.
17. Silber JH, Fridman M, DiPaola RS, et al. First-cycle blood counts and subsequent neutropenia, dose reduction, or delay in early-stage breast cancer therapy. J Clin Oncol. 1998; 16(7):2392–2400.
18. Chrischilles E, Link B, Scott S, et al. Factors associated with early termination of CHOP, and its association with overall survival among patients with intermediate-grade non-Hodgkin's lymphoma (NHL) [abstract 1539]. Proc Am Soc Clin Oncol. 2002; 21:385a.
19. Giamarellou H, Antoniadou A. Infectious complications of febrile leukopenia. Infect Dis Clin North Am 2002; 15(2):457–482.
20. Viscoli C, Varnier O, Machetti M. Infections in patients with febrile neutropenia: Epidemiology, microbiology, and risk stratification. Clin Infect Dis 2005; 40(suppl 4): S240–S245.
21. Dale DC, Crawford J, Lyman G. Chemotherapy-induced neutropenia and associated complications in randomized clinical trials: an evidence-based review [abstract 1638]. Proc Am Soc Clin Oncol 2001; 20:–410a.
22. Gomez H, Hidalgo M, Casanova L, et al. Risk factors for treatment-related death in elderly patients with aggressive non-Hodgkin's lymphoma: results of a multivariate analysis. J Clin Oncol 1998; 16(6):2065–2069.
23. Marty FM, Lee SJ, Fahey MM, et al. Infliximab use in patients with severe-graft- versus-host disease and other emerging risk factors of non-Candida invasive fungal infections in allogeneic hematopoietic stem cell transplant recipients: a cohort study. Blood 2003; 102(8):2768–2776.
24. Neth O, Turner MW, Klein NJ. Deficiency of mannose-binding lectin and burden of infection in children with malignancy: a prospective study. Lancet 2001; 358(9282): 614–618.
25. Pizzo PA. Fever in immunocompromised patients. N Engl J Med 1999; 341(12):893–900.
26. Schimpff SC. Empiric antibiotic therapy for granulocytopenic cancer patients. Am J Med 1986; 80(5c):13–20.
27. McCabe WR, Jackson GG. Gram-negative bacteremia II. Clinical, laboratory, and therapeutic observations. Arch Intern Med 1962; 110:865.
28. Bodey GP, Jadeja L, Elting L. Pseudomonas bacteremia; Retrospective analysis of 410 episodes. Arch Intern Med 1985; 145(9):1621–1629.
29. Fergie JE, Schema SJ, Lott L, et al. Pseudomonas aeruginosa bacteremia in immunocompromised children: analysis of factors associated with a poor outcome. Clin Infect Dis 1994; 18(3):390–394.
30. Schimpff S, Satterlee W, Young V, et al. Empiric therapy with carbenicillin and gentamicin for febrile patients with cancer and granulocytopenia. N Engl J Med 1971; 284(19):1061–1065.
31. Hann I, Viscoli C, Paesmans M, et al. International Antimicrobial Therapy Cooperative Group (IATCG) of the European Organization for Research and Treatment of Cancer (EORTC). A comparison of outcome from febrile neutropenic episodes in children compared with adults: results from four EORTC studies. Br J Haematol 1997; 99(3):580–588.
32. Malik IA, Khan WA, Aziz Z, et al. Self-administered antibiotic therapy for chemotherapy-induced, low-risk febrile neutropenia in patients with nonhematologic neoplasms. Clin Infect Dis 1994; 19(3):522–527.
33. Klaassen RJ, Goodman TR, Pham B, et al. 'Low-risk' prediction rule for pediatric oncology patients presenting with fever and neutropenia. J Clin Oncol 2000; 18(5):1012–1019.
34. Vidal L, Paul M, Ben-Dor I, et al. Oral versus intravenous antibiotic treatment for febrile neutropenia in cancer patients. Cochrane Database Syst Rev 2004; 18(4):CD003992.
35. Talcott JA, Finberg R, Mayer RJ, Goldman L. The medical course of cancer patients with fever and neutropenia. Clinical identification of a low-risk subgroup at presentation. Arch Intern Med 1988; 148(12):2561–2568.

36. Talcott JA, Siegel RD, Finberg R, Goldman L. Risk assessment in cancer patients with fever and neutropenia: a prospective, two-center validation of a prediction rule. J Clin Oncol 1992; 10(2):316–322.
37. Kern WV, Cometta A, De Bock R, et al. International Antimicrobial Therapy Cooperaive Group of the European Organization for Research and Treatment of Cancer. Oral versus intravenous empirical antimicrobial therapy for fever in patients with granulocytopenia who are receiving cancer chemotherapy. N Eng J Med 1999; 341(5): 312–318.
38. Freifeld A, Marchigiani D, Walsh T, et al. A double-blind comparison of empirical oral and intravenous antibiotic therapy for low-risk febrile patients with neutropenia during cancer chemotherapy. N Eng J Med 1999; 341(5):305–311.
39. Klastersky j, Paesmans M, Rubenstein EB, et al. The Multinational Association for Supportive Care in Cancer risk index: a multinational scoring system for identifying low-risk febrile neutropenic cancer patients. J Clin Oncol 2000; 18(16):3038–3051.
40. Klastersky J. Management of fever in neutropenic patients with different risk of complications. Clin Infect Dis 2004; 39(suppl 1):S32–S37.
41. Uys A, Rapoport BL, Anderson R. Febrile neutropenia: a prospective study to validate the Multinational Association of Supportive Care of Cancer (MASCC) risk-index score. Support Care Cancer. 2004; 12(8):555–560.
42. Meunier F. Infections in patients with acute leukemia and lymphoma. In: Mandel Gl, Douglas JV, Bennett JE, eds. Principles and Practice of Infections Diseases. 4th ed. Philadelphia: Churchill Livingstone Inc., 1995:2675–2686.
43. Giamarellou H, Antoniadou A. Infectious complications of febrile leucopenia. Infect Dis Clin North Am 2001; 15(2):457–482.
44. Mermel LA, Farr BM, Sherertz RJ, et al. Guidelines for the management of intravascular catheter-related infection. Clin Infect Dis 2001; 32(9):1249–1272.
45. Valdiviesco M, Gil-extremera B, Zornoza J, et al. Gram-negative bacillary pneumonia in the compromised host. Medicine (Baltimore) 1977; 56(3):241–254.
46. Heussel CP, Kauczor HU, Heussel GE, et al. Pneumonia in febrile neutropenic patients and in bone marrow and blood stem cell transplant recipients: use of high resolution computed tomography. J Clin Oncol 1999; 17(3):796–805.
47. Caillot D, Couaillier JF, Bernard A, et al. Increasing volume and changing characteristics of invasive pulmonary aspergillosis on sequential thoracic computed tomography scans in patients with neutropenia. J Clin Oncol 2001; 19(1):253–259.
48. Hauhhaard A, Ellis M, Ekelund L. Early chest radiography and CT in the diagnosis, management and outcome of invasive pulmonary Aspergillosis. Acta Radiol 2002; 43(3):292–298.
49. Gorschluter M, Mey U, Strehl J, et al. Neutropenic enterocolitis in adults: systematic analysis of evidence quality. Eur J Haematol 2005; 75(1):1–13.
50. Kontoyiannis DP, Luna MA, Samuels BI, et al. Hepatosplenic candidiasis. Infect Dis Clin North Am 2000; 14(3):721–739.
51. Sudhoff T, Giagonnidis A, Karthaus M. Evaluation of neutropenic fever: value of serum and plasma parameters in clinical practice. Chemotherapy 2000; 46(2):77–85.
52. Persson L, Soderquist B, Engervall P. Assessment of systemic inflammation markers to differentiate a stable from a deteriorating clinical course in patients with febrile neutropenia. Eur J Haematol. 2005; 74(4):297–303.
53. Muller B, Becker KL, Schachinger H, et al. Calcitonin precursors are reliable markers of sepsis in a medical intensive care unit. Crit Care Med. 2000; 28(4):977–983.
54. Tugrul S, Esen F, Celebi S, et al. Reliability of procalcitonin as a severity marker in critically ill patients with inflammatory response. Anaesth Intensive Care 2002; 30(6): 747–754.
55. Jimeno A, Garia-Velasco A, del Val O, et al. Assessment of procalcitonin as a diagnostic and prognostic marker in patients with solid tumors and febrile neutropenia. Cancer 2004; 100(11):2462–2469.
56. Giamarellos-Bourboulis EJ, Grecka P, Poulakou G, et al. Assessment of procalcitonin as a diagnostic marker of underlying infection in patients with febrile neutropenia. Clin Infect Dis 2001; 32(12):1718–1725.

57. Ruokonen E, Nousiainen T, Pulkki K, et al. Procalcitonin concentrations in patients with neutropenic fever. Eur J Clin Microbiol Infect Dis 1999; 18(4):283–285.
58. Engel A, Steinbach G, Kern P, et al. Diagnostic value of procalcitonin serum levels in neutropenic patients with fever: comparison with interleukin-8. Scand J Infect Dis 1999; 31(2):185–189.
59. Fleischhack G, Kambeck I, Cipic D, et al. Procalcitonin in paediatric cancer patients: its diagnostic relevance is superior to that of C-reactive protein, interleukin 6, interleukin 8, soluble interleukin 2 receptor and soluble tumour necrosis factor receptor II. Br J Haematol 2000; 111(4):1093–1102.
60. Persson L, Engervall P, Magnuson A, et al. Use of inflammatory markers for early detection of bacteraemia in patients with febrile neutropenia. Scand J Infect Dis 2004; 36(5):365–71.
61. Ortega M, Rovira M, Filella X, et al. Prospective evaluation of procalcitonin in adults with febrile neutropenia after haematopoietic stem cell transplantation. Br J Haematol 2004; 126(3):372–376.
62. Dornbusch HJ, Strenger V, Kerbl R, et al. Procalcitonin-a marker of invasive fungal infection? Support Care Cancer. 2005; 13(5):343–346.
63. Arber C, Passweg JR, Fluckiger U, et al. C-reactive protein and fever in neutropenic patients Scand J Infect Dis 2000; 32(5):515–520.
64. Yonemori K, Kanda Y, Yamamoto R, et al. Clinical value of serial measurement of serum C-reactive protein level in neutropenic patients. Leuk Lymphoma 2001; 41(5–6):607–614.
65. Manian FA. A prospective study of daily measurement of C-reactive protein in serum of adults with neutropenia. Clin Infect Dis 1995; 21(1):114–121.
66. Ortega M, Rovira M, Almela M, et al. Measurement of C-reactive protein in adults with febrile neutropenia after hematopoietic cell transplantation. Bone Marrow Transplant 2004; 33(7):741–744.
67. Persson L, Soderquist B, Engervall P, et al. Assessment of systemic inflammation markers to differentiate a stable from a deteriorating clinical course in patients with febrile neutropenia. Eur J Haematol 2005; 74(4):297–303.
68. Maertens J, Van Eldere J, Verhaegen J, et al. Use of circulating galactomannan screening for early diagnosis of invasive aspergillosis in allogeneic stem cell transplant recipients. J Infect Dis 2002; 186(9):1297–1306.
69. Viscoli C, Machetti M, Gazzola P. Aspergillus galactomannan antigen in the cerebrospinal fluid of bone marrow transplant recipients with probable cerebral aspergillosis. J Clin Microbiol 2002; 40(4):1496–1499.
70. Maertens J, Theunissen K, Verbeken E, et al. Prospective clinical evaluation of lower cut-offs for galactomannan detection in adult neutropenic cancer patients and haematological stem cell transplant recipients. Br J Haematol 2004; 126(6):852–860.
71. Marr KA, Balajee SA, McLaughlin L, et al. Detection of galactomannan antigenemia by enzyme immunoassay for the diagnosis of invasive aspergillosis: variables that affect performance. J Infect Dis 2004; 190(3):641–649.
72. Mennink-Kersten MA, Donnelly JP, Verveij PE. Detection of circulating galactomannan for the diagnosis and management of invasive Aspergillosis. Lancet Infect Dis 2004; 4(6):349–357.
73. Wheat LJ. Rapid diagnosis of invasive aspergillosis by antigen detection Transpl Infect Dis 2003; 5(4):158–166.
74. Mattei D, Rapezzi D, Mordini N, et al. False-positive Aspergillus galactomannan enzyme-linked immunosorbent assay results in vivo during amoxicillin-clavulanic acid treatment. J Clin Microbiol 2004; 42(11):5362–5363.
75. Husain S, Kwak EJ, Obman A, et al. Prospective assessment of Platelia Aspergillus galactomannan antigen for the diagnosis of invasive aspergillosis in lung transplant recipients. Am J Transplant. 2004 May; 4(5):796–802.
76. Blijlevens NM, Donnelly JP, Meis JF, et al. Aspergillus galactomannan antigen levels in allogeneic haematopoietic stem cell transplant recipients given total parenteral nutrition. Transpl Infect Dis 2002; 4(2):64–65.
77. Mennink-Kersten MA, Klont RR, Warris A, et al. Bifidobacterium lipoteichoic acid and false ELISA reactivity in aspergillus antigen detection. Lancet 2004; 363(9405):325–327.

78. Pinel C, Fricker-Hidalgo H, Lebeau B, et al. Detection of circulating Aspergillus fumigatus galactomannan: value and limits of the Platelia test for diagnosing invasive aspergillosis. J Clin Microbiol 2003; 41(5):2184–2186.
79. Swanink CM, Meis JF, Rijs AJ, et al. Specificity of a sandwich enzyme-linked immunosorbent assay for detecting Aspergillus galactomannan. J Clin Microbiol 1997; 35(1):257–260.
80. Kawazu M, Kanda Y, Nannya Y, et al. Prospective comparison of the diagnostic potential of real-time PCR, double-sandwich enzyme-linked immunosorbent assay for galactomannan, and a (1– > 3)-beta-D-glucan test in weekly screening for invasive aspergillosis in patients with hematological disorders. J Clin Microbiol 2004; 42(6):2733–2741.
81. Sendid B, Caillot D, Baccouch-Humbert B, et al. Contribution of the Platelia Candida-specific antibody and antigen tests to early diagnosis of systemic Candida tropicalis infection in neutropenic adults. J Clin Microbiol 2003; 41(10):4551–4558.
82. Kondori N, Edebo L, Mattsby-Baltzer I. Circulating (1-3) glucan and immunoglobulin G subclass antibodies to Candida albicans cell wall antigens in patients with systemic candidiasis. Clin Diagn Lab Immunol 2004; 11(2):344–350.
83. Pappas PG, Rex JH, Sobel JD, et al. Guidelines for the treatment of candidiasis. Clin Infect Dis 2004; 38(2):161–189.
84. Antoniadou A, Torres HA, Lewis RE, et al. Candidemia in a tertiary care cancer center: in vitro susceptibility and its association with outcome of initial antifungal therapy. Medicine (Baltimore) 2003; 82(5):309–321.
85. Hospenthal DR, Murray CK, Rinaldi MG. The role of antifungal susceptibility testing in the therapy of candidiasis. Diagn Microbiol Infect Dis 2004; 48(3):153–160.
86. Pfaller MA, Diekema DJ. International Fungal Surveillance Participant Group. Twelve years of fluconazole in clinical practice: global trends in species distribution and fluconazole susceptibility of bloodstream isolates of Candida. Clin Microbiol Infect 2004; 10(suppl 1):11–23.
87. Rolston KV. The Infectious Dieases Sociey of America 2002 guidelines for the use of antimicrobial agents in patients with cancer and neutropenia: salient features and comments. Clin Infect Dis 2004; 39(suppl 1):S44–S48.
88. Ramphal R. Changes in the etiology of bacteremia in febrile neutropenic patients and the susceptibilities of the currently isolated pathogens. Clin Infect Dis 2004; 39:(suppl 1) S25–S31.
89. Winston DJ, Lazarus HM, Beveridge RA, et al. Randomized, doubleblind, multicenter trial comparing clinafloxacin with imipenem as empirical monotherapy for febrile granulocytopenic patients. Clin Infect Dis 2001; 32(3):381–390.
90. Feld R, DePauw B, Berman S, et al. Meropenem versus ceftazidime in the treatment of cancer patients with febrile neutropenia: a randomized, double-blind trial. J Clin Oncol 2000; 18(21):3690–3698.
91. Del Favero A, Menichetti F, Martino P, et al. A multicenter, doubleblind, placebo-controlled trial comparing piperacillin-tazobactam with and without amikacin as empiric therapy for febrile neutropenia. Clin Infect Dis 2001; 33(8):1295–1301.
92. Cordonnier C, Buzyn A, Leverger G, et al. Epidemiology and risk factors for gram-positive coccal infections in neutropenia: toward a more targeted antibiotic strategy. Clin Infect Dis 2003; 36(2):149–158.
93. Rolston KV. Challenges in the treatment of infectons caused by Gram-positive and Gram-negative bacteria in patients with cancer and neutropenia. Clin Infect Dis 2005; 40:(suppl 4):S246–S252.
94. Yadegarynia D, Tarrand J, Raad I, et al. Current spectrum of bacterial infections in patients with cancer. Clin Infect Dis 2003; 37(8):1144–1145.
95. Rolston KV, Tarrand JJ. Pseudomonas aeruginosa-still a frequent pathogen in patients with cancer: 11-year experience at a comprehensive cancer center. Clin Infect Dis 1999; 29(2):463–464.
96. Raje NS, Rao SR, Iyer RS, et al. Infection analysis in acute lymphoblastic leukaemia: a report of 499 concecutive episodes in India. Pediatr Hematol Oncol 1994; 11(3): 271–280.

97. Wisplinghoff H, Seifert H, Wenzel RP, et al. Current trends in the epidemiology of noso-comial blood stream infections in patients with haematological malignancies and sold neoplasms in hospitals in the United States. Clin Infect Dis 2003; 36(9):1103–1110.

98. Tunkel AR, Sepkowitz KA. Infections caused by viridans streptococci in patients with neutropenia. Clin Infect Dis 2002; 34(11):1524–1529.

99. Gales AC, Jones RN, Turnidge J, et al. Characterization of *Pseudomonas aeruginosa* iso-lates: occurrence rates, antimicrobial susceptibility patterns, and molecular typing in the global SENTRY Antimicrobial Surveillance Program, 1997–1999. Clin Infect Dis 2001; 32(suppl 2):S146–S155.

100. Bell JM, Turnidge JD, Gales AC, et al. Prevalence of extended-spectrum beta-lactamase (ESBL)–producing clinical isolates in the Asia-Pacific region and South Africa: regional results from SENTRY Antimicrobial Surveillance Program (1998–99). Diagn Microbiol Infect Dis 2002; 42(3):193–198.

101. Fainstein V, Elting LS, Bodey GP. Bacteremia caused by non-sporulating anaerobes in cancer patients. A 12 year experience. Medicine (Baltimore) 1989; 68(3):151–162.

102. Paul M, Soares-weiser K, Leibovici L. β lactam monotherapy versus β lactam-aminoglycoside combination for fever with neutropenia: systematic review and meta-analysis. BMJ 2003; 327(7399):1111–1121.

103. Aiken SK, Wetzstein GA. Once-daily aminoglycosides in patients with neutropenic fever. Oncol Pharm 2002; 9(5):426–431.

104. Pizzo PA, Hathorn JW, Himenez J, et al. A randomized trial comparing ceftazidime alone with combination antibiotic therapy in cancer patients with fever and neutrope-nia. N Engl J Med 1986; 315(9):552–558.

105. Yamamura D, Gucalp R, Carlisle P, et al. Open randomized study of cefepime versus piperacillin-gentamicin for treatment of febrile neutropenic cancer patients. Antimi-crob Agents Chemother 1997; 41(8):1704–1708.

106. Cometta A, Calandra T, Gaya H, et al. Monotherapy with meropenem versus combination therapy with ceftazidime plus amikacin as empiric therapy for fever in granulocytopenic patients with cancer. Antimicrob Agents Chemother 1996; 40(5): 1108–1115.

107. Del Favero A, Menichetti F, Martino P, et al. A multicenter, double-blind, placebo-controlled trial comparing piperacillin/tazobactam with and without amikacin as empiric therapy for febrile neutropenia. Clin Infect Dis 2001; 33(8):1295–1301.

108. Bodey GP, Middleman E, Umsawadi T, et al. Infections in cancer patients. Results with gentamycin sulfate therapy. Cancer 1972; 29(6):1697–1701.

109. Giamarellou H, Bassaris HP, Petrikkos G, et al. Monotherapy with intravenous fol-lowed by oral high dose ciprofloxacin versus combination therapy with ceftazidime plus amikacin as initial empiric therapy for granulocytopenic patients with fever. Anti-microb Agents Chemother 2000; 44(12):3264–3271.

110. Chamilos G, Bamias A, Efstathiou E, et al. Outpatient treatment of low-risk neutropenic fever in cancer patients using oral moxifloxacin. Cancer 2005; 103(12):2629–2635.

111. Talcott JA. Out-patient management of febrile neutropenia. Intern J Antimicrob Agents 2000; 16(2):169–171.

112. European Organization for Research and Treatment of Cancer (EORTC) International Antimicrobial Therapy Cooperative Group, National Cancer Institute of Canada-Clinical Trials Group. Vancomycin added to empirical combination antibiotic therapy for fever in granulocytopenic cancer patients. J Infect Dis 1991; 163(5):951–958.

113. Raad II, Escalante C, Hachem RY, et al. Treatment of febrile neutropenic patients with cancer who require hospitalization: a prospective randomized study comparing impe-nem and cefepime. Cancer 2003; 98(5):1039–1047.

114. Rubin M, Hathorn JW, Marshall D, et al. Gram-positive infections and the use of vancomycin in 550 episodes of fever and neutropenia. Ann Intern Med 1988; 108(1): 30–35.

115. Paul M, Borok S, Fraser A, et al. Empirical antibiotics against Gram-positive infections for febrile neutropenia: systematic review and meta-analysis of randomized controlled trials. J Antimicrob Chemother 2005; 55(4):436–444.

116. Cometta A, Kern WV, De Bock R, et al. Vancomycin versus placebo for treating persistent fever in patients with neutropenic cancer receiving piperacillin-tazobactam monotherapy. Clin Infect Dis 2003; 37(3):382–389.
117. Erjavec Z, de Vries-Hospers HG, Laseur M, et al. A prospective, randomized, duble-blinded, placebo-controlled trial of empirical teicoplanin in febrile neutropenia with persistent fever after imipenem monotherapy. J Antimicrob Chemother 2000; 45(6):843–849.
118. Menichetti F. The role of teicoplanin in the treatment of febrile neutropenia J Chemother 2000; 12(suppl 5):S34–S39.
119. Wingard JR. Empirical antifungal therapy in treating febrile neutropenic patients. Clin Infect Dis 2004; 39(suppl 1):S38–S43.
120. Sipsas NV, Bodey GP, Kontoyiannis DP, et al. Perspectives for the management of febrile neutropenic patients with cancer in the 21st century. Cancer 2005; 103(6): 1103–1113.
121. Pizzo PA, Robichaud KJ, Gill FA, Witebsky FG. Empiric antibiotic and antifungal therapy for cancer patients with prolonged fever and granulocytopenia. Am J Med 1982; 72(1):101–111.
122. EORTC International Antimicrobial Therapy Cooperative Group. Empiric antifungal therapy in febrile granulocytopenic patients. Am J Med 1989; 86(6 Pt 1):668–672.
123. Walsh TJ, Finberg RW, Arndt C, et al. National Institute of Allergy and Infectious Diseases Mycoses Study Group. Liposomal amphotericin B for empirical therapy in patients with persistent fever and neutropenia. N Eng J Med 1999; 340(10):764–771.
124. Walsh TJ, Teppler H, Donowitz GR, et al. Caspofungin versus liposomal amphotericin B for empirical antifungal therapy in patients with persistent fever and neutropenia. New Engl J Med 2004; 351(14):1391–1402.
125. Walsh TJ, Pappas P, Winston DJ, et al. Voriconazole compared with liposomal amphotericin B for empirical antifungal therapy in patients with neutropenia and persistent fever. New Engl J Med 2002; 346(4):225–234.
126. Vigourouz S, Morin O, Moreau P, et al. Zygomycosis after prolonged use of voriconazole in immunocompromised patients with hematologic disease: attention required. Clin Infect Dis 2005; 40(4):e35–37.
127. Chamilos G, Marom EM, Lewis RE, et al. Predictors of pulmonary zygomycosis versus invasive pulmonary aspergillosis in patients with cancer. Clin Infect Dis 2005; 41(1):60–66.
128. Elting LS, Rubenstein EB, Rolston K, et al. Time to clinical response: an outcome of antibiotic therapy of febrile neutropenia with implications for quality and cost of care. J Clin Oncol 2000; 18(21):3699–3706.
129. Corey L, Boeckh M. Persistent fever in patients with neutropenia. N Engl J Med 2002; 346(4):222–224.
130. Kern WV. Modifications of therapy. Int J Antimicrob Agents 2000; 16(2):139–141.
131. Leather HL, Wingard JR. Infections following hematopoietic stem cell transplantation. Infect Dis Clin North Am 2001; 15(2):483–520.
132. Clark OA, Lyman G, Castro AA, et al. Colony stimulating factors for chemotherapy induced febrile neutropenia. Cochrane Database Syst Rev 2003; (3):CD003039.
133. Cheng AC, Stephens DP, Curie BJ. Granulocyte-Colony Stimulating Factor (G-CSF) as an adjunct to antibiotics in the treatment of pneumonia in adults. Cochrane Database Syst Rev 2004; (3):CD004400.
134. Özer H, Armitage JO, Bennett CL, et al. American Society of Clinical Oncology Growth Factors Expert Panel. 2000 update of recommendations for the use of hematopoietic colony-stimulating factors: evidence-based, clinical practice guidelines. J Clin Oncol 2000; 18(20):3558–3585.
135. Gafter-Gvilli A, Fraser A, Paul M, et al. Meta-analysis: Atibiotic prophylaxis reduces mortality in neutropenic patiets. Ann Intern Med 2005; 142(12 Pt 1):979–995.
136. van de Wetering MD, de Witte MA, Kremer LCM, et al. E.cacy of oral prophylactic antibiotics in neutropenic afebrile oncology patients: A systematic review of randomised controlled trials Eur J Cancer 2005; 41(10):1372–1382.

137. Engels EA, Lau J, Barza M, et al. Efficacy of quinolone prophylaxis in neutropenic cancer patients: a meta-analysis. J Clin Oncol 1998; 16(3):1179–1187.
138. Cruciani M, Rampazzor R, Malena M, et al. Prophylaxis with fluoroquinolones for bacterial infections in neutropenic patients: a meta-analysis. Clin Infect Dis 1996; 23(4):795–805.
139. Gotzsche PC, Johansen HK. Routine versus selective antifungal administration for control of fungal infections in patients with cancer. Cochrane Database Syst Rev 2002; (2):CD000026.
140. Goodman JL, Winston DJ,Greenfield RA, et al. A controlled trial of fluconazole to prevent fungal infections in patients undergoing bone marrow transplantation. N Engl J Med 1992; 326(13):845–851.
141. Kanda Y, Yamamoto R, Chizuka A, et al. Prophylactic action of oral fluconazole against fungal infection in neutropenic patients. A meta-analysis of 16 randomized, controlled trials. Cancer 2000; 89(7):1611–1625.
142. Ascioglou S, de Pauw BE, Meis J. Prophylaxis and treatment of fungal infections associated with haematological malignancies. Int J Antimicrob Agents 2000; 15(3):159–168.
143. Dykewicz CA. Hospital infection control in haematopoietic stem cell transplant recipients. Emerg Infect Dis 2001; 7(2):263–267.
144. Owczuk R, Wujtewicz MA, Sawicka W, et al. Patients with haematological malignancies reqiring invasive mechanical ventilation: differences between survivors and non-survivors in intensive care unit. Support Care Cancer 2005; 13(5):332–338.
145. Blot F, Guiguet M, Nitenberg G, et al. Prognostic factors for neutropenic patients in an intensive care unit: respective roles of underlying malignancies and acute organ failures. Eur J Cancer 1997; 33(7):1031–1037.
146. Staudinger T, Stoiser B, Mullner M. Outcome and prognostic factors in critically ill cancer patients admitted to the intensive care unit. Crit Care Med 2000; 28(5):1322–1328.
147. Price KJ, Thall PF, Susannah KK, et al. Prognostic indicators for blood and marrow transplant patients admitted to an intensive care unit. Am J Resp Crit Care Med 1998; 158(3):876–884.
148. Regazzoni CJ, Irrazabal C, Luna CM, et al. Cancer patients with septic shock: mortality predictors and neutropenia. Support Care Cancer 2004; 12(12):833–839.
149. Gruson D, Hilbert G, Vargas F. Impact of colony-stimulating factor therapy on clinical outcome and frequency rate of nosocomial infections in intensive care unit neutropenic patients. Crit Care Med 2000; 28(9):3155–3160.

7

Fever of Unknown Origin in Rheumatic Diseases

Burke A. Cunha

Infectious Disease Division, Winthrop-University Hospital, Mineola, New York, U.S.A.

OVERVIEW

Fever of unknown origin (FUO) is uncommonly due to rheumatic or collagen vascular diseases. Petersdorf, in his classic 1961 description of FUOs, described the various etiologies of prolonged undiagnosed fever. At that time, infectious diseases were the most common cause of FUO followed by malignancy, and the next most common category was that of collagen vascular diseases. Since 1961, there have been a variety of serological diagnostic tests helpful in the diagnosis of most collagen vascular diseases. The result has been that collagen vascular diseases are a relatively uncommon cause of FUO at the present time (1). Rheumatic diseases such as rheumatoid arthritis (RA) and systemic lupus erythematosus (SLE) are rare causes of FUO because of the many serological tests currently available to diagnose these disorders. The collagen vascular diseases that continue to be diagnostic problems, presenting as FUOs include those which are not readily diagnosable by simple or specific diagnostic tests. At the present time, collagen vascular diseases that are likely to remain undiagnosed after one month of fever and one week of inpatient/outpatient diagnostic testing include Kikuchi's disease, Takayasu's arteritis, late onset rheumatoid arthritis (LORA), polymyalgia rheumatica (PMR), temporal arteritis (TA), vasculitides, for example, periarteritis nodosa (PAN), and adult juvenile rheumatoid arthritis (JRA) also known as adult onset Still's disease (1,2).

Two collagen vascular diseases are special diagnostic problems, that is, sarcoidosis and SLE. Patients with SLE presenting as FUOs are either those initially clinically presenting with a flare, or fever because there is not an antecedent history of SLE and remain undiagnosed if the practitioner does not recognize the possibility of SLE and order the appropriate serological tests to confirm the diagnosis. The diagnostic difficulty is compounded in patients who have no history of SLE and present with an FUO, with clinical features uncharacteristic of SLE. Immuno-modulatory viruses, for example, cytomegalovirus (CMV), may induce a flare of SLE or, rarely, may cause such immunological pertubation of the immune system as to result in de novo SLE after following CMV infection (3).

Sarcoidosis is the other rheumatic disease that may be problematic. Sarcoidosis is basically an afebrile granulomatous disorder. There are three variations of sarcoidosis associated with fever, that is, uveoparotid fever (Heerfordt's syndrome), massive granulomatous involvement of the liver with granulomatous hepatitis secondary to sarcoidosis, and sarcoid meningitis, which is a basilar meningitis affecting the thermoregulatory center of the anterior hypothalamus. Excluding these three sarcoid variants, sarcoidosis with fever should suggest two possibilities. The first is that the diagnosis of sarcoidosis is incorrect and there is another disorder

TABLE 1   Fever of Unknown Origin: Rheumatic Causes

Common
   Adult Still's disease/ juvenile rheumatoid arthritis (JRA)
   Polymyalgia rheumatica/temporal arteritis (PMR)/(TA)
Uncommon
   Late onset rheumatoid arthritis (LORA)
   Periarteritis nodosa (PAN)
   Systemic lupus erythematosus (SLE)
Rare
   Sjogren's syndrome
   Familial Mediterranean fever (FMF)
   Behçet's disease
   Pseudogout
   Takayasu's arteritis
   Kikuchi's disease

mimicking sarcoidosis responsible for the fever. Alternately, sarcoidosis may be complicated by infectious and noninfectious disorders causing fever. If the patient truly has sarcoidosis, and in addition has fever, this may present as an FUO and be a difficult diagnostic problem. Sarcoidosis with pleural effusion and fever should suggest superimposed tuberculosis as an explanation for the patient's prolonged fevers (1). Alternately, some patients with sarcoidosis undergo malignant transformation resulting in a B-cell lymphoma, the so-called sarcoidosis-lymphoma syndrome (4). Alternately, sarcoidosis can also undergo a malignant transformation into chronic lymphatic leukemia (Richter's transformation). Although rare, sarcoidosis presenting as an FUO excluding uveal tract, hepatic, and central nervous system (CNS) involvement, should suggest the possibility of superimposed tuberculosis (TB) or malignancy, that is, B-cell lymphoma or chronic lymphatic leukemia (CLL). Similarly, whereas SLE by itself is unlikely to present as an FUO, SLE with CMV may rarely present as FUO (4) (Tables 1–3).

TABLE 2   Fever of Unkown Origin: Rheumatic Disorders—Physical Finding Clues

Anatomic region	PE findings	Rheumatic disorder
Eyes	Band keratopathy	Adult JRA
	Dry eyes	LORA
		SLE
	Watery eyes	PAN
	Conjunctivitis	SLE
	Uveitis	SLE
Lymph nodes	Lymphadenopathy	Adult JRA
		Kikuchi's disease
Spleen	Splenomegaly	Kikuchi's disease
Genitals	Epididymo-orchitis	PAN
Skeletal	Arthritis	LORA
		SLE

Abbreviations: JRA, juvenile rheumatoid arthritis; LORA, late-onset rheumatoid arthritis; PAN, periarteritis nodosa; SLE, systemic lupus erythematosus.

TABLE 3   Fever of Unknown Origin: Rheumatic Disorders—Laboratory
Test Clues

CBC	Rheumatic disorders
Leukopenia	SLE
	Kikuchi's disease
Monocytosis	SLE
	PAN
	TA
Eosinophilia	PAN
Lymphopenia	SLE
Thrombocytosis	PAN
ESR	
Highly elevated (>100 mm/hr)	Adult JRA
	SLE
	PMR/TA
	PAN
	LORA
	FMF
	Kikuchi's disease
	Takayasu's arteritis
LFTs	
↑ Alkaline phosphatase	PAN
↑ SGOT/SGPT	Adult JRA
	Kikuchi's disease
SPEP	
Polyclonal gammopathy	PAN
	Takayasu's arteritis
RFTs	
Renal insufficiency	SLE
	PAN
Ferritin	
↑ Ferritin levels	Adult JRA
	SLE

Abbreviations: CBC, complete blood count; ESR, erythrocyte sedimentation rate;
FMF, familial Mediterranean fever; JRA, juvenile rheumatoid arthritis; LFTs, liver
function tests; LORA, late onset rheumatoid arthritis; RFT, renal function tests;
PAN, periarteritis nodosa; PMR, polymyalgia rheumatica; SGOT/SGPT, serum
glutamic-oxaloacatic transaminase/serum glutamic pyruvate transaminase; SLE,
systemic lupus erythematosus; SPEP, serum protein electrophoresis; TA, temporal
arteritis.

FUO: THE MOST COMMON COLLAGEN VASCULAR DISEASE ETIOLOGIES
Polymyalgia Rheumatica/Temporal Arteritis

Polymyalgia rheumatica (PMR) is a collagen vascular disease of undetermined
etiology that is most common in the elderly. Clinically, polymyalgia presents
with fever, fatigue, and muscle stiffness in the limb girdle distribution. Importantly,
patients with PMR complain of muscle stiffness or soreness, but not muscle weakness. This is confirmed by physical examination where PMR patients do not have
demonstrable muscle weakness. Because there are no localizing signs with PMR,
it can present as an obscure cause of prolonged fevers.

Temporal arteritis (TA) is a variant of PMR with involvement of the temporal
arteries. TA is also known as giant-cell arteritis and is an uncommon cause of arteritis of mid- and large-sized extracranial arteries of the head and neck. Patients with
temporal arteritis may present with headaches, either generalized or over any part

of the scalp, but classically located over one or both temporal arteries. TA may accompany PMR. Because TA is an arteritis, there may be involvement of the ophthalmic arteries in addition to the temporal arteries. Unilateral visual impairment is a serious complication of TA and requires immediate therapy with steroids to prevent permanent blindness. Not all patients with TA demonstrate tenderness over the temporal arteries, and, in these patients, TA is a difficult diagnosis that depends on demonstrating arteritis and a temporal artery biopsy. One of the few clinical clues, if present, to TA is persistent dry cough. In addition to fever, patients with TA may also present with anorexia, weight loss, and night sweats. Physical findings include headache or scalp tenderness. Angle of the jaw pain may be noticed by the patient during mastication (1,5).

There are no specific tests for PMR or TA, although nonspecific laboratory tests may provide clues pointing towards the diagnosis of TA. The complete blood count (CBC) may show anemia and thrombocytosis in TA. The anemia in TA is the anemia of chronic disease. Thrombocytosis of TA is due to chronic inflammation. In an elderly patient, the findings of anemia and thrombocytosis are often overlooked as potentially useful diagnostic laboratory clues associated with TA. Anemia and thrombocytosis are, of course, nonspecific, but, in an obscure case, take on added diagnostic significance especially if found in conjunction with other laboratory or clinical findings. Patients with TA may also demonstrate a mild increase in the serum transaminases or alkaline phosphatase. The single most important laboratory test to suggest the possibility of either PMR or TA is a highly elevated erythrocyte sedimentation rate (ESR). The ESR, while nonspecific, is useful if highly elevated, that is, ≥ 100 mm/hour. A highly elevated ESR should suggest the possibility of collagen vascular disease, particularly PMR or TA, in an FUO patient with no other findings or localizing signs. Other nonspecific laboratory tests that may indicate TA or a variety of other abnormalities presenting with FUO include the serum protein electrophoresis (SPEP). Elevations of the alpha 1/alpha 2 globulins on the SPEP in an FUO patient should not be ascribed as being acute-phase reactants, since, by definition, the patient has a prolonged illness. Elevations of the alpha 1/2 globulins in the setting of FUO should suggest the possibility of TA or lymphoma.

The other laboratory tests useful in patients with FUO, which, although nonspecific, may also be helpful in suggesting a diagnosis, are serum ferritin levels. Elevated serum ferritin levels are often incorrectly ascribed as being acute-phase reactants. Mild transient elevations of the serum ferritin level in an acute febrile illness certainly indicate that the ferritin level is a manifestation of the acute-phase reaction. However, in FUO patients, the onset and duration of serum ferritin elevations, as well as the magnitude of ferritin levels, indicate that elevated serum ferritin levels in this clinical context is an important diagnostic finding and should not be considered as an acute-phase reactant. In the context of FUO, highly elevated ferritin levels should suggest a variety of diagnostic possibilities. In a patient with FUO and elevated ferritin levels, diagnostic possibilities that should be entertained should include malignancies, that is, myelodysplastic syndrome, lymphomas, solid tumors, lymphoreticular malignancies, adult Still's disease, and TA (1,5–7).

FUO: Adult Onset Juvenile Rheumatoid Arthritis

Arguably, adult onset juvenile rheumatoid arthritis (JRA) is the most important collagen vascular disease cause of FUO. Adult JRA presenting as an FUO has a characteristic fever pattern. Fever patterns are helpful with selected infectious and noninfectious disorders, and the more specific the fever pattern, the more likely the finding is to be of diagnostic significance. Patients with adult JRA typically have a "double quotidian" pattern. A "double quotidian" fever is one that has two fever spikes each day, separated by lower, more normal temperatures, and is not artificially induced by antipyretics. Double quotidian fever occurs in relatively few infectious-disease disorders, that is, right-sided gonococcal endocarditis, mixed malarial infections, visceral leishmaniasis, and adult JRA. Of the infectious disorders characterized by double quotidian fevers, only visceral leishmaniasis (Kala-Azar) and adult JRA can present as FUOs (1,5).

Patients with adult JRA typically have a truncal, salmon-colored, evanescent, maculopapular rash. Patients with adult JRA also demonstrate dermographia or the Koebner phenomenon. Patients with adult JRA may complain of a migratory polyarthritis or more commonly present with pauci or oligoarticular arthritis. Adult JRA patients may also complain of visual symptoms. On physical examination, adult JRA patients typically have hepatosplenomegaly as the predominant physical finding. Patients with fever, pauci articular arthritis, visual complaints, and an evanescent rash with liver or spleen involvement should be considered as having adult JRA until proven otherwise.

Routine laboratory tests are generally unhelpful in adult JRA. The CBC is unremarkable. The ESR is moderately to highly elevated. Importantly, all of the usual serological tests for RA, (rheumatoid factor, ANA) and SLE (ANA, anti double-stranded DNA) are negative. In patients with hepatomegaly, the alkaline phosphatase may be mildly elevated, but serum transaminases are usually normal. An important nonspecific test that is frequently elevated in adult JRA is the serum ferritin. Prolonged and highly elevated serum ferritin levels occur with JRA and are a nonspecific clue to the diagnosis. In a patient with FUO, an elevated ferritin level may suggest a variety of disorders ranging from malignancy to TA or adult JRA. The magnitude of the elevation of the serum ferritin is proportional to disease activity in adult JRA. Elevated serum ferritin levels in the presence of a double quotidian fever would be diagnostic of adult JRA (1,8).

Vasculitis

Although rare as a cause of FUO, the rheumatic disorders causing FUO are treatable. The collagen vascular diseases presenting as FUO that are due to vasculitis may be obscure (9,10). Takayasu's arteritis, a rare cause of arteritis and FUO, presents with diminished arterial pulses. The diagnosis of Takayasu's arteritis is made by biopsy. Takayasu's arteritis is usually treated with steroids because of their anti-inflammatory properties. The CBC in Takayasu's arteritis is usually unremarkable. Importantly, eosinophilia is not present. The ESR is typically elevated and there may be some degree of thrombocytosis (1,10). One study indicates that Takayasu's arteritis may be amenable to treatment with minocycline.

Patients with adult Still's disease present with pauciarticular and visual symptoms commonly. The most important sign of adult JRA is the presence of a double quotidian fever, which, in an FUO patient, is virtually diagnostic. Physical examination may reveal an evanescent, truncal, salmon-colored rash. More commonly, hepatosplenomegaly is present in such patients. Nonspecific laboratory tests include an elevated ESR, elevated serum ferritin levels; serum ferritin levels are also an index of disease activity and an important diagnostic clue in adult JRAs with FUO (1,5,8).

REFERENCES

1. Cunha BA. Fever of unkown origin. In: Gorbach SL, Bartlett JB, Blacklow NR, eds. Infectious Diseases in Medicine and Surgery. 4th ed. Baltimore: Lippincott Williams and Wilkins, 2005.
2. Cunha BA, Syed U, Hamid N. Fever of unknown origin (FUO) due to late onset of rheumatoid arthritis (LORA). Heart Lung 2006; 35:70–73.
3. Teglia O, Cunha BA. CMV-induced SLE presenting as fever of unknown origin. Infect Dis Pract 1993; 17:7–8.
4. DeLeon DG, Shifteh S, Cunha BA. FUO due to sarcoidosis-lymphoma syndrome. Heart Lung 2004; 33:124–129.
5. Cunha BA. Fever of unkown origin. Infect Dis Clin North Am 1996; 10:111–128.
6. Cunha BA. Fever of unknown origin in the elderly. A commentary. Infect Dis Clin Practice 1993; 2:380–383.
7. Cunha BA, Parchuri S, Mohan S. FUO: Temporal arteritis presenting with prolonged cough and elevated serum ferritin levels. Heart Lung 2000; 35:112–116.
8. Cunha BA. FUO due to adult onset juvenile rheumatoid arthritis (adult onset Still's disease): the diagnostic significance of a double quotidian fever and elevated serum ferritin levels. Heart Lung 2004; 33:417–421.
9. Bailey EM, Klein NC, Cunha BA. Kikuchi's disease with liver function presenting as fever of unknown origin. Lancet 1989; 2:986.
10. Wu YJJ, Martin BR, Ong K, et al. Takayasu's arteritis presenting as a cause of fever of unknown origin. Am J Med 1989; 87:476–477.

8 Fever of Unknown Origin in HIV Patients

Wendy S. Armstrong

Division of Infectious Diseases, Department of Medicine, Cleveland Clinic Foundation, Cleveland, Ohio, U.S.A.

Powel Kazanjian

Division of Infectious Diseases, Department of Internal Medicine, University of Michigan Medical Center, Ann Arbor, Michigan, U.S.A.

OVERVIEW
Importance
Fever of unknown origin (FUO) in human immunodeficiency virus (HIV)-infected patients is a challenging test of the acumen of the physician. The characteristics of FUO in HIV-infected persons have been published in several studies conducted prior to the advent of the new HIV therapies and published from 1992 to 1999 (Table 1). In this chapter, we will review these series on FUO in HIV (19). Since they have been reported, however, the introduction of highly active antiretroviral therapy (HAART) has resulted in a dramatic reduction in various AIDS-related illnesses that themselves cause FUO (10,11). In addition, newer manifestations of the classic AIDS-associated opportunistic infections, the immune reconstitution inflammatory syndromes (IRIS), were first described shortly following the use of HAART (12)]. This chapter will summarize the findings in the two series, which have evaluated the effect of potent antiretroviral therapy on the incidence and clinical manifestations of specific diseases that cause FUO in HIV-infected patients (13,14).

CLINICAL FEATURES
Fever of Unknown Origin in HIV-Infected Persons in the Pre-HAART Era
Prior to the HAART era, fevers $\geq 101°F$, persisting for >4 weeks as an outpatient or four days as an inpatient without an obvious source (FUO) were not an infrequent occurrence in the late stage of HIV infection. In the seven largest series published on FUO in HIV-infected persons (Table 1), the mean CD4 cell counts were all <100 cells/mm^3 (range: 40–98/mm^3). Thus, in HIV-infected persons, FUO tends to occur in the late stage of HIV infection (1–9). In these reports, the incidence of hospitalization for FUO among hospitalizations in HIV-infected persons was variable (3.4–21%) (13). Nonetheless, they each note that several HIV-associated illnesses may present with undifferentiated fever prior to the onset of specific organ-related symptoms. Examples include lymphoma, *Pneumocystis jirovecii* pneumonia (PCP), Leishmaniasis, infections due to cytomegalovirus, *Cryptococcus neoformans*, *Toxoplasma gondii*, and *Mycobacterium tuberculosis*. Other illnesses, such as disseminated mycobacterium avium intracellulare (MAI) infection and histoplasmosis, may present with constitutional symptoms alone in the absence of specific symptoms of organ involvement.

TABLE 1 Selected Reports on HIV-Associated Fever of Unknown Origin in the Pre-HAART Era

	Bissuel et al., 1994	Miralles et al., 1995	Miller et al., 1996	Lozano et al., 1996	Knobel et al., 1996	Lambertucci et al., 1999	Armstrong et al., 1999	Totals
Country	France	Spain	U.K.	Spain	Spain	Brazil	U.S.A.	
# pts	57	50	78	128	100	55	70	538
Mean CD4	94	71	40	46	56	98	58	
M tb	10	21	13	69	46	18	4	181
MAI	7	7	25	10	8	5	22	64
Other mycobacteria	6	0	3	0	15	0	1	25
PCP	3	1	6	7	5	6	10	37
CMV	5	1	2	6	6	0	8	30
Other viral	1	1	0	2	0	0	5	10
Pyogenic	2	1	14	12	5	5	4	40
Fungal	1	1	3	2	3	5	7	22
Leishmania	4	7	0	23	5	0	0	39
Toxo	2	1	0	3	5	1	1	13
Other parasites	0	0	3	1	0	3	1	6
Neoplasm	4	0	6	8	4	4	6	33
Misc	4[a]	2[b]	3[c]	0[d]	2	0[e]	3[f]	15
No Dx	8	6	7	8	10	10	14	58
>1 dx	0	0	6	0	14	38	13	

[a]Viral: HIV infection (1); pyogenic: sinusitis/bronchitis (2); fungal: cryptococcosis (1); neoplasm: lymphoma (2); misc: factitious fever, induced fever, zidovudine toxicity, and neuralgic amyotrophy each in one.

[b]Viral: Varicella-zoster encephalitis (1); pyogenic: Salmonella prostatis (1); fungal: aspergillosis (1); neoplasm: lymphoma (2); misc: drug fever (1).

[c] pyogenic: Staphylococcus aureus (3), Pseudomonas (3), Shigella enteritis (2), typhoid fever (1), Camplyobacter enteritis (1) Streptococcus pneumoniae septicemia (1), Staphylococcus epidermidis line infection (1), Corynebacterium jekeium (1) Nocardia (1); fungal: histoplasmosis (1), Penicillium marnefeii (1), crytpococcosis (1); parasites: Cryptosporidium (2), Plasmodium falciparum (1) Neoplasm: lymphoma (5), KS (1); misc: factitious fever (2), Reiter's syndrome (1).

[d]Viral: acute HIV (1), HIV (1); pyogenic: sinusitis (7), Nocardia (1), Q fever (1), brucellosis (1), parvovirus (1); fungal: cryptococcal meningitis (1), mucormycosis (1); parasitic: cryptosporidiosis (1); neoplasm: non-Hodgkin's lymphoma (8).

[e]Pyogenic sinusitis (2), Salmonella-Schistosoma mansoni association (2), syphilis (1); fungal Cryptococcal meningitis (3), histoplasmosis (2); parasitic Isosporiasis (1); neoplasm: non-Hodgkin's lymphoma (4).

[f]Viral: VZV encephalitis (1), hepatitis C (1) hepatitis B (1); adenoviral pneumonia (1); HSV esophagitis (1); pyogenic: Salmonella enteritis (1), sinusitis (1), rectal abscess (1), pyomyositis (1); fungal: histoplasmosis (5), pulmonary aspergillosis (5), disseminated cryptococcosis (1); parasitic: cryptosporidiosis (1); neoplasm: Lymphoma (5), Kaposi's sarcome (1); misc: drug fever (2), Castleman's disease (1).

Abbreviations: CMV, cytomegalovirus; HAART, highly active antiretroviral therapy; HSV, Herpes simplex virus; KS, kaposis sarcome; MAI, mycobacterium avium intracellulare; Misc, miscellaneous; PCP, Pneumocystis jirovecii; VZV, Varicella-Zoster virus.
Source: From Refs. 1–7.

Table 1 shows that infections are the most common cause of FUO, accounting for approximately 90% of cases in which a diagnosis was determined. Mycobacterial infections, both *M. tuberculosis* and *M. avium*, account for the majority of these cases. The remaining infections are due to pyogenic infections, *T. gondii*, *P. jirovecii*, *C. neoformans*, and *Leishmania* spp. Cytomegalovirus and HIV itself account for a small percentage of FUO, approximately 4% each. In several of these series, the cause of FUO was attributed to HIV alone when the diagnostic evaluation did not reveal a specific etiology and when the patient defervesced following antiretroviral therapy. The diagnosis remains unestablished in approximately 15% of cases.

The distribution of illnesses responsible for HIV-associated FUO in the United States differs from that reported in European countries (Table 1). In the United States, Disseminated mycobacterial avium infectious (DMAC) is the single most common cause of HIV-associated FUO, whereas it occurs less frequently in series from European countries. Other diagnoses that account for FUO more often in the United States than abroad include PCP, infections due to cytomegalovirus, disseminated histoplasmosis, and neoplasia. In contrast, *M. tuberculosis* is the most common cause of FUO in foreign countries, whereas this infection accounts for a smaller number of cases in series from the United States. Similarly, leishmaniasis and toxoplasmosis more commonly cause HIV-associated FUO in foreign countries than in the United States (Table 1).

Regional variations in the prevalence of these infections likely explain the different contribution they make to HIV-associated FUO according to geographic location. Tuberculosis in the general population, for example, is less common in the United States than in France or Spain. Similarly, leishmaniasis occurs more often in Spain, France, and Italy than in the United States. Moreover, toxoplasmosis is more common in France than in the United States. It is more difficult, however, to assess the influence that differences in patient risk behaviors between the United States and foreign series make to the clinical spectrum of HIV-associated FUO. Injecting drug use, for example, was the most common risk behavior in foreign series, accounting for 57% to 82% of cases, whereas this behavior was noted in only 10% to 22% of cases reported from the United States (7). Thus, the impact of the different risk behaviors on the spectrum of diseases accounting for FUO remains speculative.

Fever of Unknown Origin in HIV-Infected Persons in the HAART Era

The introduction of HAART has led to a decline in the incidence of HIV-associated FUO. In a retrospective study performed in Spain between 1997 and 1999, among 4858 patients receiving HAART, the frequency of FUO was 0.6% as compared to 3% in 2787 patients not receiving HAART (14). In addition, HAART has resulted in unique manifestations of the same illnesses reported to cause FUO in the pre-HAART era. The following sections describe how these trends have affected the patient population and the clinical manifestations of HIV-associated FUO.

Decline in Opportunistic Illnesses in the HAART Era

There has been an overall decline in opportunistic illnesses (OIs), which was initially reported after the introduction of HAART in 1996 (10,11) and sustained throughout 2002 (15). Nonetheless, some patients receiving combination antiretrovirals remain at risk for developing new OIs (16,17). Studies have identified pretreatment CD4 count <200/mm (18) as HIV RNA level >100,000 copies/mL (19) as independent predictors of progression to AIDS and death. In addition, inadequate CD4 (20) count increases and persistent viremia (21), measured after starting HIV treatment, are predictors of disease progression. Thus, several studies have shown that adequate CD4 and viral load (VL) responses to HAART provide a clinical benefit by protecting against HIV disease progression (22).

Studies of HIV-associated FUO in the HAART era have supported this data. In the two published series, the mean CD4 count at the time of FUO was low [102 cells/mm^3 (W), 68 cells/mm^3 (L)] and was similar to those noted during FUO in the pre-HAART era (13,14). Plasma viremia in these series differed, with one series reporting a mean viral load of >300,000 copies/mL and the second a mean HIV-RNA level of 1000 copies/mL. Larger studies are needed, but this data suggest that poor CD4 count responses may be a greater predictor of the development of FUO than level of viremia.

The inability to mount ample CD4 and HIV VL responses to HAART is not uncommon for patients in the later stage of HIV infection (23)]. In one study, for example, 21% of patients who started therapy with a CD4 count <200/mm^3 failed to achieve a CD4 count >200/mm^3 at 173 weeks of follow-up, in contrast to 0% of patients with baseline counts between 350 and 499 cells/mm^3 (24). In addition, a reduction in VL that cannot be maintained to low or undetectable levels, in fact, is not uncommon for patients receiving HAART. For example, virologic failure rates are especially high, varying from 20% to 70%, in those who are either treatment-experienced or have low CD4 cell counts and high VL before starting treatment (25).

Common Opportunistic Illnesses in the HAART Era That Are the Same as in the Pre-HAART Era

Studies on AIDS events have shown that PCP and MAI remain the most frequent OIs in the HAART era, as was the case in the pre-HAART era (26). For example, one study demonstrated that chemoprophylaxis failure among those with the most advanced immunosuppression was the most significant source of new PCP cases (26). Additional studies have also shown that Kaposi's sarcoma (KS) and non-Hodgkin's lymphoma (NHL) remain the major AIDS-associated malignancies in the HAART era (27,28). In contrast, another study (29) has shown that cytomegalovirus (CMV) and cerebral toxoplasmosis now occur less frequently than reported in the pre-HAART era.

These studies suggest that the most common OIs in the pre-HAART era are unchanged in the HAART era. This appears to be true in HIV-associated FUO as well (Table 2). In one U.S. study of 27 episodes of FUO after 1997, MAI and cryptococcal infection were the most commonly diagnosed OIs, with single cases of CMV, PCP, Candida infection, and herpes simplex virus (HSV). In this series, however, pyogenic infections were responsible for nearly 50% of the infectious etiologies of FUO. OIs were noted in only 36% of cases. This differs from reports from the pre-HAART era (13). In Spain, *M. tuberculosis*, visceral leishmaniasis, and MAI accounted for 69% of the infectious etiologies, again similar to the distribution and frequency of OI noted in the pre-HAART era in studies conducted in this geographic region (14). Overall, in the two series, infections accounted for 85% to 100% of diagnoses, while neoplasms accounted for 4% and 0% of diagnoses.

As noted, in the pre-HAART era, FUO attributed to HIV itself was reported in approximately 4% of cases and was diagnosed by rapid defervescence after

TABLE 2 Reports of HIV-Associated FUO in the HAART Era

Report	Lozano et al., 2002[a]	Weissman et al., 2004
Country	Spain	U.S.A.
Mean CD4/VL	68/1,000	102/301,176
Mean time on HAART	349 d (15–810d)	10.8 months[b]
Total number of patients	32	26
Mycobacterium tuberculosis	12	0
Mycobacterium avium	4[c]	5[c]
Other mycobacteria	0	0
PCP	0	1
Cytomegalovirus	1[d]	1
HIV	0	1
Pyogenic infections	3[e]	9[f]
Lymphoma	2	0
Cryptococcosis	0	2
Leishmaniasis	6	0
Toxoplasmosis	0	0
Other diagnosis	0	8[g]
Unknown	4	5
More than one causative disease	0	5

[a]Included in table are only those on HAART.
[b]17 of 26 on HAART at presentation; of these mean time on HAART was 10.8 months.
[c]One case in each series represents IRIS to MAI.
[d]CMV pneumonitis due to IRIS.
[e]Pyogenic diagnoses include Q fever, pneumonia, and pancreatic abscess (1 each).
[f]Pyogenic diagnoses include pneumonia (2) and C. difficile colitis, sinusitis with epidural empyema, pelvic inflammatory disease, sacroiliitis, soft-tissue infection of the neck, urosepsis with small bowel obstruction, urinary tract infection (1 each).
[g]Other diagnoses are: Candida esophagitis, HSV esophagitis, secondary syphilis, encephalitis, adverse drug reaction to TMP/SMX (1 pt) and phenytoin (1 pt), polyclonal plasmacytic lymphoproliferative disorder.
Abbreviations: HAART, highly active antiretroviral therapy; HSV, herpes simplex virus; IRIS, immune reconstitution inflammatory syndrome; MAI, Mycobacterium avium intracellulare; PCP, *Pneumocytis jirovecii* pnenmonia; TMP/SMX, trimethoprim-sulfamethoxazole; VL, viral load.

initiation of antiretroviral therapy, without emergence of an alternate etiology. In the HAART era, fever caused by HIV is reported in a single case described as an acute retroviral rebound syndrome, which represents a new and different manifestation of fever caused by the virus than that noted previously (13).

Immune Reconstitution Inflammatory Syndrome: Newer Manifestations of Classic Opportunistic Illnesses

Focal manifestations of opportunistic illnesses caused by a variety of organisms, such as *M. tuberculosis*, *M. avium* complex, or *C. neoformans*, may occur in AIDS patients with severe immune suppression who have an exuberant response to HAART initiation (12). When reconstitution of the immune system occurs shortly after the use of HAART, an inflammatory reaction can occur at sites of occult infection with a variety of pathogens (30–32). These abnormalities are the result of an inflammatory reaction to the infecting organism as HAART restores cell-mediated immune responses. The syndrome, referred to as the immune reconstitution inflammatory syndrome (IRIS), may reflect an unmasking of subclinical disease, or worsen the intensity of an infection that was already apparent at the time of HAART initiation.

Studies have identified IRIS as a focal inflammatory condition, which classically involves specific organ systems depending on the inciting organism.

Manifestations most commonly occur within three months of initiating HAART (75% of cases) (12). Furthermore, most patients have advanced immune suppression at the time of starting HAART (CD4 $\sim 30/mm^3$) and a CD4 response to HAART at the time of IRIS diagnosis (CD4 $\sim 70/mm^3$). In these cases, focal involvement of IRIS differs from the classic presentation of disseminated multiorgan disease in patients with advanced immunodeficiency. For example, in IRIS due to MAI, blood cultures taken from patients usually do not grow mycobacteria, unlike in disseminated disease; rather, a biopsy of an involved focal organ, such as lymph node, GI tract, or liver, may be required to establish a diagnosis (31). In the two series published in the HAART era, four cases of IRIS (3 due to MAI, 1 due to CMV) were reported to cause FUO (7% of the total cases) (13,14).

DIFFERENTIAL DIAGNOSIS
Diagnostic Pitfalls
There are both similarities and differences in FUO in HIV-infected persons and the general population. In both populations, conditions that may present with prolonged, undifferentiated fever prior to the onset of specific organ involvement tend to account for FUO. PCP and infections due to cytomegalovirus, *C. neoformans*, and *Histoplasma capsulatum* are examples of such diseases in HIV-infected persons, while lymphoma and *M. tuberculosis* may result in prolonged undifferentiated fever in either population. In addition, in either population, an unusual presentation of a common disease is more likely to occur than a classic manifestation of more rare illnesses. [In an HIV-infected person, for example, a variant presentation of PCP is more likely to account for FUO than is Castleman's disease]. In contrast, a feature of FUO in HIV-infected patients—multiple etiologies accounting for a significant number of cases 19% in one series (7), differs from FUO in the general population. This feature has not been described in FUO series conducted in the general population, but has been noted in one of the European reports on HIV-associated FUO published abroad; multiple etiologies were responsible for 14% of cases in that series (Table 1).

The laborious process of investigating FUOs is difficult to accomplish in today's medical environment. The process of carefully listening to and examining a patient, contemplating the problem in a quiet environment, and collaborating with others is an arduous task. Frustration, weariness, and impatience intervene when a diagnosis is not promptly reached, and they render the physician vulnerable to overlooking the appearance of a valuable new finding. The physician must expect to devote a large amount of time to pacifying impatient relatives of the patient and justifying the length of stay to responsible insurers and institutional administrators who are desirous of a more expeditious solution. The physician must pay attention to the patient's fear of imagined diagnoses and assure the individual's compliance with the diagnostic plan. Despite such pressure, both external and self-imposed, the physician will be rewarded by recognizing that the patient has benefited from his/her approach: meticulous attention and logically pursuing available diagnostic tests.

DIAGNOSTIC APPROACH
Value of Exposure History
In the evaluation of prolonged, unexplained fevers in HIV-infected patients, the patient's previous exposures, stage of HIV infection, and epidemiologic setting

often provide important clues (1–9). For example, tuberculosis should be suspected in any person who has had a recent or remote exposure to an infected individual or who has resided in an endemic region. Similarly, histoplasmosis or coccidiomycosis may occur in persons who have had an exposure to endemic regions within the United States. Leishmaniasis should be considered in persons who have had prior exposure to South America or the Mediterranean region. Infections due to *Penicillium marneffei* should be considered in persons who lived in Southern Asia. Also, extrapulmonic *Pneumocystis* may be identified in a patient who is in the late stage of infections and has been receiving aerosolized pentamidine. Infections due to *Bartenella henselae* should be considered in individuals who have had exposure to cats; the organism may be identified by isolator cultures of blood. Finally, lymphoma should be suspected in a patient without an exposure history to a particular pathogen.

Value of Physical Findings

In the evaluation of prolonged, unexplained fevers, diagnostic testing in HIV-infected patients is guided by notable findings on the physical examination or abnormal values in a routine laboratory test. The careful evaluation of patients necessary to reach a diagnosis cannot be replaced by the early use of new diagnostic tests. One study in the general population showed that diagnosis required a mean time of 19 days (range: 1 day to 8 months), 11 days of hospitalization (range: 3 days to 5 weeks), and four outpatient visits (range: 0–11 outpatient visits) (33). Since an average hospital length of stay of 19 days for FUO exceeds that which is federally allotted by Medicare for this illness by 13 days (34), a substantial portion of the evaluation must take place in an outpatient setting, if the patient's condition allows. This fact supports the revised definition of the diagnostic criteria for FUO stipulating that the evaluation of a patient by a physician may be performed outside of a hospital setting.

The approach to FUO in HIV-infected patients is influenced by whether abnormal findings are present in the early or later stages of FUO. Several studies in the general population have reaffirmed the paramount importance of protracted study of patients in the evaluation of FUO for those cases in which no abnormal findings are present in the early stages of the illness. Prolonged, meticulous observation yields crucial findings that do not become evident until a late stage of the illness. In one series of classic FUO in 86 patients, repetition of the physical examination, selected laboratory tests, or observation after specific therapeutic intervention led to a diagnosis in 28 of 86 cases (33).

Noninvasive Tests

Cultures of blood for bacteria, mycobacteria, and fungi using an isolator technique are valuable diagnostic tests in the evaluation of FUO in HIV-infected persons. In one report, isolator blood cultures had a sensitivity of 75% for disseminated *M. avium* infection; other reports suggest a sensitivity of 64% to 85% for mycobacteria. Available technology of isolator cultures includes Bactec, Dupont Isolator, and lysis-centrifugation systems; the comparative yield for each of these systems for FUO in HIV-infected persons is unknown (35). In contrast, quantitative CMV antigen testing or polymerase chain reaction (PCR) testing for cytomegalovirus has not been proven to be a reliable test in establishing the diagnosis of disseminated cytomegaloviral infection, because patients may be viremic without having disease due to CMV infection (36). Diagnosis of CMV esophagitis, colitis, gastritis, or pneumonia requires pathological evidence of the virus effects; retinitis may be diagnosed by fundoscopic examination.

Serum and urine antigen techniques are useful in identifying certain fungal and viral infections. The serum cryptococcal antigen is sensitive and specific for detecting dissemination with *C. neoformans,* and is therefore a useful test for this purpose (37). Detecting *Histoplasma* antigen in urine or serum is very sensitive and specific in diagnosing disseminated histoplasmosis; serial antigen assessments were also found useful to monitor response to therapy (38).

For the diagnosis of PCP, expectorated sputum is rarely diagnostic, as the cough is nonproductive in most cases. Nebulizer-induced sputum is available as a diagnostic aid in many cases because of the high number of organisms present in alveoli (39). The technique involves centrifugation of liquefied sputum and staining the specimen with a direct fluorescent monoclonal antibody that reacts with the cyst wall (40). This test may establish the diagnosis of PCP in a noninvasive fashion and obviate the need to perform bronchoscopy for the diagnosis of PCP.

Thus, many cases of FUO in HIV-infected patients may be identified by a variety of noninvasive tests, as was shown to be the case in one series (Table 3). This table lists the diagnostic methods according to the number of times they yielded the diagnosis that was taken from one series (7). Overall, in that series, the diagnosis was established by noninvasive means as often as invasive

TABLE 3   Diagnostic Method According to the Number of Times It Yielded a Diagnosis

Method	Instances FUO identified no. (%)
Noninvasive methods	
Blood isolator cultures	16 (22)
Respiratory specimen[a]	7 (10)
Clinical course/exam	5 (7)
Noninvasive radiologic procedure	3 (4)
Blood smear	3 (4)
Stool culture	1 (1)
Serology	1 (1)
Total	36 (50)
Invasive testing	
Respiratory specimen[b]	11 (15)
Bone marrow examination	5 (7)
Lymph node biopsy	4 (6)
Liver biopsy	4 (6)
Lung biopsy	3 (5)
Intestinal biopsy	2 (3)
Skin biopsy	2 (3)
Lumbar puncture	2 (3)
Esophageal biopsy	1 (1)
Brain biopsy	1 (1%)
Mediastinal biopsy	1 (1%)
Total	36 (50%)

[a]Specimen obtained as a result of expectoration or induction of sputum.
[b]Specimen obtained by bronchoscopy; includes brushings and bronchoalveolar lavage.
Abbreviation: FUO, fever of unknown origin.
Source: From Ref. 7.

methods. Several factors, including advances in diagnostic capabilities, may account for this observation. As outlined above, blood cultures with use of the lysis-centrifugation technique may identify mycobacteria and obviate the performance of a bone marrow aspiration. The demonstration that isolator blood culture yielded the greatest number of diagnoses in one series (22%) (7) supports this hypothesis. In other instances, available molecular techniques have supplanted the need for pathologic analyses of surgically obtained tissue; for example, presence of JC viral PCR in spinal fluid may establish the diagnoses of progressive multifocal leukoencephalopathy and prevent the need to perform invasive procedures. In some cases, serology has supplanted the need for pathologic analysis of surgically obtained tissue as well, such as avoiding a brain biopsy in a patient with reactive serologies to *T. gondii* or in a patient with multifocal enhancing brain masses (35).

It is possible that the number of cases of FUO diagnosed by noninvasive techniques may increase in the future if new noninvasive diagnostic tests are introduced. The development of potential adjunctive diagnostic assays, such as the polymerase chain reaction for disseminated *M. avium* (MAI) infection, may further reduce the need for invasive procedures by identifying the organism far in advance of the time that is required to isolate it from blood cultures (35). Finally, advances in obtaining expectorated sputum and analyzing it for the presence of *P. jirovecii* by PCR will drastically reduce the need for bronchoscopy for the diagnosis of PCP in persons with AIDS who have had prolonged fevers (35). Caution must be exercised when interpreting results from newer technology, however. For example, PCR for Epstein-Barr virus in the CSF has been promoted as obviating the need for brain biopsy in patients with mass lesions in the brain by indicating a presumptive diagnosis of central nervous system (CNS) lymphoma. Additional data suggests that the positive predictive value of this study was 29% in one series (41). Therefore, judicious use of invasive procedures when the likelihood of obtaining a diagnosis is high remains appropriate.

When the initial and subsequent evaluation for FUO has been unrevealing, abdominal computed tomography (CT) scan occasionally proves to be a useful diagnostic tool (7,42). Occasionally, peritoneal masses or a group of enlarged retroperitoneal lymph nodes may be identified on the scan; a directed CT-guided biopsy of these abnormal areas on CT scan may reveal the cause of fevers. Gallium scans and indium-labeled white blood cells (WBC) scans are frequently performed in the setting of prolonged unexplained fevers (43), but the utility of these tests for the evaluation of FUO in HIV-infected patients remains to be established; as many as 50% of abnormalities detected in one study were unconfirmed. This high rate of false-positive results, which may lead to unnecessary additional tests, diminishes enthusiasm for these studies at present (44). Fluorodeoxyglucose (FDG)-positron emission tomography (PET) scanning may be more promising, but additional studies are needed. Brain scans in 23 patients with space-occupying lesions showed a sensitivity and specificity of 100% for differentiating lymphoma from infectious etiologies [progressive multifocal leukoencephalopathy (PML), toxoplasmosis] in one study (45).

Invasive Testing

Although sensitive, noninvasive tests for providing the diagnosis of many conditions responsible for FUO in HIV-infected persons has reduced the need to perform invasive procedures, some invasive measures continue to play a major role in identifying causes of FUO. For example, in one series, respiratory specimens that led to a diagnosis were obtained invasively in 11 of 18 times (7). Other useful diagnostic methods in that series included bone marrow examination (7%), and biopsy of lymph node (6%) and liver (6%). Thus, procedures such as bone marrow examination and biopsies of liver and abnormal lymph nodes continue to play an especially important role when patients remain febrile despite a prolonged noninvasive evaluation.

The yields of bone marrow exam and liver biopsy have been addressed in several papers, and, in HIV-infected patients, exceed the yield in FUO in the general population (35). The yield of bone marrow examination has ranged from 32% to 42% (46–48). One series showed that in 86% of cases in which an etiology for the fever was identified by base marrow exam (BME), the same diagnosis had been established by a noninvasive diagnostic modality. This series also showed that the diagnosis was made by BME as rapidly or sooner than other modalities in 53% of cases and that the diagnosis was made exclusively by BME in 16% of cases. The paper concluded that BME is indicated when a diagnosis is urgently sought or when an evaluation with other diagnostic modalities has been unsuccessful. The yield of liver biopsy has varied between 40% and 58% in evaluating FUO in HIV-infected persons (46,49,50). Liver biopsy acid-fast stains and mycobacterial cultures were able to identify seven of eight patients with mycobacterial disease (46). Biopsy of enlarged lymph nodes has been reported to have a high yield (51). In a high-risk population for HIV, the yield of lymph node biopsy for tuberculosis was 57%. A thorough evaluation of FUO (outlined above), that may include a combination of noninvasive as well as invasive tests, yields a diagnosis in most (approximately 85%) cases. As outlined earlier, multiple causes for FUO will be identified in 2% to 10% of cases—the feature that distinguishes FUO in HIV-infected persons from those who are not infected with HIV.

Clinical Approach

An initial approach in the evaluation of FUO in HIV-infected persons should be to discontinue medications, especially certain antiviral agents (such as abacavir) and sulfa agents. Accompanying clinical features of opportunistic infections causing prolonged fever often overlap with those associated with drug reactions—cytopenias, elevation of liver enzyme tests. If there is no response after two to three days, blood cultures using the lysis-centrifugation technique is a sensitive method of identifying organisms that cause disseminated infections and are located intracellularly (*H. capsulatum, M. avium*). However, because the mean time for cultures to turn positive is 18 to 25 days for *M. avium*, other noninvasive tests should be performed simultaneously. Induced sputum for *P. jirovecii* and *M. tuberculosis* should be obtained, because prolonged fevers may precede the onset of respiratory symptoms in PCP and tuberculosis respectively. Tuberculin skin testing and antigen testing for *H. capsulatum* in serum and urine also should be performed. If the serum cryptococcal antigen is reactive at a titer of >1:8, a lumbar puncture should be performed even if the patient does not complain of headache or demonstrate nuchal rigidity. A dilated ophthalmologic examination should be performed to investigate retinitis due to cytomegalovirus.

The subsequent evaluation, indicated if the initial approach does not yield a specific diagnosis, should include repeated physical examinations and routine laboratory work. Because abnormal findings of diagnostic importance (skin nodules, asymmetric and enlarging lymphadenopathy, rapid and significant rise of alkaline phosphates) may make their first appearance long after the onset of undifferentiated fever, a biopsy of an abnormal organ—bone marrow, lymph node, skin, or liver—should be performed as it may identify an organism by a special stain of the organ. Other invasive procedures should not be performed while waiting for an organism to be isolated from lysis-centrifugation cultures if the patient remains stable, because cultures of material aspirated from bone marrow, lymph nodes, or biopsied from the liver are not more sensitive than isolator blood cultures. If cultures of blood remain negative in three weeks, a bone marrow examination should be performed even if the patient is stable because the bone marrow examination may be the sole method of identifying an illness (5% of cases in one series) when all noninvasive testing has been unrevealing.

THERAPY
Therapeutic Interventions
Blind therapeutic trials should also be discouraged in most instances. The purpose of such trials is to establish a diagnosis by noticing defervescence following use of a therapeutic agent, such as antibiotics, corticosteroids or nonsteroidal anti-inflammatory agents (NSAIAs). The empiric use of these agents may be misleading for several reasons. Medical intervention would make it difficult to determine whether a new finding resulted from the treatment of the underlying disease. Also, fall of temperature may be fortuitous or result from the antipyretic effects of steroids or NSAIAs. Improper use of antibiotics may lead to a false sense of therapeutic and diagnostic security and only interfere with finding a diagnosis. The spontaneous resolution of fever in stable patients is another reason against the empiric use of therapeutic trials. Employing empiric antibiotics except in the most urgent situation is to ultimately create more frustration, confusion, and despair between the physician and the patient.

Prolonged empiric therapy may have multiple deleterious consequences beyond unnecessary expense and inconvenience for the patient. When fever in patients with self-limited illnesses coincidentally abates while receiving antimycobacterial therapy for possible tuberculosis or mycobacterial infection, the patient may be exposed to unnecessary iatrogenic complications resulting from the adverse reactions of the intervention. In addition, complications resulting from unnecessary interventions may confuse further diagnostic strategies based on abnormalities in physical examination or laboratory findings. For these reasons, therapeutic interventions should be discouraged in stable patients.

SUMMARY

This chapter reviews papers that describe the clinical features of HIV-associated FUO; it occurs in late-stage HIV infection, multiple etiologies of FUO are present in a significant number of cases, and MAI is the most likely infection in the United States. In comparison with foreign series, MAI is present more often in the United States, and leishmania and tuberculosis are more common abroad, reflecting geographic variations in these infections in different locations. In addition, noninvasive testing frequently leads to a diagnosis, supporting the notion that invasive testing should be reserved for those who are unstable or in whom no etiology has been identified. Indirect evidence reviewed in this article suggests that HAART has influenced both the incidence of FUO as well as resulted in unique manifestations of illnesses causing FUO that were identified in the pre-HAART era. However, whether decreases in AIDS-related illnesses resulting in fever that are now observed as a result of the introduction of new antiretroviral agents will persist remains to be seen.

Continued series investigating HIV-associated FUO in the United States and other countries are indicated to determine how the clinical spectrum is impacted by new therapies, available rapid diagnostic tests, and geographic location. It is possible that new conditions, both infectious and neoplastic, may occur in persons who fail treatment with the new active antiviral agents. Furthermore, rapid tests, such as PCR for *M. tuberculosis* or *M. avium*, could possibly permit the detection of these infections early in the course of fever and before FUO develops. Finally, additional papers conducted in locations such as Southeast Asia or South America may identify illnesses endemic in those regions, such as *P. marneffei* in Southeast Asia or Chagas disease in South America, as causes of HIV-associated FUO. These papers will help clarify the shape that FUO, which will continue to be a challenge for clinicians caring for HIV-infected patients, will take in future years.

REFERENCES

1. Bissuel F, Leport C, Perronne C, et al. Fever of unknown origin in HIV-infected patients: a critical analysis of a retrospective series of 57 cases. J Intern Med 1994; 236: 529–535.
2. Miralles P, Moreno S, Perez-Tascon M, et al. Fever of uncertain origin in patients infected with the human immunodeficiency virus. Clin Infect Dis 1995; 20:872–875.
3. Miller RF, Hingorami AD, Foley NM. Pyrexia of undetermined origin in patients with human immunodeficiency virus infection and AIDS. Int J STD AIDS 1996; 7: 170–175.
4. Lozano F, Torre-Cisneros J, Bascunana A, et al. Grupo Andaluz para el Estudio de las Enfermedades Infecciosas. Prospective evaluation of fever of unknown origin in patients infected with the human immunodeficiency virus. Eur J Clin Microbiol Infect Dis 1996; 15:705–711.
5. Knobel H, Supevía A, Salvadó M, et al. Fiebre de origen desconocido en pacientes con infección por el virus de la immunodeficiencia humana. Estudio de 100 casos. Rev Clin Esp 1996; 196: 349–353.
6. Lambertucci JR, Rayes AA, Nunes F, et al. Fever of undetermined origin in patients with the acquired immunodeficiency syndrome in Brazil: report on 55 cases. Rev Inst Med Trop Sao Paulo 1999; 41:27–32.
7. Armstrong W, Katz J, Kazanjian P. Human immunodeficiency virus-associated fever of unknown origin: A study of 70 patients. Clin Infect Dis 1999; 28:341345.
8. Sepkowitz KA, Telzak EE, Carrow M, et al. Fever among outpatients with advanced human immunodeficiency virus infection. Arch Intern Med 1993; 153:1909–1912.
9. Genne D, Chave JP, Glaser MP. Fievre d'origine indeterminee dans un collectif de patients HIV positifs. Schweiz Med Wochenschr 1992; 122:1797–1802.
10. Palella F, Delaney K, Moorman A. Declining morbidity and mortality among patients with advanced HIV infection. N Engl J Med 1998; 338:853–860.
11. Ledergerber B, Egger B, Erard V, et al. AIDS-related opportunistic illnesses occurring after initiation of potent antiretroviral therapy. JAMA 1999; 282:2220–2226.
12. Shelburne SA, Visnegarwala F, Darcourt J. Incidence and risk factors for immune reconstitution inflammatory syndrome during highly active antiretroviral therapy. AIDS 2005; 19:399–406.
13. Weissman S, Golden MP, Jain S. FUO in the HIV-positive patients in the era of HAART. Infect Med 2004; 21:335–340.

14. Lozano F, Torre-Cisneros J, Santos J, et al. Impact of highly active antiretroviral therapy on fever of unknown origin in HIV-infected patients. Eur J Clin Microbiol Infect Dis 2002; 21:137–139.

15. Cohn DL, Breese PS, Burman WJ, et al. Continued benefit from HAART: trends in AIDS-related opportunistic illnesses in a public health care system, 1990-2001. Abstracts from the XIV International AIDS Conference, Barcelona, Spain, July 11, 2002. (Abstract ThOrC1443).

16. Van Sighem AI, van de Wiel MA, Ghani A, et al, on behalf of the ATHENA cohort study group. Mortality and progression to AIDS after starting highly active antiretroviral therapy. AIDS 2003; 17:2227–2236.

17. Egger M, May M, Chene G, et al. ART Cohort Collaboration. Prognosis of HIV-1 infected patients starting highly active antiretroviral therapy: A collaborative analysis of prospective studies. Lancet 2002; 360:119–129.

18. Wood E, Hogg R, Yip B, et al. Higher baseline levels of plasma HIV type 1 RNA are associated with increased mortality after initiation of triple drug antiretroviral therapy. J Infect Dis 2003; 188:1421.

19. Tarwater PM, Gallant JE, Mellors JW, et al. Prognostic value of plasma HIV RNA among highly active antiretroviral users. AIDS 2004; 18:2419–2423.

20. ART Cohort Collaboration. Prognostic importance of initial response in HIV-1 infected patients starting patent antiretroviral therapy: analysis of prospective studies. Lancet 2003; 362:679–686.

21. Raffanti SP, Fusco JS, Sherrill BH, et al. Effect of persistent moderate viremia on disease progression during HIV therapy. J Acquir Immune Defic Syndr 2004; 37:1147–1154.

22. Olsen CH, Gatel J, Ledergerber B, et al. Risk of AIDS and death at given HIV-RNA and CD4 cell counts, in relation to specific antiretroviral drugs in the regimen. AIDS 2005; 19:319–330.

23. Koletar SL, Williams PL, Wu J, et al, for the AIDS Clinical Trials Group 362 Study Team. Long-Term follow-up of HIV-infected individuals who have significant increases in CD4 cell counts during antiretroviral therapy. Clin Inf Dis 2004; 39:1500–1506.

24. Garcia F, de Lazzari E, Plana M, et al. Long-term CD4 T cell response to highly active antiretroviral therapy according to baseline CD4 T cell count. J Acquir Immune Defic Syndr 2004; 36:702–713.

25. Paredes R, Mocroft A, Kirk O, et al. Predictors of virologic success and ensuing failure in HIV-positive patients starting highly active antiretroviral therapy in Europe. Arch Intern Med 2000; 160:1123–1132.

26. Moorman AC, Von Bargen JC, Palella FJ, et al. HIV Outpatient Study (HOPS) Investigators. Pneumocystis carinii pneumonia incidence and chemoprophylaxis failure in ambulatory HIV-infected patients. J Acquir Immune Defic Syndr Hum Retrovirol 1998; 19:182–188.

27. Mocroft A, Lederberger B, Katlama C, et al. EuroSIDA Study Group. Decline in AIDS and death rates in the EuroSIDA study: an observational study. Lancet 2003; 362:22–39.

28. Ives N, Gazzard BG, Easterbrook PJ. Changing pattern of AIDS defining illnesses with introduction of highly active antiretroviral therapy in a London clinic. J Infect 2001; 42:134–139.

29. Kazanjian P, Weiw, Gandhi T, Amin K, Viral load responses to HAART is an independent predictor of a new AIDS event in late stage HIV infected patients. J Trans Med 2005; 3:40–49.

30. Desimone JA, Babinchak TJ, Kaulback KR, et al. Treatment of mycobacterium avium complex immune reconstitution disease in HIV-1 infected individuals. AIDS Patient Care STDs 2003; 17(17):617–622.

31. Price L, O'Mahony C. Focal adentitis developing after immune reconstitution with HAART. Int J STD AIDS 2000; 11(10):85–86.

32. Cunningham CO, Selwyn PA. Mastitis due to mycobacterium avium complex in an HIV-infected woman taking highly active antiretroviral therapy. AIDS Patient Care STDS 2003; 17(11):547–550.

33. Kazanjian PH. Fever of unknown origin: review of 86 patients treated in community hospitals. Clin Infect Dis 1992; 15:968–973.

34. Jacobs C, Lamprey J. The criteria for intensity of service, severity of illness and discharge screens–a review system with adult criteria. In: Dahlgren R, Clark S, eds. Westboro, Massachusetts: Interqual, 1998:28–32.
35. Armstrong W, Kazanjian P. Fever of unknown origin in the general population and in HIV-infected persons. In: Cohen J and Powderly W, eds. Infectious Diseases. London: Mosby Co., 1997:871–881.
36. Wetherill P, Landry M, Alcobes P, et al. Use of quantitative CMV antigenemia test in evaluating HIV infected patients with and without CMV disease. J Acquir Immune Defic Syndr 1996; 12:33–37.
37. Powderly W, Clioud G, Dismukes W, et al. Measurement of cryptococcal antigen in serum and CSF: value in the management of AIDS-associated cryptococcal meningitis. Clin Infect Dis 1994; 18:789–792.
38. Wheat LJ, Kohler RB, Tewari RP. Diagnosis of disseminated histoplasmosis by detection of histoplasma capsulatum antigen in serum and urine specimens. N Engl J Med 1986; 314:83–88.
39. Ng VL, Garner I, Weymouth LA, et al. The use of mucolysed induced sputum for the identification of pulmonary pathogens associated with HIV infection. Arch Pathol Lab Med 1989; 113:488.
40. Kovacs JA, Ng VL, Leong G, et al. Diagnosis of pneumocystis pneumonia: Improved detection in sputum with use of monoclonal antibodies. N Engl J Med 1988; 318:589.
41. Ivers LC, Kim AY, Sax PE. Predictive value of polymerase chain reaction of cerebrospinal fluid for detection of Epstein-Barr virus to establish the diagnosis of HIV-related primary central nervous system lymphoma. Clin Infect Dis 2004; 38:1629–1632.
42. Sansom H, Seddon B, Padley SP. Clinical utility of abdominal CT scanning in patients with HIV disease. Clin Radiol 1997; 52:698–703.
43. Knockaert DC, Mortelmans LA, De Roo MC, et al. Clinical value of gallium-67 scintigraphy in evaluation of fever of unknown origin. Clin Infect Dis 1994; 18:601–605.
44. Fineman DS, Palestro CJ, Kim CK, et al. Detection of abnormalities in febrile AIDS patients with In-111-labeled leukocyte and Ga-67 scintigraphy. Radiol 1989; 170:677–680.
45. O'Doherty MJ, Barrington SF, Campbell M, et al. PET scanning and the human immunodeficiency virus-positive patient. J Nucl Med 1997; 38:1575–1583.
46. Prego V, Glatt AE, Roy V, et al. Comparative yield of blood culture for fungi and mycobacteria, liver biopsy, and bone marrow biopsy in the diagnosis of fever of undetermined origin in human immunodeficiency virus-infected patients. Arch Intern Med 1990; 150:333–336.
47. Benito N, Nunez A, de Gorgolas M, et al. Bone marrow biopsy in the diagnosis of fever of unknown origin in patients with acquired immunodeficiency syndrome. Arch Int Med 1997; 157:1577–1580.
48. Engels E, Marks PW, Kazanjian P. Usefulness of bone marrow examination in the evaluation of unexplained fevers in patients infected with human immunodeficiency virus. Clin Infect Dis 1995; 21:427–428.
49. Cavicchi M, Pialoux G, Carnot F, et al. Value of liver biopsy for the rapid diagnosis of infection in human immunodeficiency virus-infected patients who have unexplained fever and elevated serum levels of alkaline phosphatase and γ-glutamyl transferase. Clin Infect Dis 1995; 20:606–610.
50. Oehler R, Loos U, Ferber J, et al. Diagnostic value of liver biopsy in HIV patients with unexplained fever. 8th International AIDS Conference, 8(2):B211, Amsterdam, Netherlands, 19–24 July 1992 (Abstract POB3722).
51. Bottles K, McPhaul LW, Volberding P. Fine needle aspiration biopsy of patients with AIDS; experience in an outpatient clinic. Ann Intern Med 1988; 108:42–45.

9 Fever of Unknown Origin in Solid Organ Transplant Recipients

Emilio Bouza, Belén Loeches, and Patricia Muñoz

Servicio de Microbiología Clínica y E. Infecciosas, Hospital General Gregorio Marañón, University of Madrid, Madrid, Spain

INTRODUCTION

Organ transplantation has been known for many years, but the introduction of drug regimens using azathioprine and corticosteroids in 1960 and cyclosporine in 1980 meant a great expansion of the field. The advent of tracolimus, mycophenolate mofetil (MMF), and a variety of therapeutic monoclonal antibodies has revolutionized organ transplantation.

Fever is a common clinical manifestation in transplant patients, and it may be due to many different reasons, including the underlying disease of the patient, the surgical intervention, rejection episodes, drugs administered, or intercurrent infections.

Our task is to review fever of unknown origin (FUO) in transplant patients, but we must clarify that there is not a clear and widely accepted definition of FUO for transplant patients. From the seminal work on FUO of Petersdorf and Beeson (1), the practice of medicine has evolved enormously. Petersdorf and Beeson required that fever was prolonged (≥ 3 weeks) because, by the end of that period, most common fevers have been identified or have self-resolved. This long evolution period cannot be witnessed passively in many circumstances at present and particularly in immunosuppressed transplant patients. The methodology of diagnosis has also been speeded up and made more accurate not only for the image diagnosis, but also for microbiology. This led Durack and Street (2) to offer new definitions for different subsets of populations with FUO (Table 1) as follows: Classic FUO, Nosocomial FUO, Neutropenic FUO, and HIV-associated FUO. Most unfortunately, transplant patients were not included, and the situation remains that way.

In our opinion, the term FUO in transplant patients should be used only for prolonged fevers that do not result in an obvious cause after three consecutive outpatient visits or after three days of hospital evaluation, provided that commonly used image and microbiologic tests are reported negative by that time. In transplant recipients, fever has been defined as an oral temperature of $37.8°C$ or greater on at least two occasions during a 24-hour period (3). Antimetabolite immunosuppressive drugs, MMF and azathioprine, are associated with significantly lower maximum temperatures and leukocyte counts (4).

Consideration should be given to the specific type of transplant patient, the results of the physical examination, and the epidemiological antecedents. After that, a syndromic approach, followed by an etiologically oriented differential diagnosis, is pertinent in our opinion.

TABLE 1 Diagnostic Criteria for Fever of Unknown Origin in Different Population Groups

Classic FUO
  Fever 101°F (≥38.3°C) on several occasions.
  Fever of more than three weeks duration.
  Diagnosis uncertain, despite appropriate investigations, after at least three outpatient visits or
    at least 3 days in hospital.
Nosocomial FUO
  Fever 101°F (≥38.3°C) on several occasions in a hospitalized patient receiving acute care.
  Infection not present or incubating on admission.
  Diagnosis uncertain after three days despite appropriate investigation, including at least two days
    incubation of microbiologic cultures.
Neutropenic FUO
  Fever 101°F (≥38.3°C) on several occasions.
  Patient has less than 500 neutrophils/μL in peripheral blood or expected to fall below
    within one to two days.
  Diagnosis uncertain after three days despite appropriate investigation, including at least two days
    incubation of microbiologic cultures.
HIV-associated FUO
  Fever 101°F (≥38.3°C) on several occasions.
  Confirmed positive serology for HIV infection.
  Fever of more than four weeks duration for outpatients or more than three days' duration in
    hospital.
  Diagnosis uncertain after three days, despite appropriate investigation, including at least two days
    incubation of microbiologic cultures.

Abbreviations: FUO, fever of unknown origin; HIV, human immunodeficiency virus.
Source: From Ref. 2.

INCIDENCE OF FEVERS IN DIFFERENT TRANSPLANT PATIENTS

The precise incidence of fever in different transplant patients is not well known. In a prospective evaluation of febrile episodes in liver transplant recipients, Chang et al. (5) reported that fever was due to infections in 78% of the episodes and to noninfectious causes in 22%. The predominant sources of fever were bacterial (62%) and viral infections (6%), while rejection accounted for only 4% of the episodes. Nevertheless, 40% of the infections were unaccompanied by fever, particularly fungal infections. Overall, six of the seven febrile viral infections were due to viruses other than cytomegalovirus (CMV), of which human herpes virus-6 (HHV-6) was the predominant pathogen, a cause particularly prone to infections fulfilling our definition of FUO in transplant patients. Episodes of fever in liver transplant recipients were most likely to occur within 12 weeks (58%) or one year (29%) after transplantation. In the latter case, 100% were due to episodes of recurrent hepatitis, malignancy, or chronic hemodialysis.

In a later report by the same group of authors, the sources of fever in liver transplant patients were due to infections in 87% of the cases admitted to the intensive care unit (ICU) and in 80% of those occurring out of the ICU (6). The main causes of infectious fevers included pneumonia, catheter-related bacteremia, biliary tract, peritonitis, intra-abdominal or wound infections, *Clostridium difficile*-associated colitis (CDAD), and other causes. Among the noninfectious episodes, rejection, malignancy, adrenal insufficiency, drug fever, post-transfusion, and postprocedural were the most common. The episodes presented as FUO only in 5 out of the 40 episodes occurring out of the ICU and in no single case of the 38 episodes of fever appearing during ICU admission.

The incidence of infection after heart transplantation (HT) ranges from 30% to 60% (with a related mortality of 4–15%) and the rate of infectious episodes per patient is 1.73 in a recent series. Infections are more frequent and severe than those occurring in renal transplant recipients, but less frequent than those occurring after liver or lung transplantation. We were unable, however, to find reports on the incidence of febrile episodes in those patients and particularly on the frequency in which febrile episodes present clinically as FUOs. In any case, episodes of prolonged fever or unknown origin are distinctly uncommon in heart transplant patients. Reports include cases with infections such as visceral leishmaniasis (7), intestinal tuberculosis (8), or respiratory syncytial virus (RSV) pneumonia (9). Everolimus has been reported on one occasion as a presumptive cause of a long-term fever in a heart transplant recipient (10).

In a report of 74 outpatient febrile episodes in 22 pediatric heart transplant patients, only 22 episodes (30%) resulted in hospital admission. The duration of fever was predictive of a more serious disease (11).

In kidney transplantation, fever is no longer a frequent presentation of rejection, and prolonged FUO episodes are uncommon. In a series of 61 renal transplant patients, 90 acute rejection episodes occurred during the first six postoperative months. The vast majority of them (83%) were not associated with fever. Of the 37 patients with episodes of fever in this series of patients, only 15 were ascribed to acute rejection, 17 to infection, 11 to antibody therapy, and 4 to other causes. Fever in the first 16 days was significantly more likely to be due to rejection than to infection. Episodes of fever due to infection tended to occur after the first month, coincident with the peak incidence of CMV infection. However, with the exception of CMV disease, fever was not a reliable guide for the presence of infection, including septicemia (12).

Different infectious diseases can present with FUO in renal transplant patients, including HSV with or without esophagitis (13,14), CMV disease, particularly cases with ischemic colitis (15,16), bacillary angiomatosis (17), nocardiosis (18), tuberculosis (19–22), visceral leishmaniasis (23–28), disseminated microsporidiosis (29), and disseminated strongyloidiasis (30).

Noninfectious causes of prolonged fever in kidney transplant patients include drug fever caused by mycophenolate (31) and systemic lupus erythematosus (16).

SYNDROMIC APPROACH TO TRANSPLANT PATIENTS WITH FEVER OF UNKNOWN ORIGIN

Risk factors for infection should be carefully sought in all solid organ transplant (SOT) patients. The pretransplantation history, for example, serological status against microorganisms such as CMV, hepatitis virus, *Toxoplasma*, and so on, may yield valuable information. Previous infections or colonization, exposure to tuberculosis, contact with animals, raw food ingestion, gardening, prior antimicrobial therapy or prophylaxis, vaccines or immunosuppressors, and contact with contaminated environment or persons should be recorded (32,33). History of residence or travel to endemic areas of regional mycosis (34) or *Strongyloides stercoralis* may be essential to recognize these diseases (35). Exposure to ticks may be essential to diagnose entities such as human monocytic ehrlichiosis, which may be potentially lethal in immunosuppressed patients (36).

Fever in most transplant recipients should be considered an emergency. In our opinion, a basic tenet of the management of a SOT with fever is that physical examination data should be directly obtained by the ID consultant, not relying on second-hand information. This may be more useful than many expensive and time-consuming tests.

The oral cavity is frequently forgotten and may disclose previously unnoticed herpetic gingivostomatitis or ulcers. Within the exploration of the thoracic area, the consultant should visualize the entry sites of all intravascular devices, even if they "have just been cleansed." It should be remembered that the presence of inflammatory signs is suggestive of infection, although their absence does not exclude infection. Fever and sepsis, without local signs, may be the initial sign of post-surgical mediastinitis in heart transplant recipients. Although unusual after SOT, cardiac auscultation and echography may help to detect endocarditis (37) and physical examination may occasionally disclose the existence of pneumonia or empyema before abnormal radiological signs become evident.

The abdominal examination is always essential, especially in liver transplant (LT) recipients. The surgical wound is also a common site of infection and a cause of fever. Its presence requires rapid debridement and effective antimicrobial therapy and should prompt the exclusion of adjacent cavities or organ infection. If ascites is present, it should be immediately analyzed and properly cultured to exclude peritonitis. We recommend bedside inoculation in blood-culture bottles due to its higher yield of positive results. Examination of the lower abdomen is particularly important after kidney transplantation. Tenderness, erythema, and fluctuance or increase in the allograft size may indicate the presence of a deep infection or rejection. Ultrasound or computed tomography (CT)-guided aspiration may facilitate the diagnosis. The possibility of colonic perforation in steroid-treated patients or gastro-intestinal CMV disease should always be considered in intra-abdominal infections. It is important to remember that even very severe intestinal CMV disease may occur in patients with negative blood antigen, especially in patients on MMF (38).

Finally, skin and retinal examination are "windows" through which the physician may look to obtain quite useful information on the possible etiology of a previously unexplained febrile episode. We have analyzed the value of ocular lesions in the diagnosis and prognosis of patients with tuberculosis, bacteremia, and sepsis (39,40). Cutaneous or subcutaneous lesions are a valuable source of information and frequently allow a rapid diagnosis. Viral and fungal infections are the leading causes of skin lesions in this setting. The entire skin surface should be inspected and palpated in SOT recipient with unexplained fever. The biopsy of nodules, subcutaneous lesions or collections may lead to the immediate diagnosis of invasive mycoses and infections caused by Nocardia or Mycobacteria, among others.

An aggressive diagnostic attitude is necessary when dealing with febrile SOT patients. It has been proved that a high rate of infectious complications remains undiagnosed in patients dying in the ICU in the transplant population. The majority of the missed diagnoses were fungal infections. Several syndromic situations deserve a particular mention.

Pneumonia

Pneumonia accounts for 30% to 80% of infections suffered by SOT recipients and for a great majority of episodes of fever (41). Pneumonia is among the leading causes of infectious mortality in this population. The incidence of pneumonia is higher in the early postoperative period, especially in the patients who require prolonged ventilation.

The incidence of bacterial pneumonia is highest in recipients of heart–lung (22%) and liver transplants (17%), intermediate in recipients of heart transplants (5%), and lowest in renal transplant patients (1–2%). The crude mortality of bacterial pneumonia in solid organ transplantation has exceeded 40% in most series (42).

Singh (41) has recently analyzed 40 LT who developed lung infiltrates in the ICU. The etiology was: pulmonary edema 40%, pneumonia 38%, atelectasias 10%, acute respiratory distress syndrome (ARDS) 8%, contusion 3%, and unknown 3%. The signs that suggest an infectious origin were: Clinical Pulmonary Infection Score (CPIS) score >6 (73% vs. 6%), abnormal temperature (73% vs. 28%), and creatinine level >1.5 mg/dL (80% vs. 50%) (41). Methicillin-resistant *Staphylococcus aureus* (MRSA), *Pseudomonas aeruginosa*, and *Aspergillus* caused 70% of all pneumonias in the ICU. All *Aspergillus* and 75% of MRSA pneumonias, but only 14% of the gram-negative pneumonias occurred within 30 days of transplantation. *Legionella*, *Toxoplasma gondii*, and CMV may also cause pneumonia in this setting (43,44).

Pneumonia is the most common infection, following HT. Gram-negative pneumonia in the early post-transplant period is associated with significant mortality. In a recent multicentric prospective study performed in Spain, the incidence of pneumonia after HT was 15.6 episodes/100 HT (45). Most cases occurred in the first month after transplantation. Etiology could be established in 61% of the cases. Bacteria caused 91% of the cases, fungi 9%, and virus 6%. In another study, opportunistic microorganisms caused 60% of the pneumonias, nosocomial pathogens 25%, and community-acquired bacteria and mycobacteria 15% (46). Gram-negative rods caused early pneumonias (median 9 days), gram-positive cocci (11 days), fungi (80 days), *Mycobacterium tuberculosis* and *Nocardia* spp. (145 days), and virus (230 days). *Legionella* should always be included in the differential diagnosis (47–50). Pneumonia increases the risk of mortality after HT (Odds ratio 3.7, IC 95% 1.5–8.1, $P < 0.01$).

Lung infections are very common in lung and heart–lung transplant recipients. In fact, the anastomosis is especially vulnerable to invasion with opportunistic pathogens, including gram-negative bacilli (*Pseudomonas*), staphylococci, or fungus. Lung transplant recipients with underlying cystic fibrosis may be prone to suffer infections caused by multiresistant microorganisms such as *Burkholderia cepacia*. Pathogens transmitted from the donor may also cause pneumonia in this setting.

Pneumonia is less common after renal transplantation (8–16%), although it remains a significant cause of morbidity (51–54).

Postsurgical Infections

Complications in the proximity of the surgical area must always be investigated in SOT patients with fever. In the early post-transplantation period, renal and pancreas transplant recipients may develop perigraft hematomas, lymphoceles, and urinary fistula. Liver transplant recipients are at risk for portal vein thrombosis, hepatic vein occlusion, hepatic artery thrombosis, and biliary stricture formation and leaks. Heart transplant recipients are at risk for mediastinitis and infection at the aortic suture line, with resultant mycotic aneurysm, and lung transplantation recipients are at risk for disruption of the bronchial anastomosis.

In LT recipients, intra-abdominal infections may be responsible of 50% of bacterial complications and cause significant morbidity (55); they include intra-abdominal abscesses, biliary tree infections, and peritonitis. In nonabdominal transplantations, intra-abdominal infections may be caused by pre-existing problems such as biliary tract litiasis, diverticulitis, CMV disease, and so on.

Hepatic abscess is frequently associated with hepatic artery thrombosis (56). Clinical presentation of hepatic abscess includes fever, but with nowadays image technology it rarely becomes a cause of FUO. In fact 40% to 45% of the liver abscesses are associated with bacteremia.

Ultrasonography or CT of the abdomen is the normal technique to identify intra-abdominal or biliary infections. However, sterile fluid collections are exceedingly common after liver transplantation, so an aspirate is necessary to establish infection.

In heart and lung transplant recipients, the possibility of mediastinitis (2–9%) should be considered. HT patients have a higher risk of postsurgical mediastinitis and sternal osteomyelitis than other heart surgical patients (57). Mediastinitis may initially appear merely as fever or bacteremia of unknown origin. Inflammatory signs in the sternal wound, sternal dehiscence, and purulent drainage may appear later. The most commonly involved microorganisms are *Staphylococcus spp.*, but gram-negative rods represent at least a third of our cases. Mycoplasma, mycobacteria, and other less common pathogens should be suspected in "culture-negative" wound infections (58,59). A bacteremia of unknown origin during the first month after HT should always suggest the possibility of mediastinitis. Risk factors are prolonged hospitalization before surgery, early chest re-exploration, low-output syndrome in adults, and the immature state of immune response in infants.

Urinary Tract Infections

Urinary tract infections (UTIs) are the most common form of bacterial complication affecting renal transplant recipients (60,61). The incidence in patients not receiving prophylaxis has been reported to vary from 5% to 36% in recent series (62). However, it is not a common cause of FUO. Unless another source of fever is readily apparent, any febrile kidney transplant patient with an abrupt deterioration of renal function should be treated with empiric antibacterial therapy aimed at gram-negative bacteria, including *P. aeruginosa*, after first obtaining blood and urine cultures (63). Prolonged administration of antimicrobial therapy has been classically recommended for the treatment of early infections, although no double-blind, comparative study is available (60).

Gastrointestinal Infections

Gastrointestinal symptoms are present in up to 51% of HT patients in recent series, although only 15% are significant enough to warrant endoscopic, radiologic, or surgical procedures.

Peritonitis, intra-abdominal infections, and *C. difficile* colitis accounted for 5% of all febrile episodes in OLT in the ICU (6). Abdominal pain and/or diarrhea are detected in up to 20% of organ transplant recipients (64,65). CMV and *C. difficile* are the most common causes of infectious diarrhea in SOT patients (66–69).

CMV may involve the whole gastrointestinal tract, although duodenum and stomach are the most frequent sites involved (70), and they may occasionally behave as an FUO or as gastrointestinal bleeding. Differential diagnosis should include diverticulitis, intestinal ischemia, cancer, and Epstein-Barr virus (EBV)-associated lymphoproliferative disorders. A particular gastric lymphoma called mucosa-associated lymphoid tissue (MALT) lymphoma may develop in renal transplant patients. It usually responds to the eradication of *Helicobacter pylori* (71).

C. difficile should be suspected in patients who present with nosocomial diarrhea and occasionally may present with fever and leukocytosis without evident diarrhea (72–75). Most episodes of *C. difficile*-associated diarrhea in SOT patients occur early after transplantation, but they fulfill criteria of FUO only anecdotally. In these cases, significant leukocytosis may be a very useful clue.

Immunosuppressive drugs, such as MMF, cyclosporine A (CSA), tacrolimus, and sirolimus, are all known to be associated with diarrhea and occasionally present with fever.

Focal Neurological Manifestations

The detection of central nervous system (CNS) symptoms in a SOT recipient should immediately arouse the suspicion of an infection (76,77). Fever, headache, altered mental status, seizures, focal neurological deficit, or a combination of them should prompt a neuroimaging study. Some causes of CNS infections in these patients, which are very uncommon in general population, can present as an FUO (Table 2).

Noninfectious causes include immunosuppressive-associated leukoencephalopathy, toxic and metabolic etiologies, and stroke and malignancies (77,78).

Most common cause of meningoencephalitis in organ transplant recipients is herpes virus, followed by *Listeria monocytogenes, Cryptococcus neoformans*, and *T. gondii*. In a recent review, HHV-6 encephalitis occurred a median of 45 days (range 10 days to 15 months) after transplantation. Mental status changes, ranging from confusion to coma (92%), seizures (25%), and headache (25%), were the predominant clinical presentations. Focal neurologic findings were present in only 17% of the patients. Only 25% of the patients had fever, occasionally reaching 40°C, but the criteria of FUO is rarely fulfilled (79–86).

CMV infection of the CNS is quite uncommon in SOT recipients and rarely fulfills FUO criteria if proper diagnostic methodology is used.

Among causes of encephalitis, West Nile virus has emerged as an important cause of several outbreaks of febrile illness and encephalitis in North America over the past few years, with particular incidence in SOT patients (87–97).

L. monocytogenes infections can occur at almost any time, although the most common occurrence is two to six months post-transplant (98–103). Patients with listeriosis commonly have fever but not a prolonged undiagnosed FUO, if proper etiologic workup is performed.

Cryptococcosis is mostly a cause of meningitis, pneumonia, and skin lesions in transplant recipients but rarely a cause of FUO (104–114).

Focal brain lesions may be caused by *Listeria, T. gondii*, fungi (*Aspergillus, Mucorales*, pheohyphomycetes or dematiaceous fungi), post-transplantation lymphoproliferative disease, or *Nocardia* (115–121), but modern technology and approach avoid the evolution of these diseases as causes of FUOs.

Toxoplasmosis was more prevalent when prophylaxis with cotrimoxazole was not provided (122,123). The incidence is higher in heart transplant recipients. The disease usually occurred within three months post-transplantation, with fever, neurological disturbances, and pneumonia as the main clinical features. It may also behave as a prolonged FUO if not clinically suspected and proper microbiological tests are not performed (124–128). Diagnosis is established by serology

TABLE 2 Pathogens and Clinical Syndromes in Transplants

Syndrome	Common etiologies in transplantation
Acute meningitis	*Listeria monocyogenes*
Acute chronic meningitis	*Crytococcus neoformans*
	Mycobacterium tuberculosis
	Coccidioides immitis
	Histoplasma capsulatum
Focal brain infection	*Aspergillus fumigatus*
	Nocardia asteroides
	Listeria monocytogenes
	Toxoplasma gondii
Progressive dementia	*Progressive multifocal leukoencephalopaty (JC virus)*

and by direct examination, culture, or polymerase chain reaction (PCR) of biological samples. In heart transplant recipients, the diagnosis may be provided by the endomyocardial biopsy (129).

Other parasitic infections such as Chagas disease, neurocysticercosis, schistosomiasis, and strongyloidiasis are exceedingly less common (35,130–135).

Bloodstream Infections, Catheter-Related Infections, and Infective Endocarditis

Bloodstream infections are common among SOT, particularly during their postoperative period or during episodes requiring intensive care, but obviously they do not constitute a cause of FUO. Infective endocarditis is a rare event in HT population (1.7–6%), but it may be an underappreciated sequela of hospital-acquired infection in transplant patients (37). The spectrum of organisms causing infective endocarditis was clearly different in transplant recipients than in the general population; 50% of the infections were due to *Aspergillus fumigatus* or *S. aureus*, but only 4% were due to *viridans streptococci*.

FUO may be a form of presentation in patients with infective endocarditis caused by microorganisms not easily recovered in blood, as is the case with *Aspergillus* (37,136–140).

Toxoplasma and parvovirus B19 may cause myocarditis in this population, and they may behave as FUOs.

Fever Without an Evident Portal of Entry

Undoubtedly, the most common alarm signal suggesting infection in SOT is fever. The major difference with immunocompetent patients is that the list of potential etiological agents is much longer and is influenced by time elapsed from transplantation. CMV (as main offender or as co-pathogen) should be considered in practically all-infectious complications in this population. Accordingly, a sample for CMV antigenemia (or PCR if available) should always be obtained. Other viruses such as adenovirus, influenza A, or HHV-6 may also cause severe infections after SOT and can be recovered from respiratory samples or blood. If indicated, invasive diagnostic procedures should be performed rapidly and a serum sample stored.

Bacterial infections must always be considered and urine and blood cultures obtained before starting therapy. The first steps for diagnosis of pneumonia should include a chest X-ray and culture of expectorated sputum or bronchoaspirate (submitted for virus, bacteria, mycobacteria, and fungus). A CT scan or ultrasonography may also be ordered to exclude the presence of collections in the proximity of the surgical area. Lumbar puncture and cranial CT (including the paranasal sinus) must be performed if neurological symptoms or signs are detected. In case of diarrhea, *C. difficile* should be investigated. Cultures and PCR for detection of *M. tuberculosis* should be ordered for all transplant recipients with suspicion of infection.

Fungal infections should be aggressively pursued in colonized patients and in patients with risk factors.

Parasitic infections are uncommon, but toxoplasmosis and leishmaniasis should be considered if diagnosis remains elusive. Serology or bone marrow cultures usually provide the diagnosis. HT recipients are more susceptible to toxo-plasmosis, which may be transmitted with the allograft. The risk of primary toxo-plasmosis (R-D+) in over 50% in HT, 20% after liver transplantation, and <1% after kidney transplantation. Leishmaniasis is a parasitic infection that should be excluded, although it is exceedingly uncommon after SOT. It may present as fever, pancytopenia, and splenomegaly.

Multimodality imaging, such as the use of combined indium-labeled WBC scintigraphy and CT, allowed the detection of infection within retained left ventricular assist device tubing in a heart transplant recipient with a diagnosis of FUO (142).

ETIOLOGIC APPROACH TO FEVER OF UNKNOWN ORIGIN IN TRANSPLANT PATIENTS
Viruses

Most life-threatening viral infections occur within the first three months post-transplantation. CMV is the most common pathogen after SOT. When no prophylaxis is given, 30% to 90% of patients will show laboratory data of "CMV infection" and 10% to 50% may develop associated clinical manifestations (CMV disease). CMV may involve the whole gastrointestinal tract, although duodenum and stomach are the most frequent sites involved (49,70,143). Differential diagnosis should include diverticulitis, intestinal ischemia, cancer, and EBV-associated lymphoproliferative disorders. Fever is a common manifestation of CMV disease, but nowadays a very uncommon cause of FUO (15,144).

Herpes simplex (145,146) and Varicella-Zoster-Virus (VZV) (may cause soft tissue infections and pneumonia in the transplant population. HHV-6 has been reported to cause diverse clinical symptoms, including fever, skin rash, pneumonia, bone marrow suppression, encephalitis, and rejection. HHV-6 is a neurotropic ubiquitous virus known to cause febrile syndromes and exanthema subitum in children. Less commonly, and particularly in organ transplant recipients, it may cause hepatitis, bone marrow suppression, interstitial pneumonitis, and meningoencephalitis (79). Mental status changes, ranging from confusion to coma (92%), seizures (25%), and headache (25%), were the predominant clinical presentations. Focal neurologic findings were present in only 17% of the patients. Twenty-five percent of the patients had fever, occasionally reaching 40°C (76). A growing body of evidence suggests that the more important effect of HHV-6 and HHV-7 reactivation on the outcomes of liver transplantation may be mediated indirectly by their interactions with CMV (147). HHV-6 viremia is an independent predictor of invasive fungal infection (148).

Due to the unawareness of HHV-6 and the unavailability of diagnostic methods in many institutions, HHV-6 may present as prolonged or unexplained fevers (80,82,149).

Both hepatitis B virus (HBV) and hepatitis C virus (HCV) are very common in transplant patients but not a cause of FUO.

Community-acquired respiratory viruses, particularly influenza, parainfluenza, adenoviruses, and RSV and human metapneumovirus, are important pathogens in the transplant patient, but, again, almost never behave as FUOs (89,150–158). Respiratory viruses may be associated with high morbidity, particularly in lung transplant recipients, and may appear as "culture-negative" pneumonia.

In a recent report, 11 transplant recipients with naturally acquired West Nile encephalitis were identified (4 kidney, 2 stem cell, 2 liver, 1 lung, and 2 kidney/pancreas). Nine of eleven patients survived infection, but three had significant residual deficits. This viral infection should be considered in all transplant recipients who present with a febrile illness associated with neurological symptoms. Fever in this situation is usually transient (159–161).

Papovaviruses may be implicated in a variety of clinical syndromes in transplant patients. Papillomaviruses may cause warts and squamous cell carcinomas of the skin. JC virus causes progressive leukoencephalopathy, and BK virus causes transplant nephropathy in kidney recipients (162–166).

Bacteria

Bacteria are the most common causes of infection in transplant patients, with a pathogenesis and microbial etiology quite similar to that observed in general population. Due to the acuteness of most bacterial diseases and the simplicity of bacterial isolation, the vast majority of bacterial diseases in transplant patients do not present clinically as FUOs.

M. tuberculosis is a well-known cause of FUO both in normal and in immunocompromised patients, including solid organ transplantation. In transplant patients living in areas of high-level endemicity, it might reach up to 15% (167–169). Although there is a huge regional variability, in general, SOT incidence is 20 to 74 times higher than in the general population, with a mortality rate of up to 30%. The most frequent form of acquisition of tuberculosis after transplantation is the reactivation of latent tuberculosis in patients with previous exposure. Tuberculosis develops a mean of nine months after transplantation (0.5 to 13 months). Risk factors for early onset are nonrenal transplant, allograft rejection, immunosuppressive therapy with OKT3 or anti-T cell antibodies and previous exposure to *M. tuberculosis*. Clinical presentation is frequently atypical and diverse, with unsuspected and elusive sites of involvement. A large series of TBC in transplant recipients described pulmonary involvement in 51% of patients, extrapulmonary tuberculosis in 16%, and disseminated infection in 33% (169). In lungs, radiographic appearance may vary between focal or diffuse interstitial infiltrates, nodules, pleural effusion, or cavitary lesions. Manifestations include FUO, allograft dysfunction, gastrointestinal bleeding, peritonitis, or ulcers. In transplant patients, *M. tuberculosis* infection was also described in skin, muscle, osteoarticular system, CNS, genitourinary tract, lymph nodes, larynx, adrenal glands, and thyroid (169,170). Ocular lesions may be an early way to detect dissemination (39).

Fungal Infections

Fungal infections should be aggressively pursued in colonized patients and in patients with risk factors. Early stages of fungal infection may be very difficult to detect (171,172). Isolation of *Candida* or *Aspergillus* from even superficial sites may indicate infection and should be considered with caution. Retinal examination, blood and respiratory cultures, and *Aspergillus* and *Cryptococcus* antigen detection tests must be performed.

Different types of transplantations imply differences in fungal infections (173). In a recent series prospectively collected in Spain, the reported incidence of invasive aspergillosis in SOT recipients ranged from 0.3% in kidney transplant to 3.9% in pancreas recipients (174). In lung and heart–lung transplantation, the incidence of fungal infections, most notably aspergillosis, ranges from 14% to 35% if no prophylaxis is provided, but has significantly decreased since aerosolized amphotericin B is provided to these patients (175).

In liver transplantation, *Aspergillus* infection is less common when compared to lung or heart–lung transplant recipients, and is more commonly found than in kidney transplant recipients. In liver transplant recipients, IA usually is an early event and most patients were still in the ICU with evidence of organ dysfunction when the disease was diagnosed (176,177).

Aspergillus brain abscesses usually occur in the early post-transplantation period. Most of the patients present with simultaneous lung lesions that allow an easier diagnostic way. Overall, disseminated *Aspergillus* disease has been described in 9% to 36% of kidney recipients, 15% to 20% of lung recipients, 20% to 35% of heart recipients, and 50% to 60% of liver recipients with IA (172,178).

Scedosporium and *Blastoschyzomyces* species are increasingly recognized as significant pathogens, particularly in immunocompromised hosts. These fungi now account for ~25% of all non-Aspergillus mould infections in organ transplant recipients (179–184).

Pneumocystic jiroveci (formerly *P. carinii*) is now rarely seen in SOT receiving prophylaxis. Before prophylaxis, incidence was around 5%, although it has been described to reach up to 80% in lung transplant recipients (51,185–187).

Incidence of cryptococcosis after organ transplantation is 0.3% to 6% (109,114,188–190). *Cryptococcus* is mostly a cause of meningitis, pneumonia, and skin lesions (105,107,108,111,113,114,191–193). However, more uncommon sites of infection have been also described in immunocompromised patients, such as hepatic cryptococcosis in a heart transplant recipient (108). Cryptococcosis is usually a late disease after transplantation, although rare, fulminant, early cases have been reported. Once more, fungal opportunistic infections rarely present as FUOs in the SOT population.

Histoplamosis can present as a prolonged febrile illness with subacute pulmonary symptoms in these patients, despite the absence or a regional outbreak (194–197).

Parasites

Parasitic infections are uncommon, but toxoplasmosis and leishmaniasis should be particularly considered in SOT patients. Serology or bone marrow cultures usually provide the diagnosis. The possibility of a *Toxoplasma* primary infection should be considered when a seronegative recipient receives an allograft from a seropositive donor. HT recipients are more susceptible to toxoplasmosis, which may be transmitted with the allograft, and occasionally requires ICU admission. The risk of primary toxoplasmosis (R-D+) is over 50% in HT, 20% after liver transplantation, and <1% after kidney transplantation. Patients with toxoplasmosis have fever, altered mental status, focal neurological signs, myalgias, myocarditis, and lung infiltrates. Allograft-transmitted toxoplasmosis is more often associated with acute disease (61%) than with reactivation of latent infection (7%). Lethal cases associated with hemophagocytic syndrome have been described (141). Disseminated toxoplasmosis should be considered in the differential diagnosis of immunocompromised patients with culture-negative sepsis syndrome, particularly if combined with neurologic, respiratory, or unexplained skin lesion (198).

Leishmaniasis is another parasitic infection that should be excluded, although it is exceedingly uncommon after SOT. It may present as fever, pancytopenia, and splenomegaly.

Chagas disease and other parasites infections are very uncommon (199).

Noninfectious Causes of Fever

Both infectious and noninfectious causes of fever should be considered when approaching a febrile SOT patient. In a recent series, 87% of the febrile episodes detected in OLT in the ICU were due to infections and 13% were noninfectious (6). Rejection, malignancy, adrenal insufficiency, and drug fever were the most common noninfectious causes.

Fever is common in the first 48 hours after surgery and after certain procedures. If it is not persistent or is accompanied by other signs or symptoms, it should not trigger any diagnostic action. Acute rejection accounts for 4% to 17% of the noninfectious febrile episodes (5). It is usually related to an impairment of the allograft function and requires histological confirmation. It is more common in the first six months, especially in the first 16 days after transplantation in one study (12). It is important to remember that severe graft rejection and increased immunosuppression could stimulate cooperatively active CMV (200,201).

Malignancy, mainly lymphoproliferative disease, is relatively common after SOT and may initially present as a febrile episode (80%) (202). It usually occurs later after transplantation (5). Acute adrenal insufficiency should be excluded in SOT patients admitted to an ICU because of sepsis or surgery, mainly when corticosteroids have been withdrawn and drugs that accelerate the degradation of cortisol (phenytoin, rifampin) are administered (203).

However, although analytical adrenal insufficiency is frequent in SOT patients, prospective studies suggest that supplemental steroids are not needed in most cases even under stress (204,205). Another setting of potential adrenal insufficiency are renal transplants that return to dialysis (206,207). Occasionally, lymphoproliferative disease may present with adrenal insufficiency after liver transplantation (208).

Drugs such as OKT3, ATG, everolimus, antimicrobials, interferon, anticonvulsants, etc. may also cause fever in this population (10). The temporal relationship with the drug is usually a diagnostic clue. New induction therapies, such as basiliximab, are related to fewer side effects and fewer CMV infections (209).

Other causes of noninfectious fever include thromboembolic disease, hematoma reabsorption, pericardial effusions, tissue infarction, hemolytic uremic syndrome, and transfusion reaction. Noncardiogenic pulmonary edema (pulmonary reimplantation response) is a common finding after lung transplantation (50–60%) and may occasionally lead to a differential diagnosis with pneumonia. It conditions prolonged mechanical ventilation and ICU stay, but does not affect survival (210).

MANAGEMENT AND OUTCOME

Fever is not harmful by itself, and accordingly it should not be systematically elimi-nated. In fact, it has been demonstrated that fever enhances several host defense mechanisms (chemotaxis, phagocytosis, and opsonization) (65,211). Besides, anti-biotics may be more active at higher body temperatures. If provided, antipyretic drugs should be administered at regular intervals to avoid recurrent shivering and an associated increase in metabolic demand.

After obtaining the previously mentioned samples, empiric antibiotics should be promptly started in all transplant patients with suspicion of infection and a toxic or unstable situation. They are also recommended if a focus of infection is apparent in the early post-transplant setting in which nosocomial infection is very common, or when there has been a recent increase of immunosuppression. In a stable patient without a clear source of infections, further diagnostic testing should be carried out and noninfectious causes considered.

REFERENCES

1. Petersdorf RO, Beeson PB. Fever of unexplained origin: report on 100 cases. Medicine (Baltimore) 1961; 40:1–30.
2. Durack DT, Street AC. Fever of unknown origin—reexamined and redefined. In: Remington JS SM, ed. Curr Clin Top Infect Dis. Blackwell Scientific Publications, 1991:35–51.
3. Singhal S, Mehta J. Reimmunization after blood or marrow stem cell transplantation. Bone Marrow Transplant 1999; 23(7):637–646.
4. Sawyer RG, Crabtree TD, Gleason TG, Antevil JL, Pruett TL. Impact of solid organ transplantation and immunosuppression on fever, leukocytosis, and physiologic response during bacterial and fungal infections. Clin Transplant 1999; 13(3):260–265.
5. Chang FY, Singh N, Gayowski T, Wagener MM, Marino IR. Fever in liver transplant recipients: changing spectrum of etiologic agents. Clin Infect Dis 1998; 26(1): 59–65.
6. Singh N, Chang FY, Gayowski T, Wagener M, Marino IR. Fever in liver transplant recipients in the intensive care unit. Clin Transplant 1999; 13(6):504–511.
7. Zorio GE, Blanes JM, Martinez Ortiz de Urbina L, Almenar BL, Peman GJ. Persistent fever, pancytopenia and spleen enlargement in a heart transplant carrier as presen-tation of visceral leishmaniasis. Rev Clin Esp 2003; 203(3):164–165.
8. Zedtwitz-Liebenstein K, Podesser B, Peck-Radosavljevic M, Graninger W. Intestinal tuberculosis presenting as fever of unknown origin in a heart transplant patient. Infection 1999; 27(4–5):289–290.
9. Berbari N, Johnson DH, Cunha BA. Respiratory syncytial virus pneumonia in a heart transplant recipient presenting as fever of unknown origin diagnosed by gallium scan. Heart Lung 1995; 24(3):257–259.
10. Dorschner L, Speich R, Ruschitzka F, Seebach JD, Gallino A. Everolimus-induced drug fever after heart transplantation. Transplantation 2004; 78(2):303–304.
11. Crandall WV, Norlin C, Bullock EA, et al. Etiology and outcome of outpatient fevers in pediatric heart transplant patients. Clin Pediatr (Phila) 1996; 35(9):437–442.
12. Toogood GJ, Roake JA, Morris PJ. The relationship between fever and acute rejection or infection following renal transplantation in the cyclosporin era. Clin Transplant 1994; 8(4):373–377.
13. Gelman R, Khankin E, Ben-Itzhak A, Finkelshtein R, Nakhoul F. Herpes simplex viral infection presenting as fever of unknown origin and esophagitis in a renal transplant patient. Isr Med Assoc J 2002; 4(suppl 11):970–971.
14. Katafuchi R, Saito S, Yanase T, et al. A case of fever of unknown origin with severe stomatitis in renal transplant recipient resulting in graft loss. Clin Transplant 2000; 14(suppl 3):42–47.

15. Lee CJ, Lian JD, Chang SW, et al. Lethal cytomegalovirus ischemic colitis presenting with fever of unknown origin. Transpl Infect Dis 2004; 6(3):124–128.
16. Kaaroud H, Beji S, Jebali A, et al. A rare cause of fever associated with leukopenia in a renal transplant patient. Nephrol Dial Transplant 2004; 19(8):2140–2141.
17. Juskevicius R, Vnencak-Jones C. Pathologic quiz case: a 17-year-old renal transplant patient with persistent fever, pancytopenia, and axillary lymphadenopathy. Bacillary angiomatosis of the lymph node in the renal transplant recipient. Arch Pathol Lab Med 2004; 128(1):e12–e14.
18. Case records of the Massachusetts General Hospital. Weekly clinicopathological exercises. Case 29-2000. A 69-year-old renal transplant recipient with low grade fever and multiple pulmonary nodules. N Engl J Med 2000; 343(12):870–877.
19. Yilmaz E, Balci A, Sal S, Cakmakci H. Tuberculous ileitis in a renal transplant recipient with familial Mediterranean fever: Gray-scale and power Doppler sonographic findings. J Clin Ultrasound 2003; 31(1):51–54.
20. Parry RG, Playford EG, Looke DF, Falk M. Soft-tissue abscess as the initial manifestation of miliary tuberculosis in a renal transplant recipient with prolonged fever. Nephrol Dial Transplant 1998; 13(7):1860–1863.
21. Muñoz P, Rodriguez C, Bouza E. Mycobacterium tuberculosis infection in recipients of solid organ transplants. Clin Infect Dis 2005; 40(4):581–587; Epub Jan 25, 2005.
22. Munoz P, Palomo J, Munoz R, Rodriguez-Creixems M, Pelaez T, Bouza E. Tuberculosis in heart transplant recipients. Clin Infect Dis 1995; 21(2):398–402.
23. Sipsas NV, Boletis J. Fever, hepatosplenomegaly, and pancytopenia in a renal transplant recipient. Transpl Infect Dis 2003; 5(1):47–52.
24. Rajaram KG, Sud K, Kohli HS, Gupta KL, Sakhuja V. Visceral leishmaniasis: a rare cause of post-transplant fever and pancytopenia. J Assoc Physicians India 2002; 50:979–980.
25. Apaydin S, Ataman R, Serdengect K, et al. Visceral leishmaniasis without fever in a kidney transplant recipient. Nephron 1997; 75(2):241–242.
26. Moulin B, Ollier J, Bouchouareb D, Purgus R, Olmer M. Leishmaniasis: a rare cause of unexplained fever in a renal graft recipient. Nephron 1992; 60(3):360–362.
27. Kher V, Ghosh AK, Gupta A, Arora P, Dhole TN. Visceral leishmaniasis: an unusual case of fever in a renal transplant recipient. Nephrol Dial Transplant 1991; 6(10):736–738.
28. Fernandez-Guerrero ML, Aguado JM, Buzon L, et al. Visceral leishmaniasis in immunocompromised hosts. Am J Med 1987; 83(6):1098–1102.
29. Mahmood MN, Keohane ME, Burd EM. Pathologic quiz case: a 45-year-old renal transplant recipient with persistent fever. Arch Pathol Lab Med 2003; 127(4):e224–e226.
30. Soman R, Vaideeswar P, Shah H, Almeida AF. A 34-year-old renal transplant recipient with high-grade fever and progressive shortness of breath. J Postgrad Med 2002; 48(3):191–196.
31. Chueh SC, Hong JC, Huang CY, Lai MK. Drug fever caused by mycophenolate mofetil in a renal transplant recipient—a case report. Transplant Proc 2000; 32(7): 1925–1926.
32. Papanicolaou GA, Meyers BR, Meyers J, et al. Nosocomial infections with vancomycin-resistant *Enterococcus faecium* in liver transplant recipients: risk factors for acquisition and mortality. Clin Infect Dis 1996; 23(4):760–766.
33. Duchini A, Goss JA, Karpen S, Pockros PJ. Vaccinations for adult solid-organ transplant recipients: current recommendations and protocols. Clin Microbiol Rev 2003; 16(3):357–364.
34. Braddy CM, Heilman RL, Blair JE. Coccidioidomycosis after renal transplantation in an endemic area. Am J Transplant 2006; 6(2):340–345.
35. Martín-Rabadán P, Muñoz P, Palomo J, Bouza E. Strongyloidiasis: The Harada-Mori test revisited. Clin Microbiol Infect 1999; 5:374–376.
36. Tan HP, Stephen Dumler J, Maley WR, et al. Human monocytic ehrlichiosis: an emerging pathogen in transplantation. Transplantation 2001; 71(11):1678–1680.
37. Paterson DL, Dominguez EA, Chang FY, Snydman DR, Singh N. Infective endocarditis in solid organ transplant recipients. Clin Infect Dis 1998; 26(3):689–694.

38. Mugnani G, Bergami M, Lazzarotto T, Bedani PL. Intestinal infection by cytomegalovirus in kidney transplantation: diagnostic difficulty in the course of mycophenolate mofetil therapy. G Ital Nefrol 2002; 19(4):483–484.

39. Bouza E, Merino P, Muñoz P, Sánchez-Carrillo C, Yáñez J, Cortés C. Ocular tuberculosis: a prospective study in a General Hospital. Medicine (Baltimore) 1997; 76: 53–61.

40. Bouza E, Cobo-Soriano R, Rodriguez-Creixems M, Munoz P, Suarez-Leoz M, Cortes C. A prospective search for ocular lesions in hospitalized patients with significant bacteremia. Clin Infect Dis 2000; 30(2):306–312.

41. Singh N, Gayowski T, Wagener MM, Marino IR. Pulmonary infiltrates in liver transplant recipients in the intensive care unit. Transplantation 1999; 67(8):1138–1144.

42. Mermel LA, Maki DG. Bacterial pneumonia in solid organ transplantation. Semin Respir Infect 1990; 5(1):10–29.

43. Singh N, Yu VL, Wagener MM, Gayowski T. Cirrhotic fever in the 1990s: a prospective study with clinical implications. Clin Infect Dis 1997; 24(6):1135–1138.

44. Jensen WA, Rose RM, Hammer SM, et al. Pulmonary complications of orthotopic liver transplantation. Transplantation 1986; 42(6):484.

45. Jimenez-Jambrina M, Hernandez A, Cordero E, et al. Pneumonia after Heart Transplantation in the XXI Century: a Multicenter Prospective Study. 45th Interscience Conference on Antimicrobial Agents and Chemoterapy 2005:(K-1561/370).

46. Cisneros JM, Muñoz P, Torre-Cisneros J, et al. Pneumonia after heart transplantation: a multiinstitutional study. Clin Infect Dis 1998; 27:324–331.

47. Fraser TG, Zembower TR, Lynch P, et al. Cavitary Legionella pneumonia in a liver transplant recipient. Transpl Infect Dis 2004; 6(2):77–80.

48. Singh N, Gayowski T, Wagener M, Marino IR, Yu VL. Pulmonary infections in liver transplant recipients receiving tacrolimus. Changing pattern of microbial etiologies. Transplantation 1996; 61(3):396–401.

49. Nichols L, Strollo DC, Kusne S. Legionellosis in a lung transplant recipient obscured by cytomegalovirus infection and Clostridium difficile colitis. Transpl Infect Dis 2002; 4(1):41–45.

50. Horbach I, Fehrenbach FJ. Legionellosis in heart transplant recipients. Infection 1990; 18(6):361–363.

51. Gupta RK, Jain M, Garg R. Pneumocystis carinii pneumonia after renal transplantation. Indian J Pathol Microbiol 2004; 47(4):474–476.

52. Renoult E, Georges E, Biava MF, et al. Toxoplasmosis in kidney transplant recipients: report of six cases and review. Clin Infect Dis 1997; 24(4):625–634.

53. Renoult E, Georges E, Biava MF, et al. Toxoplasmosis in kidney transplant recipients: a life-threatening but treatable disease. Transplant Proc 1997; 29(1–2):821–822.

54. Chang GC, Wu CL, Pan SH, et al. The diagnosis of pneumonia in renal transplant recipients using invasive and noninvasive procedures. Chest 2004; 125(2):541–547.

55. Ho MC, Wu YM, Hu RH, et al. Surgical complications and outcome of living related liver transplantation. Transplant Proc 2004; 36(8):2249–2251.

56. Stange BJ, Glanemann M, Nuessler NC, Settmacher U, Steinmuller T, Neuhaus P. Hepatic artery thrombosis after adult liver transplantation. Liver Transpl 2003; 9(6):612–620.

57. Munoz P, Menasalvas A, Bernaldo de Quiros JC, Desco M, Vallejo JL, Bouza E. Postsurgical mediastinitis: a case-control study. Clin Infect Dis 1997; 25(5):1060–1064.

58. Thaler F, Gotainer B, Teodori G, Dubois C, Loirat P. Mediastinitis due to Nocardia asteroides after cardiac transplantation. Intensive Care Med 1992; 18(2):127–128.

59. Levin T, Suh B, Beltramo D, Samuel R. Aspergillus mediastinitis following orthotopic heart transplantation: case report and review of the literature. Transpl Infect Dis 2004; 6(3):129–131.

60. Muñoz P. Management of urinary tract infections and lymphocele in renal transplant recipients. Clin Infect Dis 2001; 33(suppl 1):S53–S57.

61. Tolkoff RNE, Rubin RH. Urinary tract infection in the immunocompromised host. Lessons from kidney transplantation and the AIDS epidemic. Infect Dis Clin North Am 1997; 11(3):707–717.

62. Kahana L, Baxter J. OKT3 rescue in refractory renal rejection. Nephron 1987; 46(suppl 1):34–40.
63. Peterson PK, Anderson RC. Infection in renal transplant recipients. Current approaches to diagnosis, therapy, and prevention. Am J Med 1986; 81(1A):2–10.
64. Singh G. The study of prolonged fevers. J Assoc Physicians India 2000; 48(4):454–455.
65. Singh N. Post-transplant fever in critically ill transplant recipients. In: Singh N, Aguado JM, eds. Infectious Complications in Transplant Patients. Kluwer Academic publishers, 2000:113–132.
66. Keven K, Basu A, Re L, et al. Clostridium difficile colitis in patients after kidney and pancreas-kidney transplantation. Transpl Infect Dis 2004; 6(1):10–14.
67. Ginsburg PM, Thuluvath PJ. Diarrhea in liver transplant recipients: etiology and management. Liver Transpl 2005; 11(8):881–890.
68. Altiparmak MR, Trablus S, Pamuk ON, et al. Diarrhea following renal transplantation. Clin Transplant 2002; 16(3):212–216.
69. Kottaridis PD, Peggs K, Devereux S, Goldstone AH, Mackinnon S. Simultaneous occurrence of Clostridium difficile and Cytomegalovirus colitis in a recipient of autologous stem cell transplantation. Haematologica 2000; 85(10):1116–1117.
70. Kaplan B, Meier-Kriesche HU, Jacobs MG, et al. Prevalence of cytomegalovirus in the gastrointestinal tract of renal transplant recipients with persistent abdominal pain. Am J Kidney Dis 1999; 34(1):65–68.
71. Ponticelli C, Passerini P. Gastrointestinal complications in renal transplant recipients. Transpl Int 2005; 18(6):643–650.
72. Bouza E, Burillo A, Munoz P. Antimicrobial therapy of Clostridium difficile-associated diarrhea. Med Clin North Am 2006; 90(6):1141–1163.
73. Munoz P, Palomo J, Yanez J, Bouza E. Clinical microbiological case: a heart transplant recipient with diarrhea and abdominal pain. Recurring C. difficile infection. Clin Microbiol Infect 2001; 7(8):8–9, 451–452.
74. West M, Pirenne J, Chavers B, et al. Clostridium difficile colitis after kidney and kidney-pancreas transplantation. Clin Transplant 1999; 13(4):318–323.
75. Apaydin S, Altiparmak MR, Saribas S, Ozturk R. Prevalence of clostridium difficile toxin in kidney transplant recipients. Scand J Infect Dis 1998; 30(5):542.
76. Singh N, Paterson DL. Encephalitis caused by human herpesvirus-6 in transplant recipients: relevance of a novel neurotropic virus. Transplantation 2000; 69(12):2474–2479.
77. Singh N, Husain S. Infections of the central nervous system in transplant recipients. Transpl Infect Dis 2000; 2(3):101–111.
78. Ponticelli C, Campise MR. Neurological complications in kidney transplant recipients. J Nephrol 2005; 18(5):521–528.
79. Nash PJ, Avery RK, Tang WH, Starling RC, Taege AJ, Yamani MH. Encephalitis owing to human herpesvirus-6 after cardiac transplant. Am J Transplant 2004; 4(7):1200–1203.
80. Deborska-Materkowska D, Lewandowski Z, Sadowska A, et al. Fever, human herpes-virus-6 (HHV-6) seroconversion, and acute rejection episodes as a function of the initial seroprevalence for HHV-6 in renal transplant recipients. Transplant Proc 2006; 38(1):139–143.
81. Cervera C, Marcos MA, Linares L, et al. A prospective survey of human herpesvirus-6 primary infection in solid organ transplant recipients. Transplantation 2006; 82(7):979–982.
82. Ward KN. Human herpesviruses-6 and -7 infections. Curr Opin Infect Dis 2005; 18(3):247–252.
83. Benito N, Ricart MJ, Pumarola T, Marcos MA, Oppenheimer F, Camacho AM. Infection with human herpesvirus 6 after kidney-pancreas transplant. Am J Transplant 2004; 4(7):1197–1199.
84. Yoshikawa T, Yoshida J, Hamaguchi M, et al. Human herpesvirus 7-associated meningitis and optic neuritis in a patient after allogeneic stem cell transplantation. J Med Virol 2003; 70(3):440–443.
85. Yoshida H, Matsunaga K, Ueda T, et al. Human herpesvirus 6 meningoencephalitis successfully treated with ganciclovir in a patient who underwent allogeneic bone

marrow transplantation from an HLA-identical sibling. Int J Hematol 2002; 75(4): 421–425.

86. Tokimasa S, Hara J, Osugi Y, et al. Ganciclovir is effective for prophylaxis and treatment of human herpesvirus-6 in allogeneic stem cell transplantation. Bone Marrow Transplant 2002; 29(7):595–598.

87. Murtagh B, Wadia Y, Messner G, Allison P, Harati Y, Delgado R. West Nile virus infection after cardiac transplantation. J Heart Lung Transplant 2005; 24(6):774–776.

88. Kusne S, Smilack J. Transmission of West Nile virus by organ transplantation. Liver Transpl 2005; 11(2):239–241.

89. Kumar D, Humar A. Emerging viral infections in transplant recipients. Curr Opin Infect Dis 2005; 18(4):337–341.

90. Hoekstra C. West Nile virus: a challenge for transplant programs. Prog Transplant 2005; 15(4):397–400.

91. Hayes EB, Komar N, Nasci RS, Montgomery SP, O'Leary DR, Campbell GL. Epidemiology and transmission dynamics of West Nile virus disease. Emerg Infect Dis 2005; 11(8):1167–1173.

92. Cairoli O. The West Nile virus and the dialysis/transplant patient. Nephrol News Issues 2005; 19(12):73–75.

93. Bragin-Sanchez D, Chang PP. West Nile virus encephalitis infection in a heart transplant recipient: a case report. J Heart Lung Transplant 2005; 24(5):621–623.

94. Weiskittel PD. West Nile virus infection in a renal transplant recipient. Nephrol Nurs J 2004; 31(3):327–329.

95. Shepherd JC, Subramanian A, Montgomery RA, et al. West Nile virus encephalitis in a kidney transplant recipient. Am J Transplant 2004; 4(5):830–833.

96. Rosenberg RN. West Nile virus encephalomyelitis in transplant recipients. Arch Neurol 2004; 61(8):1181.

97. Roos KL. West Nile encephalitis and myelitis. Curr Opin Neurol 2004; 17(3): 343–346.

98. Wiesmayr S, Tabarelli W, Stelzmueller I, et al. Listeria meningitis in transplant recipients. Wien Klin Wochenschr 2005; 117(5–6):229–233.

99. Rettally CA, Speeg KV. Infection with Listeria monocytogenes following orthotopic liver transplantation: case report and review of the literature. Transplant Proc 2003; 35(4):1485–1487.

100. Hofer CB, Melles CE, Hofer E. Listeria monocytogenes in renal transplant recipients. Rev Inst Med Trop Sao Paulo 1999; 41(6):375–377.

101. Limaye AP, Perkins JD, Kowdley KV. Listeria infection after liver transplantation: report of a case and review of the literature. Am J Gastroenterol 1998; 93(10):1942–1944.

102. Stamm AM, Smith SH, Kirklin JK, McGiffin DC. Listerial myocarditis in cardiac transplantation. Rev Infect Dis 1990; 12(5):820–823.

103. Ascher NL, Simmons RL, Marker S, Najarian JS. Listeria infection in transplant patients. Five cases and a review of the literature. Arch Surg 1978; 113(1):90–94.

104. Summers SA, Dorling A, Boyle JJ, Shaunak S. Cure of disseminated cryptococcal infection in a renal allograft recipient after addition of gamma-interferon to anti-fungal therapy. Am J Transplant 2005; 5(8):2067–2069.

105. Rakvit A, Meyerrose G, Vidal AM, Kimbrough RC, Sarria JC. Cellulitis caused by Cryptococcus neoformans in a lung transplant recipient. J Heart Lung Transplant 2005; 24(5):642.

106. Geusau A, Sandor N, Messeritsch E, Jaksch P, Tintelnot K, Presterl E. Cryptococcal cellulitis in a lung-transplant recipient. Br J Dermatol 2005; 153(5):1068–1070.

107. Akamatsu N, Sugawara Y, Nakajima J, Kishi Y, Kaneko J, Makuuchi M. Cryptococcosis after living donor liver transplantation: report of three cases. Transpl Infect Dis 2005; 7(1):26–29.

108. Utili R, Tripodi MF, Ragone E, et al. Hepatic cryptococcosis in a heart transplant recipient. Transpl Infect Dis 2004; 6(1):33–36.

109. Singh N, Husain S, De Vera M, Gayowski T, Cacciarelli TV. Cryptococcus neoformans infection in patients with cirrhosis, including liver transplant candidates. Medicine (Baltimore) 2004; 83(3):188–192.

110. Lee YA, Kim HJ, Lee TW, et al. First report of Cryptococcus albidus-induced disseminated cryptococcosis in a renal transplant recipient. Korean J Intern Med 2004; 19(1):53–57.
111. Vilchez R, Shapiro R, McCurry K, et al. Longitudinal study of cryptococcosis in adult solid-organ transplant recipients. Transpl Int 2003; 16(5):336–340; Epub Mar 04, 2003.
112. Bag R. Fungal pneumonias in transplant recipients. Curr Opin Pulm Med 2003; 9(3):193–198.
113. Singh N, Gayowski T, Marino IR. Successful treatment of disseminated cryptococcosis in a liver transplant recipient with fluconazole and flucytosine, an all oral regimen. Transpl Int 1998; 11(1):63–65.
114. Singh N, Gayowski T, Wagener MM, Marino IR. Clinical spectrum of invasive cryptococcosis in liver transplant recipients receiving tacrolimus. Clin Transplant 1997; 11(1):66–70.
115. Wiesmayr S, Stelzmueller I, Tabarelli W, et al. Nocardiosis following solid organ transplantation: a single-centre experience. Transpl Int 2005; 18(9):1048–1053.
116. Peraira JR, Segovia J, Fuentes R, et al. Pulmonary nocardiosis in heart transplant recipients: treatment and outcome. Transplant Proc 2003; 35(5):2006–2008.
117. John GT, Shankar V, Abraham AM, Mathews MS, Thomas PP, Jacob CK. Nocardiosis in tropical renal transplant recipients. Clin Transplant 2002; 16(4):285–289.
118. Tripodi MF, Adinolfi LE, Andreana A, et al. Treatment of pulmonary nocardiosis in heart-transplant patients: importance of susceptibility studies. Clin Transplant 2001; 15(6):415–420.
119. Tan SY, Tan LH, Teo SM, Thiruventhiran T, Kamarulzaman A, Hoh HB. Disseminated nocardiosis with bilateral intraocular involvement in a renal allograft patient. Transplant Proc 2000; 32(7):1965–1966.
120. Reddy SS, Holley JL. Nocardiosis in a recently transplanted renal patient. Clin Nephrol 1998; 50(2):123–127.
121. Kursat S, Ok E, Zeytinoglu A, et al. Nocardiosis in renal transplant patients. Nephron 1997; 75(3):370–371.
122. Munoz P, Arencibia J, Rodriguez C, et al. Trimethoprim-sulfamethoxazole as toxoplasmosis prophylaxis for heart transplant recipients. Clin Infect Dis 2003; 36(7):932–933.
123. Baden LR, Katz JT, Franck L, et al. Successful toxoplasmosis prophylaxis after orthotopic cardiac transplantation with trimethoprim-sulfamethoxazole. Transplantation 2003; 75(3):339–343.
124. Wulf MW, van Crevel R, Portier R, et al. Toxoplasmosis after renal transplantation: implications of a missed diagnosis. J Clin Microbiol 2005; 43(7):3544–3547.
125. Conrath J, Mouly-Bandini A, Collart F, Ridings B. Toxoplasma gondii retinochoroiditis after cardiac transplantation. Graefes Arch Clin Exp Ophthalmol 2003; 241(4):334–338; Epub Mar 22, 2003.
126. Aboul-Hassan S, el-Shazly AM, Farag MK, Habib KS, Morsy TA. Epidemiological, clinical and laboratory studies on parasitic infections as a cause of fever of undetermined origin in Dakahlia Governorate, Egypt. J Egypt Soc Parasitol 1997; 27(1):47–57.
127. Ionescu DN, Dacic S. Persistent fever in a lung transplant patient. Arch Pathol Lab Med 2005; 129(6):e153–e154.
128. Ortonne N, Ribaud P, Meignin V, et al. Toxoplasmic pneumonitis leading to fatal acute respiratory distress syndrome after engraftment in three bone marrow transplant recipients. Transplantation 2001; 72(11):1838–1840.
129. Wagner FM, Reichenspurner H, Uberfuhr P, et al. How successful is OKT3 rescue therapy for steroid-resistant acute rejection episodes after heart transplantation? J Heart Lung Transplant 1994; 13(3):438–442; discussion 42–43.
130. Nowicki MJ, Chinchilla C, Corado L, et al. Prevalence of antibodies to Trypanosoma cruzi among solid organ donors in Southern California: a population at risk. Transplantation 2006; 81(3):477–479.
131. Walker M, Zunt JR. Parasitic central nervous system infections in immunocompromised hosts. Clin Infect Dis 2005; 40(7):1005–1015; Epub Mar 2, 2005.
132. Bryan CF, Tegtmeier GE, Rafik N, et al. The risk for Chagas' disease in the Midwestern United States organ donor population is low. Clin Transplant 2004; 18(suppl 12):12–15.

133. Barsoum RS. Parasitic infections in organ transplantation. Exp Clin Transplant 2004; 2(2):258–267.
134. Orlent H, Crawley C, Cwynarski K, Dina R, Apperley J. Strongyloidiasis pre and post autologous peripheral blood stem cell transplantation. Bone Marrow Transplant 2003; 32(1):115–117.
135. Stolf NA, Higushi L, Bocchi E, et al. Heart transplantation in patients with Chagas' disease cardiomyopathy. J Heart Transplant 1987; 6(5):307–312.
136. Scherer M, Fieguth HG, Aybek T, Ujvari Z, Moritz A, Wimmer-Greinecker G. Disseminated Aspergillus fumigatus infection with consecutive mitral valve endocarditis in a lung transplant recipient. J Heart Lung Transplant 2005; 24(12):2297–2300; Epub Sep 28, 2005.
137. Ruttmann E, Bonatti H, Legit C, et al. Severe endocarditis in transplant recipients—an epidemiologic study. Transpl Int 2005; 18(6):690–696.
138. Sherman-Weber S, Axelrod P, Suh B, et al. Infective endocarditis following orthotopic heart transplantation: 10 cases and a review of the literature. Transpl Infect Dis 2004; 6(4):165–170.
139. Bishara J, Robenshtok E, Weinberger M, Yeshurun M, Sagie A, Pitlik S. Infective endocarditis in renal transplant recipients. Transpl Infect Dis 1999; 1(2):138–143.
140. Chim CS, Ho PL, Yuen ST, Yuen KY. Fungal endocarditis in bone marrow transplantation: case report and review of literature. J Infect 1998; 37(3):287–291.
141. Segall L, Moal MC, Doucet L, Kergoat N, Bourbigot B. Toxoplasmosis-associated hemophagocytic syndrome in renal transplantation. Transpl Int 2006; 19(1):78–80.
142. Roman CD, Habibian MR, Martin WH. Identification of an infected left ventricular assist device after cardiac transplant by indium-111 WBC scintigraphy. Clin Nucl Med 2005; 30(1):16–17.
143. Sarkio S, Halme L, Arola J, Salmela K, Lautenschlager I. Gastroduodenal cytomegalovirus infection is common in kidney transplantation patients. Scand J Gastroenterol 2005; 40(5):508–514.
144. Huang HP, Chien YH, Huang LM, et al. Viral infections and prolonged fever after liver transplantation in young children with inborn errors of metabolism. J Formos Med Assoc 2005; 104(9):623–629.
145. Liebau P, Kuse E, Winkler M, et al. Management of herpes simplex virus type 1 pneumonia following liver transplantation. Infection 1996; 24(2):130–135.
146. Weiss RL, Colby TV, Spruance SL, Salmon VC, Hammond ME. Simultaneous cytomegalovirus and herpes simplex virus pneumonia. Arch Pathol Lab Med 1987; 111(3): 242–245.
147. Razonable RR, Paya CV. The impact of human herpesvirus-6 and -7 infection on the outcome of liver transplantation. Liver Transpl 2002; 8(8):651–658.
148. Rogers J, Rohal S, Carrigan DR, et al. Human herpesvirus-6 in liver transplant recipients: role in pathogenesis of fungal infections, neurologic complications, and outcome. Transplantation 2000; 69(12):2566–2573.
149. Persson L, Dahl H, Linde A, Engervall P, Vikerfors T, Tidefelt U. Human cytomegalovirus, human herpesvirus-6 and human herpesvirus-7 in neutropenic patients with fever of unknown origin. Clin Microbiol Infect 2003; 9(7):640–644.
150. Friedrichs N, Eis-Hubinger AM, Heim A, Platen E, Zhou H, Buettner R. Acute adenoviral infection of a graft by serotype 35 following renal transplantation. Pathol Res Pract 2003; 199(8):565–570.
151. Wright JJ, O'Driscoll G. Treatment of parainfluenza virus 3 pneumonia in a cardiac transplant recipient with intravenous ribavirin and methylprednisolone. J Heart Lung Transplant 2005; 24(3):343–346.
152. Kumar J, Shaver MJ, Abul-Ezz S. Long-term remission of recurrent parvovirus-B associated anemia in a renal transplant recipient induced by treatment with immunoglobulin and positive seroconversion. Transpl Infect Dis 2005; 7(1):30–33.
153. Kumar D, Erdman D, Keshavjee S, et al. Clinical impact of community-acquired respiratory viruses on bronchiolitis obliterans after lung transplant. Am J Transplant 2005; 5(8):2031–2036.
154. Barton TD, Blumberg EA. Viral pneumonias other than cytomegalovirus in transplant recipients. Clin Chest Med 2005; 26(4):707–720, viii.

155. Slifkin M, Doron S, Snydman DR. Viral prophylaxis in organ transplant patients. Drugs 2004; 64(24):2763–2792.
156. Mazzone PJ, Mossad SB, Mawhorter SD, Mehta AC, Mauer JR. Cell-mediated immune response to influenza vaccination in lung transplant recipients. J Heart Lung Transplant 2004; 23(10):1175–1181.
157. Vilchez RA, McCurry K, Dauber J, et al. Influenza virus infection in adult solid organ transplant recipients. Am J Transplant 2002; 2(3):287–291.
158. Ison MG, Hayden FG. Viral infections in immunocompromised patients: what's new with respiratory viruses? Curr Opin Infect Dis 2002; 15(4):355–367.
159. Wadei H, Alangaden GJ, Sillix DH, et al. West Nile virus encephalitis: an emerging disease in renal transplant recipients. Clin Transplant 2004; 18(6):753-758.
160. Kleinschmidt-DeMasters BK, Marder BA, Levi ME, et al. Naturally acquired West Nile virus encephalomyelitis in transplant recipients: clinical, laboratory, diagnostic, and neuropathological features. Arch Neurol 2004; 61(8):1210–1220.
161. DeSalvo D, Roy-Chaudhury P, Peddi R, et al. West Nile virus encephalitis in organ transplant recipients: another high-risk group for meningoencephalitis and death. Transplantation 2004; 77(3):466–469.
162. Khaled AS. Polyomavirus (BK virus) nephropathy in kidney transplant patients: a pathologic perspective. Yonsei Med J 2004; 45(6):1065–1075.
163. Lipshutz GS, Flechner SM, Govani MV, Vincenti F. BK nephropathy in kidney transplant recipients treated with a calcineurin inhibitor-free immunosuppression regimen. Am J Transplant 2004; 4(12):2132–2134.
164. de Bruyn G, Limaye AP. BK virus-associated nephropathy in kidney transplant recipients. Rev Med Virol 2004; 14(3):193–205.
165. Ramos E, Drachenberg CB, Portocarrero M, et al. BK virus nephropathy diagnosis and treatment: experience at the University of Maryland Renal Transplant Program. Clin Transpl 2002; 143–153.
166. Hirsch HH. Polyomavirus associated nephropathy. A new opportunistic complication after kidney transplantation. Internist (Berl) 2003; 44(5):653–655.
167. Munoz P, Rodriguez C, Bouza E. Mycobacterium tuberculosis infection in recipients of solid organ transplants. Clin Infect Dis 2005; 40(4):581–587; Epub Jan 25, 2005.
168. Muñoz P, Palomo J, Muñoz R, Rodríguez-Creixéms M, Pelaez T, Bouza E. Tuberculosis in heart transplant recipients. Clin Infect Dis 1995; 21:398–402.
169. Singh N, Paterson DL. Mycobacterium tuberculosis infection in solid-organ transplant recipients: impact and implications for management. Clin Infect Dis 1998; 27(5): 1266–1277.
170. Aguado JM, Herrero JA, Gavalda J, et al. Clinical presentation and outcome of tuberculosis in kidney, liver, and heart transplant recipients in Spain. Spanish Transplantation Infection Study Group, GESITRA. Transplantation 1997; 63(9):1278–1286.
171. Muñoz P, de la Torre J, Bouza E, et al. Invasive Aspergillosis In Transplant Recipients. A Large Multicentric Study. 36th Interscience Conference of Antimicrobial Agents and Chemotherapy American Society for Microbiology 1996.
172. Paterson DL, Singh N. Invasive aspergillosis in transplant recipients. Medicine 1999; 78(2):123–138.
173. Munoz P, Alcala L, Sanchez Conde M, et al. The isolation of Aspergillus fumigatus from respiratory tract specimens in heart transplant recipients is highly predictive of invasive aspergillosis. Transplantation 2003; 75(3):326–329.
174. Gavalda J, Len O, Rovira M, et al. Epidemiology of Invasive Fungal Infections (IFI) in Solid Organ (SOT) and Hematopoeitic Stem Cell (HSCT) Transplant Recipients: a Prospective Study from RESITRA. 45th Interscience Conference on Antimicrobial Agents and Chemoterapy 2005:(M-990/461).
175. Dummer JS, Lazariashvilli N, Barnes J, Ninan M, Milstone AP. A survey of antifungal management in lung transplantation. J Heart Lung Transplant 2004; 23(12): 1376–1381.
176. Singh N, Gayowski T, Wagener MM. Intensive care unit management in liver transplant recipients: beneficial effect on survival and preservation of quality of life. Clin Transplant 1997; 11(2):113–120.
177. Paterson DL, Singh N, Gayowski T, Marino IR. Pulmonary nodules in liver transplant recipients. Medicine 1998; 77(1):50–58.

178. Bonham CA, Dominguez EA, Fukui MB, et al. Central nervous system lesions in liver transplant recipients: prospective assessment of indications for biopsy and implications for management. Transplantation 1998; 66(12):1596–1604.
179. Vagefi MR, Kim ET, Alvarado RG, Duncan JL, Howes EL, Crawford JB. Bilateral endogenous Scedosporium prolificans endophthalmitis after lung transplantation. Am J Ophthalmol 2005; 139(2):370–373.
180. Husain S, Munoz P, Forrest G, et al. Infections due to Scedosporium apiospermum and Scedosporium prolificans in transplant recipients: clinical characteristics and impact of antifungal agent therapy on outcome. Clin Infect Dis 2005; 40(1):89–99; Epub Dec 08, 2004.
181. Bouza E, Munoz P. Invasive infections caused by Blastoschizomyces capitatus and Scedosporium spp. Clin Microbiol Infect 2004; 10(suppl 1):76–85.
182. Munoz P, Marin M, Tornero P, Martin RP, Rodriguez-Creixems M, Bouza E. Successful outcome of Scedosporium apiospermum disseminated infection treated with voriconazole in a patient receiving corticosteroid therapy. Clin Infect Dis 2000; 31(6):1499–1501.
183. Bouza E, Munoz P, Vega L, Rodriguez-Creixems M, Berenguer J, Escudero A. Clinical resolution of Scedosporium prolificans fungemia associated with reversal of neutropenia following administration of granulocyte colony-stimulating factor. Clin Infect Dis 1996; 23(1):192–193.
184. Husain S, Alexander BD, Munoz P, et al. Opportunistic mycelial fungal infections in organ transplant recipients: emerging importance of non-Aspergillus mycelial fungi. Clin Infect Dis 2003; 37(2):221–229; Epub Jul 09, 2003.
185. Rodriguez M, Sifri CD, Fishman JA. Failure of low-dose atovaquone prophylaxis against Pneumocystis jiroveci infection in transplant recipients. Clin Infect Dis 2004; 38(8):e76–e78; Epub Mar 29, 2004.
186. Radisic M, Lattes R, Chapman JF, et al. Risk factors for Pneumocystis carinii pneumonia in kidney transplant recipients: a case-control study. Transpl Infect Dis 2003; 5(2):84–93.
187. Muñoz P, Muñoz RM, Palomo J, Rodríguez Creixéms M, Muñoz R, Bouza E. Pneumocystis carinii infections in heart transplant patients. Twice a week prophylaxis. Medicine (Baltimore) 1997; 76:415–422.
188. Husain S, Wagener MM, Singh N. Cryptococcus neoformans infection in organ transplant recipients: variables influencing clinical characteristics and outcome. Emerg Infect Dis 2001; 7(3):375–381.
189. Singh N, Lortholary O, Alexander BD, et al. Allograft loss in renal transplant recipients with cryptococcus neoformans associated immune reconstitution syndrome. Transplantation 2005; 80(8):1131–1133.
190. Singh N, Lortholary O, Alexander BD, et al. An immune reconstitution syndrome-like illness associated with Cryptococcus neoformans infection in organ transplant recipients. Clin Infect Dis 2005; 40(12):1756–1761; Epub Apr 29, 2005.
191. Gupta RK, Khan ZU, Nampoory MR, Mikhail MM, Johny KV. Cutaneous cryptococcosis in a diabetic renal transplant recipient. J Med Microbiol 2004; 53(Pt 5):445–449.
192. Singh N, Rihs JD, Gayowski T, Yu VL. Cutaneous cryptococcosis mimicking bacterial cellulitis in a liver transplant recipient: case report and review in solid organ transplant recipients. Clin Transplant 1994; 8(4):365–368.
193. Basaran O, Emiroglu R, Arikan U, Karakayali H, Haberal M. Cryptococcal necrotizing fasciitis with multiple sites of involvement in the lower extremities. Dermatol Surg 2003; 29(11):1158–1160.
194. Freifeld AG, Iwen PC, Lesiak BL, Gilroy RK, Stevens RB, Kalil AC. Histoplasmosis in solid organ transplant recipients at a large Midwestern university transplant center. Transpl Infect Dis 2005; 7(3–4):109–115.
195. Nath DS, Kandaswamy R, Gruessner R, Sutherland DE, Dunn DL, Humar A. Fungal infections in transplant recipients receiving alemtuzumab. Transplant Proc 2005; 37(2):934–936.
196. McGuinn ML, Lawrence ME, Proia L, Segreti J. Progressive disseminated histoplasmosis presenting as cellulitis in a renal transplant recipient. Transplant Proc 2005; 37(10):4313–4314.
197. Jha V, Sree Krishna V, Varma N, et al. Disseminated histoplasmosis 19 years after renal transplantation. Clin Nephrol 1999; 51(6):373–378.

198. Arnold SJ, Kinney MC, McCormick MS, Dummer S, Scott MA. Disseminated toxoplasmosis. Unusual presentations in the immunocompromised host. Arch Pathol Lab Med 1997; 121(8):869–873.

199. Walker M, Kublin JG, Zunt JR. Parasitic central nervous system infections in immunocompromised hosts: malaria, microsporidiosis, leishmaniasis, and African trypanosomiasis. Clin Infect Dis 2006; 42(1):115–125; Epub Nov 23, 2005.

200. von Muller L, Schliep C, Storck M, et al. Severe graft rejection, increased immunosuppression, and active CMV infection in renal transplantation. J Med Virol 2006; 78(3):394–399.

201. Toupance O, Bouedjoro-Camus MC, Carquin J, et al. Cytomegalovirus-related disease and risk of acute rejection in renal transplant recipients: a cohort study with case-control analyses. Transpl Int 2000; 13(6):413–419.

202. Heo JS, Park JW, Lee KW, et al. Post-transplantation lymphoproliferative disorder in pediatric liver transplantation. Transplant Proc 2004; 36(8):2307–2308.

203. Singh N, Gayowski T, Marino IR, Schlichtig R. Acute adrenal insufficiency in critically ill liver transplant recipients. Implications for diagnosis. Transplantation 1995; 59(12):1744–1745.

204. Hummel M, Warnecke H, Schüler S, Luding K, Hetzer R. Risk of adrenal cortex insufficiency following heart transplantation. Klin Wochenschr 1991; 69(6):269–273.

205. Bromberg JS, Alfrey EJ, Barker CF, et al. Adrenal suppression and steroid supplementation in renal transplant recipients. Transplantation 1991; 51(2):385–390.

206. Rodger RS, Watson MJ, Sellars L, Wilkinson R, Ward MK, Kerr DN. Hypothalamic-pituitary-adrenocortical suppression and recovery in renal transplant patients returning to maintenance dialysis. Q J Med 1986; 61(235):1039–1046.

207. Sever MS, Turkmen A, Yildiz A, Ecder T, Orhan Y. Fever in dialysis patients with recently rejected renal allografts. Int J Artif Organs 1998; 21(7):403–407.

208. Khan A, Ortiz J, Jacobson L, Reich D, Manzarbeitia C. Post-transplant lymphoproliferative disease presenting as adrenal insufficiency: case report. Exp Clin Transplant 2005; 3(1):341–344.

209. Mourad G, Rostaing L, Legendre C, Garrigue V, Thervet E, Durand D. Sequential protocols using basiliximab versus antithymocyte globulins in renal-transplant patients receiving mycophenolate mofetil and steroids. Transplantation 2004; 78(4):584–590.

210. Khan SU, Salloum J, PB OD, et al. Acute pulmonary edema after lung transplantation: the pulmonary reimplantation response. Chest 1999; 116(1):187–194.

211. Singh N, Paterson DL, Gayowski T, Wagener MM, Marino IR. Predicting bacteremia and bacteremic mortality in liver transplant recipients. Liver Transpl 2000; 6(1):54–61.

10   Nosocomial Fever of Unknown Origin

Burke A. Cunha

Infectious Disease Division, Winthrop-University Hospital, Mineola, New York, U.S.A.

INTRODUCTION

The first work on prolonged fevers was by Keefer, entitled *Prolonged and Perplexing Fevers*; it was the first compilation of infectious and noninfectious disorders characterized by prolonged fevers (1). The term fever of unknown origin (FUO) was first used by Petersdorf in 1961 to define prolonged febrile illnesses that were not easily diagnosed. Petersdorf defined FUO as an obscure fever with a duration ≥3 weeks, temperatures ≥101°F (38.3°C) on multiple occasions during three weeks, remaining undiagnosed after a week of hospitalization. These FUO criteria have remained useful (2–5).

Some authors have tried to define FUOs in special populations, for example, FUO in the HIV population, nosocomial FUO, FUO in travelers, and FUO in the elderly. Bryan has suggested that instead of considering such patients as FUO subtypes, they should really be considered as subsets of patients (3).

Nosocomial FUO was one of the four subtypes suggested by Durack and Street in their 1991 article (6). The term prolonged, undiagnosed fevers in the hospital may be preferable to nosocomial FUO (5,7).

NOSOCOMIAL FUOs

Prolonged fevers acquired in hospitalized patients may be due to a variety of noninfectious and infectious disorders. The diagnostic approach to nosocomial prolonged fevers depends on the magnitude of the fever, the duration of the fever, the fever pattern, the relationship of the pulse to the fever, and the presence or absence of localizing signs. Many common noninfectious disease disorders present as fever in the hospital, for example, pulmonary embolism/infarction, myocardial infarction, acute pancreatitis, gastrointestinal hemorrhage, IV-line infections, nosocomial pneumonias, adrenal insufficiency, a flare of systemic lupus erythematosus (SLE), or drug fevers. The noninfectious causes of fever may be divided into those that may exceed 101°F (38.8°C) and those that do not exceed 101°F (38.8°C) (8–10).

The noninfectious causes of fever acquired in the hospital setting ≤102°F (38.8°C) include myocardial infarction, pulmonary embolus, gastrointestinal hemorrhage, and acute pancreatitis. Noninfectious disorders with temperatures ≥102°F (38.8°C) include adrenal insufficiency and drug fever. Drug fevers may also be present with temperatures ≤102 °F (38.8°C) or may generate temperatures ≥106 °F (41.1°C) (9,10).

Infectious causes of hospital-acquired fever in the intensive care unit (ICU) include nosocomial pneumonia, IV-line infections, *Clostridium difficile* diarrhea/colitis, or postoperative abscesses. The height of the fever, that is, ≥102°F

(38.8°C), provides a good way to clinically approach infectious/noninfectious fevers. Temperatures ≥102°F (38.8°C) without an obvious explanation should suggest the possibility of abscess in a postoperative surgical patient. Temperatures are also ≥102°F with C. *difficile* colitis and IV-line infections. Phlebitis, uncomplicated wound infections, catheter-associated bacteriuria, and simple cellulitis do not ordinarily exceed 102°F (38.8°C).

Extreme hyperpyrexia, that is, temperature 106°F (≥41.1°C) virtually excludes an infectious etiology. Central fevers following craniotomy, drug-induced malignant neuroleptic syndromes, and drug fevers are disorders likely to present with extreme hyperpyrexia (10–12).

Nosocomial FUO should convey to the physician that the cause of the prolonged fever is not apparent after a week in the hospital. Hospital-acquired prolonged fevers are associated with relatively few disorders that can evade detection for a prolonged period and include nosocomial endocarditis (from central IV lines, implanted pacemakers, or defibrillators), nosocomial sinusitis in patients who have had prolonged nasotracheal intubation, fungemias or disseminated/invasive fungal infections, postsurgical abscesses particularly of the pelvis or abdomen, C. *difficile* colitis, ischemic colitis, central fevers, postperfusion syndrome following open heart procedures, herpes simplex virus (HSV)-1 nosocomial pneumonia, adrenal insufficiency, fat emboli syndrome, and drug fevers (10,13,14).

FEVERS OF SHORT DURATION

As with prolonged fever, the challenge for the clinician is to differentiate infectious from noninfectious disorders. Most febrile disorders are self-limited, for example, fevers secondary to transfusion reactions of blood or blood products, cerebrovascular accidents (CVA) (not associated with massive intracranial hemorrhage), acute attack of gout precipitated by stress, superficial phlebitis, deep vein thrombosis (DVTs), acute flare of systemic lupus erythematosus (SLE), extremity gangrene of the digits, Dressler's syndrome, acute myocardial infarction, acute gastrointestinal hemorrhage, acute pulmonary embolus/infarction, acute pancreatitis, and acute adrenal insufficiency. These noninfectious disorders are usually readily diagnosable from the clinical presentation combined with laboratory/X-ray findings. The undiagnosed noninfectious disease disorders most likely to be confused with infectious disorders include an SLE flare, acute adrenal insufficiency, and repeated showers of small pulmonary emboli; fever from a CVA will decrease within days after the embolic/thrombotic event. Gastrointestinal hemorrhage unless massive and prolonged, will rapidly lose its febrile component. In acute myocardial infarction, the fever peaks two to three days after the event and the patient rapidly becomes afebrile. The fever of acute pancreatitis usually lasts only a few days unless complicated by infected pseudocyst or abscess (10–12).

Among the infectious disorders that are common in the hospital setting are sacral decubiti with/without accompanying osteomyelitis. Sacral decubiti may cause low-grade fevers that are not diagnostic problems. Septic thrombophlebitis presents as phlebitis with temperatures ≥102°F (38.8°C). The common causes of prolonged fevers are septic thrombophlebitis, arteriovenous (AV) shunt infections, central line infections, and procedure-related nosocomial endocarditis (15–18) (Table 1).

TABLE 1 Causes of Acute Nosocomial Fevers

Noninfectious causes	Infectious causes
Acute myocardial infarction	Nosocomial pneumonia
Acute pulmonary embolus/infarction	IV central line infections
Acute gastrointestinal bleed	Septic thrombophlebitis
Transfusion reactions	
Dressler's syndrome	
SLE flare	
Acute gout flare	
CVA/massive intracranial bleed	

Abbreviations: CVA, cerebrovascular accident; IV, intravenous; SLE, systemic lupus erythematosus.

NOSOCOMIAL LOW-GRADE FEVERS

Most commonly encountered noninfectious disorders are essentially afebrile disorders, but may be accompanied by low-grade fever, usually in the range of 99°F to 100°F (37.2°C–37.7°C). The temperatures associated with these disorders rarely exceed 102°F (38.8°C), and include catheter-associated bacteriuria (CAB), atelectasis, dehydration, noninfectious (non-*C. difficile*) diarrhea, uncomplicated wound infections, infected drain tube sites, infected ascites or pleural fluid, and tracheobronchitis. Noninfectious and infectious disorders are usually accompanied by some degree of leukocytosis. Because syndromic diagnosis is the primary means of approaching clinical infectious-disease problems, it is important that the correct associations should be made between various signs/symptoms before ascribing them to a particular syndrome complex. The importance of the noninfectious disorders mentioned is that they may mislead the clinician into believing that fever/leukocytosis are due to these conditions, when they should prompt a search for an alternate explanation for the patient's fever, particularly if ≥102°F (38.8°C) (9–11) (Table 2).

FEVER OF UNKNOWN ORIGIN IN THE INTENSIVE CARE UNIT SETTING

Disorders that could present as FUO in the ICU are relatively limited. As with acute fevers, the conditions potentially presenting as an FUO consist of both infectious and noninfectious disorders. Among the disorders that often escape diagnosis and persist long enough to present as an FUO include cholesterol-emboli syndrome

TABLE 2 Causes of Prolonged Low-Grade Nosocomial Fevers

Noninfectious causes	Infectious causes
Atelectasis	Tracheobronchitis
Dehydration	Wound infections
Pleural effusion	Sacral decubitus ulcers (grade III/IV/
Ascites	chronic osteomyelitis)
Dry (ischemic) gangrene	
Noninfectious diarrhea (non-*Clostridium difficile*)	
Phlebitis	
Deep vein thrombosis	

following open heart surgery, "postperfusion syndrome" due to cytomegalovirus (CMV) following open heart surgery, sternal osteomyelitis, mediastinitis, and nosocomial pneumonia.

Postperfusion Syndrome

Postperfusion syndrome due to CMV usually presents weeks after the surgery and temperatures may persist for extended periods of time, presenting as an FUO during recovery. Postperfusion syndrome was formerly known as "40-day postoperative fever" because of its delayed incubation period after being acquired by the host via multiple blood transfusions associated with open heart surgical procedures. The risk of acquiring CMV postoperatively is directly related to the number of units transfused during the open heart procedure. Patients with postperfusion syndrome present with a CMV infectious mononucleosis-like syndrome following open heart surgery. The clue to the diagnosis is the finding of leukopenia, thrombocytopenia, lymphopenia, or atypical lymphocytes in the peripheral smear. Serum transaminases are minimally elevated. Unlike nonsurgically acquired CMV infectious mononucleosis, such patients do not have a sore throat or peripheral adenopathy (9,10,19).

Postperfusion syndrome must be differentiated from Dressler's syndrome (postpericardiotomy syndrome). Dressler's syndrome, in contrast to postperfusion syndrome, occurs approximately two weeks after myocardial infarction or open heart surgery. Dressler's syndrome is a noninfectious disorder characterized by autoimmune phenomena, for example, splinter hemorrhages, Roth's spots, shoulder pain, and increased erythrocyte sedimentation rate (ESR). Atypical lymphocytes and increase in serum transaminases are not part of Dressler's syndrome, nor are leukopenia, lymphopenia, or thrombocytopenia.

Cholesterol Emboli Syndrome

Cholesterol emboli syndrome occurs following open heart procedures secondary to cholesterol embolization from clamping off major vessels to go on cardiopulmonary bypass. Cholesterol emboli released into the circulation can result in multiorgan manifestations and dysfunction. Emboli frequently go to the central nervous system (CNS), the kidneys, the pancreas, the extremities, and, uncommonly, even the coronary arteries. Patients present clinically with livedo reticularis of the lower extremities and a peripheral eosinophilia accompanied by fever. The diagnosis is clinical and is suggested by the time relationship between the open heart procedure and the finding of otherwise unexplained multiorgan dysfunction, accompanied by fever, eosinophilia, and a livedo reticularis extremity rash (10,20).

Invasive/Disseminated Fungal Infections

Patients in the ICU will receive corticosteroids for a variety of reasons. If the stay in the ICU or the critical care unit (CCU) is prolonged and steroid therapy is continued throughout the patient's stay, then the possibility of invasive or disseminated fungal infections should be entertained. Patients who are receiving broad-spectrum antimicrobial therapy, steroids and/or who have undergone major surgical procedures, have additional risk factors for invasive/disseminated fungal infections. If a patient has been maintained on prolonged broad-spectrum antimicrobial therapy or corticosteroids that spike temperatures without explanation, the possibility of invasive/disseminated fungal infection should be entertained. Patients with candidemia usually have positive blood cultures to suggest the diagnosis. Invasive aspergillosis is not usually accompanied by positive blood cultures. Diagnosis is made by tissue biopsy of the affected organ, demonstrating tissue and vessel invasion by *Aspergillus* or other fungi. Treatment is based on identifying the organism in tissue biopsy/culture (10–12).

Nosocomial Sinusitis

Nosocomial sinusitis may rarely complicate extended nasotracheal intubation. Such patients present without clinical signs relating to sinusitis, but with otherwise unexplained fevers. Nosocomial sinusitis is a diagnosis of exclusion in patients with prolonged nasotracheal intubation. Diagnosis is confirmed by obtaining a head computed tomography (CT) or magnetic resonance imaging (MRI) demonstrating sinusitis. Treatment is to remove the nasotracheal tube, which usually results in sufficient drainage (21).

Intra-abdominal or Pelvic Abscesses

An intra-abdominal or pelvic abscess may complicate any surgical procedure/perforation. The possibility of an intra-abdominal or pelvic abscess depends on the nature of the antecedent surgical procedure and a high index of suspicion. Indium or gallium scans are unhelpful because postoperative changes cannot be differentiated from infection. The best diagnostic technique is an abdominal/pelvic CT or MRI scan to rule out postoperative pelvic or abdominal abscess. Treatment is appropriate antimicrobial therapy to cover common coliforms and *Bacteroides fragilis*, and surgical drainage (9,11,18,22).

Arteriovenous Shunt Infections

Shunt infections, particularly peripheral shunts or hemodialysis catheter infections can be difficult to diagnose if they are not thought of. The catheter entry site or the graft site is not always tender and erythematous. The only clue to an otherwise occult graft infection may be the intermittently or constantly positive bacteremia, and prolonged, otherwise unexplained fevers. Diagnosis is made by indium or gallium scan showing an uptake in the area of the graft or dialysis catheter (12,23).

Infected Implanted Pacemakers/Defibrillators

Some patients in the ICU have an implantable defibrillator or pacemaker inserted. Persistent and otherwise unexplained fevers in the absence of another explanation for the fever should suggest the possibility of an infected device. Diagnosis is made by gallium or indium scanning, which may show uptake on the wire pacemaker/generator or pocket. Cure usually requires removal of the pacemaker wire/generator or defibrillator (24).

Nosocomial Endocarditis

Nosocomial endocarditis may complicate/follow central IV-lines (PICC, short-term central IV catheters) or Swan-Ganz catheter placement. Diagnosis is made by positive blood cultures and demonstrating a vegetation by echocardiography. Treatment is to remove the IV device/line if still in place, and treat the endocarditis with appropriate therapy.

Clostridium difficile Colitis

Nosocomial diarrhea may be either infectious or noninfectious. The more common causes of nosocomial noninfectious diarrhea are overzealous enteral feeds, drug-induced changes in the patient's microflora, or drug-induced intestinal peristalsis. If the nosocomial diarrhea is infectious, it is invariably due to *C. difficile*. Patients receiving enteral feeds are protected somewhat from getting *C. difficile* diarrhea. Diarrhea due to enteral feeds may be eliminated by either decreasing the infusion rate per hour, or by changing to another formulation. *C. difficile* diarrhea may result from exposure to cancer-chemotherapeutic agents, or selected but not any anti-biotics. Antibiotics differ in their *C. difficile* potential, and the antibiotics most commonly associated with *C. difficile* include clindamycin and β-lactam antibiotics. Quinolones are a less common cause of *C. difficile* diarrhea. Daptomycin, linezolid, quinupristin/dalfopristin, polymyxin B, aztreonam, carbapenems, aminoglyco-sides, and TMP-SMX, doxycycline rarely cause *C. difficile* diarrhea. Unrecognized, untreated *C. difficile* diarrhea may progress to *C. difficile* colitis. *C. difficile* colitis in a patient with *C. difficile* diarrhea is heralded by an abrupt increase in the white blood cell count (WBC) (WBC 25–50 k/mm^3) a temperature that $\geq 102°F$ (38.8°C), new acute abdominal pain, or an abrupt stop in diarrhea. In contrast, uncompli-cated *C. difficile* diarrhea is associated with temperatures $\leq 102°F$ (38.8°C). The diag-nosis of *C. difficile* colitis may be confirmed by abdominal CT/MRI or sigmoidoscopy. Rarely, *C. difficile* colitis may occur without preceding *C. difficile* diarrhea. Such cases of *C. difficile* colitis without antecedent *C. difficile* diarrhea may present as a nosocomial FUO. Treatment of *C. difficile* colitis is with metronida-zole. The addition of oral vancomycin offers no benefit. In severe cases, partial or total colectomy may be necessary (11,25).

Central Fever

Central fevers occur in patients following neurosurgical procedures or CNS trauma. Clinicians unfamiliar with neurosurgical patients will have difficulties diagnosing obscure fevers in such patients if they are not aware of the clinical fea-tures of central fever. The diagnosis of central fever depends on having a CNS cause for the fever, that is, hemorrhage, trauma, granuloma, tumor, and so on. Central fevers characteristically are high, plateau-like, and may be accompanied by relative bradycardia. Central fevers are relatively resistant to antipyretics. The clinical clue to central fever is that the temperatures are not accompanied by perspiration. The diagnosis of central fever requires analysis of CNS fluid, which usually shows a pleocytosis and RBCs but no organisms on Gram stain or culture. Treatment is supportive (8,11,12).

Drug Fever

Drug fevers are the sole manifestation of a hypersensitivity reaction to a medi-cation. Drug rash is a hypersensitivity reaction that causes fever and is accompanied by rash. There is no diagnostic difficulty when rash/fever are present, but in the absence of a rash, the diagnosis of drug fever can be difficult. Because most patients in the ICU have multisystem disease, multiple interventions (surgically/medically), and numerous drugs, it is easy to overlook the possibility that the patient's prolonged fevers are due to a drug. Most medications are capable of causing a hypersensitivity reaction, but the potential varies considerably. Most drug fevers in the ICU setting are not caused by antibiotics but by common medications. Common causes of drug fever in the ICU setting include antiarrhythmics, antiseizure medications, pain medications, or sulfa-based stool softeners. Among the antibiotics, sulfa-containing antibiotics, for example, TMP-SMX, β-blockers, calcium channel blockers, ACE inhibitors, or the β-lactams are the commonest causes of antibiotic-caused drug fever. Steroid, multivitamins, and digitalis preparations do not cause drug fevers. Importantly, certain antibiotics rarely, if ever, are the cause of drug fever, for example, quinolones, monobactams, carbapenems, aminoglycosides, tetracyclines, macrolides, TMP/SMX, daptomycin, linezolid, quinupristin/dalfopristin, antifungals, and polymyxin B. The diagnosis of drug fever is a diagnosis of exclusion. With drug fever, blood cultures are negative, excluding contaminants. Patients on sensitizing medications do not necessarily have an atopic/allergy history. WBC count is usually increased with a shift to the left, mimicking an infectious disease process. Serum transaminases are modestly/transiently elevated early and such subtle changes are often missed by clinicians taking care of ill individuals. Eosinophils are common in the peripheral smear, but eosinophilia is uncommon.

Relative bradycardia regularly accompanies drug fever and is a clue to the diagnosis. Relative bradycardia may also occur with tumors, central fevers, and a variety of infectious diseases. Relative bradycardia is also present in febrile patients on β-blockers (not with digitalis preparations, ACE inhibitors, or calcium channel blockers). Therefore, an obscure fever occurring in the ICU accompanied by pulse temperature deficit in a patient not on β-blocker medication should suggest the possibility of drug fever.

With multiple medications, it is often difficult to determine which drug is responsible for the drug fever. The most likely drug/drugs should be discontinued, and if they are the offending agents, temperature will decrease to near normal levels within 72 hours. Alternately, if clinically feasible, all nonlife-supporting medication can be withdrawn and the patient observed for 72 hours. Patients may also have an infectious disease and a drug fever due to one of the medications that the patient is receiving. If the antibiotic being used to treat the infection is the cause of the drug fever, then a hypoallergenic agent with the same spectrum and pharmacokinetic profile should be substituted, for example, a carbapenem in place of a β-lactam. Patients with drug fevers appear relatively well for the degree of fever. Drug fevers often are between $102°F–104°F$ ($38.8–40°C$), but may exceed $106°F$

TABLE 3 Causes of Nosocomial FUO

Noninfectious causes	Infectious causes
Relative adrenal insufficiency	Endocarditis ($2°$ to central IV lines,
Central fever	Swan Ganz catheters, etc.)
Post craniotomy	Infected pacemaker/defibrillator
(postperfusion syndrome)	Invasive/disseminated fungal infections
Drug fever	*Clostridium difficile* colitis
	Postoperative intraabdominal/pelvic abscess
	Postoperative heart surgery
	(postperfusion syndrome $2°$ to CMV)
	Cholesterol emboli syndrome
	AV shunt infections
	Nosocomial sinusitis

Abbreviations: AV, arteriovenous; CMV, cytomegalovirus; FUO, fever of unknown origin; IV, intravenous.

(41.1°C). The main diagnostic difficulty with drug fever is failure to consider the diagnosis. A second problem is failure to carefully review the medication list, looking for nonantibiotic agents that are the most likely causes of drug fever (12–14) (Table 3).

REFERENCES

1. Keefer CS, Leard SE. Prolonged and Perplexing Fevers. Boston, MA: Little Brown and Co, 1955.
2. Petersdorf RO, Beeson PB. Fever of unexplained origin: report on 100 cases. Medicine (Baltimore) 1961; 40:1–30.
3. Bryan CS. Fever of unknown origin. Arch Intern Med 2003; 163:1003–1004.
4. Vanderschueren S, Knockaert D, Adrienssens T, et al. From prolonged febrile illness to fever of unkown origin: the challenge continues. Arch Intern Med 2003; 163:1033–1041.
5. Cunha BA. Fever of unknown origin. In: Gorbach SL, Bartlett JB, Blacklow NR, eds. Infectious Diseases in Medicine and Surgery, 3rd ed. Philadelphia: W. B. Saunders, 2004:1568–1577.
6. Durack DT, Street AC. Fever of unknown origin—reexamined and redefined. Curr Clin Top Infect Dis 1991; 11:35–51.
7. Arbo MJ, Fine MJ, Hanusa BH, et al. Fever of nosocomial origin: etiology, risk factors, and outcomes. Am J Med 1993; 95:505–512.
8. Gabbay DS, Cunha BA. Pseudosepsis secondary to bilateral adrenal hemorrhage. Heart Lung 1998; 27:348–351.
9. Vincent J-L. Nosocomial infections in adult intensive-care units. Lancet 2003; 361: 2068–2077.
10. Cunha BA. Fever in the intensive care unit. Intensive Care Med 1999; 25:648–651.
11. Cunha BA. Fever in the critical care unit. In: Cunha BA, ed. Infectious Diseases in Critical Care Medicine, 2nd ed. New York: Informa; 2007; 41–72.
12. Cunha BA. The clinical significance of fever patterns. Infect Dis Clin North Am 1996; 10:33–44.
13. Mackowiak PA, LeMaistre CF. Drug fever: a critical appraisal of conventional concepts. Ann Intern Med 1987; 106:728–733.
14. Johnson DH, Cunha BA. Drug fever. Infect Dis Clin North Am 1996; 10:85–92.
15. Legras A, Malvy D, Quinioux AI, et al. Nosocomial infections: prospective survey of incidence in five French intensive care units. Intensive Care Med 1998; 24:1040–1046.
16. Richards MJ, Edwards JR, Culver DH, Gaynes RP. Nosocomial infections in combined medical-surgical intensive care units in the United States. Infect Control Hosp Epidemiol 2000; 2110–2115.
17. Cunha BA. Clinical approach to fever. In: Gorbach SL, Bartlett JB, Blacklow NR, eds. Infectious Diseases in Medicine and Surgery, 3rd ed. Philadelphia: W. B. Saunders, 2004:54–63.
18. Papia G, McLellan BA, El Helou P, et al. Infection in hospitalized trauma patients: incidence, risk factors, and complications. J Trauma 1999; 47:923–927.
19. Cunha BA. Postoperative fever in the post-open heart surgical patient. Infect Dis Pract 1997; 21:47–48.
20. Lazar J, Marzo KM, Bonoan JT, Cunha BA. Cholesterol emboli syndrome following cardiac catheterization. Heart Lung 2002; 42:452–454.
21. George DL, Falk PS, Umberto MG, et al. Nosocomial sinusitis in patients in the medical intensive care unit: a prospective epidemiological study. Clin Infect Dis 1998; 27: 463–470.
22. Donowitz LG, Wenzel RP, Hoyt JW. High risk of hospital-acquired infection in the ICU patient. Crit Care Med 1982; 10:355–357.
23. Minnaganti V, Cunha BA. Infections associated with uremia and dialysis. Infect Dis Clin North Am 2001; 16:385–406.
24. Cunha BA. Nosocomial diarrhea. Crit Care Clin 1998; 14:329–338.

11 Fever of Unknown Origin in Older Persons

Dean C. Norman

UCLA Geffen School of Medicine and VA Greater Los Angeles Healthcare System, Los Angeles, California, U.S.A.

Megan Bernadette Wong

VA Greater Los Angeles Healthcare System, Los Angeles, California, U.S.A.

OVERVIEW

Infections in older persons may present in atypical, nonclassical fashions. This is important because of the high impact of infectious diseases on this vulnerable population. Older persons are more susceptible to infections and, in turn, infectious diseases are associated with higher morbidity and mortality rates compared to a younger population. Multiple factors are thought to be responsible for the higher incidence and elevated morbidity and mortality rates for infections in older persons. These include decremental biologic changes with age, including changes in renal and hepatic function, which alter the pharmacokinetics and pharmacodynamics of drugs and comorbidities that diminish host defenses and mask the clinical presentation of infections. The geriatric patient is likely to suffer from more than one chronic disease and is usually taking multiple medications that may affect host defenses and increase the risk of adverse drug reactions, including-drug induced fever. An atypical presentation of an infection in the older patient may delay diagnosis and delay the initiation of empiric antimicrobial therapy in a patient who is already compromised by aging and chronic diseases.

The most important clinical diagnostic clue to the presence of infection is fever, and this cardinal sign of infection may be blunted or absent in up to a third of infected older persons. Conversely, the presence of a fever and/or the presence of a leukocytosis in a geriatric patient are more likely to be associated with a serious bacterial or viral infection than it is in a younger febrile patient (1,2).

Fever of unknown origin (FUO) may occur in the elderly but differs significantly in etiology. It is difficult to ascertain the incidence or prevalence of FUO in the elderly. However, the prevalence of FUO in hospitalized patients is estimated to be 2.9% (3), and in one prospective study of 167 hospitalized patients with FUO, 28% of cases occurred in patients over the age of 65 years (4). The importance of aggressively determining the etiology of FUO in geriatric patients is that FUO in this population is often treatable.

The traditional definition of FUO is a fever >101°F (38.3°C) on several occasions over a period of at least three weeks, the etiology of which remains undetermined after one week of intensive study in the hospital. Given the ready availability of diagnostic tests and procedures in the ambulatory care setting, the last part of the definition maybe generalized to one week of intensive study in any care setting. However, this definition may not work as well for geriatric patients due to the blunted or absent febrile response to infection observed in this age group (5). This is because, as noted earlier, approximately 20% to 30% of infected geriatric patients will present with a blunted or even absent fever response (5–7). Studies looking at bacteremia (8,9), endocarditis (10–12), pneumonia (13–16), tuberculosis (17), and meningitis (18) demonstrated that infected older persons may present with diminished fever compared to younger adults. Based on these studies and careful studies done by Castle et al. (19,20), fever in older persons should be defined as persistent oral or tympanic membrane temperatures of $\geq$99°F (37.2°C) or persistent rectal temperatures of $\geq$99.5°F (37.5°C) (5). Moreover, a change of temperature over a baseline of $\geq$2.4°F (1.3°C) would also indicate that a fever is present.

In summary, given the above, the definition of FUO in the elderly should be changed to reflect current understanding of fever in this population; instead of 101°F (38.3°C) criterion for fever, an oral or tympanic membrane of 99°F or a rectal temperature of 99.5°F should be considered to be a fever. Any change in functional status associated with a change in temperature reinforces the significance of this finding and increases the likelihood that an infection is present.

As mentioned earlier, FUO in older persons differs from FUO in younger individuals both in etiology and because a diagnosis can be made in a higher percentage of cases. A precise etiologic diagnosis can be made in substantial majority of cases (>80%) of older persons with FUO (21–23). Table 1 summarizes this comparative data and supports aggressively investigating the etiology of FUO in older persons since many of the causative diseases are treatable.

In many cases, FUO in older persons is due to atypical presentations of common diseases (24). Similar to the frequency observed in young patients, infection is the most common etiology of FUO in older persons and occurs in 25% to 35% of cases. There are differences in etiology of these infections, because tuberculosis (TB) is much more likely to be a cause of FUO in older persons compared to the young. TB, similar to endocarditis, may present particular diagnostic challenges.

TB is a more common disease in the older patient with FUO compared to younger patients with FUO and was responsible for 50% of infections in the older age group in the most recent FUO study comparing old and young FUO patients (25). A more recent study of 94 FUO patients reported from Taiwan found that TB was the cause in 23% of cases overall and was more likely to be

TABLE 1 Etiology of Fever of Unknown Origin in the Elderly vs. Younger Patients

	Elderly[a] n (%)	Young[a] n (%)	Recent studies (all adult ages) n (%)
Total patients	204	152	200[b]
Infections	72 (35)	33 (21)	54 (25)
Viral	1 (.05)	8 (5)	7 (3)
TB	20 (10)	4 (3)	4 (2)
Abscess	25 (12)	6 (4)	6 (3)
Endocarditis	14 (7)	2 (1)	5 (2)
Other	12 (6)	13 (9)	32 (15)
Noninfectious inflammatory			
Diseases	57 (28)[c]	27 (17)[c]	52 (24)
Neoplasms	38 (19)	8 (5)	31 (14)
Miscellaneous	17 (8)	39 (26)	17 (8)
No diagnosis	18 (9)	45 (29)	66 (30)

[a]Adapted from the comparative study in Ref. 23 and includes subjects from the 1970s to the 1980s.
[b]Adapted from Refs. 4 and 25 and includes cases from the late 1980s to the early 1990s.
[c]In descending order of frequency (23): Temporal arteritis, polymyalgia rheurnatica, Wegener's granulomatosis, periarteritis nodosa, rheumatoid arthritis, and sarcoidosis.
Abbreviation: TB, tuberculosis.

present in older patients with FUO (26). In a prospective comparison study of TB, elderly patients were less likely to have fever, hemoptysis, cough, and a positive response to 5TU purified protein derivative (PPD) but were more likely to have disseminated disease (17).

Endocarditis in older patients presents with less severe clinical symptoms (e.g., blunted or absent fever) compared to younger patients and may present with vague, nonspecific constitutional symptoms such as lethargy, malaise, anorexia, and weight loss. However, transesophageal echocardiography (TEE) facilitates diagnosis and reduces diagnostic delays caused by the differences in clinical presentation between old and younger persons with infective endocarditis (11,12). Obviously, any heart murmur in an older FUO patient should lead to the consideration that endocarditis is present. Similar to endocarditis, intra-abdominal infections may present in a nonspecific manner; even mild symptoms and findings (minimal tenderness and distention) may indicate an intra-abdominal infection (27,28).

Human immunodeficiency virus (HIV) may occur in older persons and should be considered if no other etiology of FUO is found, or if the history of sexual activity becomes a potential diagnostic clue.

Noninfectious inflammatory diseases such as temporal arteritis, rheumatoid arthritis, and polymyalgia rheumatica are second to infection as a cause of FUO and are responsible for 25% to 31% of cases in older persons (29). A new localized headache, temporal artery abnormality (decreased pulse, tenderness, or nodules), elevated erythrocyte sedimentation rate, especially if ≥ 50 mm/hr Westergren, a high C-reactive protein are potentially diagnostic clues that should lead to a prompt, confirmatory, temporal-artery biopsy.

Finally, malignancies, usually hematological in origin, account for 12% to 23% of cases of FUO in older persons (21,23). Rapid weight loss might suggest the presence of a neoplasm but may also occur with depression, dementia, and any systemic disease or adverse drug reaction in the elderly.

CLINICAL FEATURES

A thorough clinical history and physical examination is very important in establishing the etiology of an FUO in the older patient and potential diagnostic clues should be carefully elucidated. Historical data should be obtained from the patient, but even if the patient appears to be cognitively intact, verification and supplemental information should be obtained from caregivers and family, when appropriate. Occupational exposures, pets, travel, family history, and prior medical illnesses should be thoroughly explored. Medical records should be reviewed carefully, and it is useful to have the patient bring in all of the medications he or she is taking including over-the-counter medications and any herbal supplements. Noncompliance with medications is common in older persons, and an attempt should be made to review each medication with the patient to determine the actual dosage and frequency of administration that the patient is using. The patient should be queried about alcohol and drug use and a sexual-activities history should also be performed. The widespread availability of drugs for the treatment of erectile dysfunction makes the latter an important component of the history. Inquiries should also be made about the presence of any implanted devices such as artificial heart valves.

The physical examination is also very important and for older persons should include a neurological examination and an assessment of cognitive function with the Mini-Mental State Examination (MMSE) or its equivalent test. The temporal arteries should be viewed for swelling and palpated, feeling for thickening, tenderness, and nodules. In the geriatric patient, careful attention should be paid to the oropharynx; especially the condition of the dentition and the sinuses should be examined for tenderness. The abdomen should be carefully palpated, remembering that the elderly with intra-abdominal infections such as biliary tract infection, diverticulitis, and intra-abdominal abscess may present with nonspecific symptoms and blunted signs (27,28). Digital rectal examination should be performed on male patients to determine whether or not the prostate is boggy, tender, or has nodules. All immobile patients with fever should undergo a careful examination of the skin for infected pressure ulcers. Small, sacral ulcers in obese patients maybe difficult to detect unless the patient is turned over and carefully examined. The responsible clinician should not rely on the reports of others but should personally examine the patient for skin ulceration himself or herself. Moreover, the lower extremities should be examined, looking for the presence of deep venous thrombosis. Examination of the muscles of the shoulder girdle for tenderness or observation of pain on motion may indicate polymyalgia rheumatica, a disease commonly associated with temporal arteritis. Finally, the physical examination should be repeated at intervals to determine if new signs developed over time (30).

The list of drugs capable of causing FUO is extensive, and it should be assumed that any drug or drug combination is capable of causing FUO in older persons. Pulmonary embolism may also be a cause of FUO and particularly should be considered for immobile patients, especially those with chest pain. Hyperthyroidism may rarely cause FUO and has a very different presentation in the elderly versus younger persons. Older patients with hyperthyroidism may present atypically with weight loss, depression, or "failure to thrive" symptoms.

DIAGNOSTICS

Patients with FUO have already undergone an intensive diagnostic work up, which minimally would include basic laboratory testing and imaging. Supplemental tests would depend on potential diagnostic clues, but if none are present, should include laboratory testing for thyroid function, erythrocyte sedimentation rate, C-reactive protein, and repeated blood cultures. Abdominal ultrasound would be the next step and, if negative, computed tomography (CT) of the abdomen and chest should be performed.

Transthoracic followed by TEE should be considered if diagnostic clues point toward the possibility of endocarditis or after other tests are exhausted. It should be noted that heart murmurs are a frequent occurrence in older persons and may commonly be present, secondary to aging-related aortic valve sclerosis.

Nonessential drugs should be eliminated, and essential drugs discontinued one by one. Usually the fever, if the drug is the cause, resolves within two days (31).

Finally, one study determined that when potentially diagnostic clues are found, certain nuclear medicine scans may be helpful in localizing inflammation and should be considered (32). A recent FUO study found that a cause for the FUO could be found in 12 of 19 patients (67%). Indium 111 labeled-granulocyte scintigraphy was superior to fluorine-18 fluorodeoxyglucose (FDG) positron emission tomography (PET), because FDG-PET was associated with a much higher false-positive rate (33).

Liver and bone marrow biopsy may be considered but are most useful when diagnostic clues such as abnormal liver function tests or scans or abnormalities in blood component counts point to pathology in these organ systems.

THERAPY

A trial of antibiotics is rarely indicated and only would be considered in patients with rapid clinical deterioration. A trial of steroids may be considered even prior to temporal artery biopsy where temporal arteritis is a strong consideration and vasculitis complications such as visual loss are occurring. A trial of "watch and wait" is indicated for stable patients. A prospective study of 61 FUO patients discharged from the hospital without an etiologic diagnosis and followed for a mean of 5.8 years, found that, in most patients, fevers resolved. The age range of these study participants was between 16 and 75 years and a diagnosis was eventually made in 12 patients during the follow-up period, and all were successfully treated. Although 10% of the cases died during the follow-up period, it was determined that only in two cases (3%) was death thought to have resulted from the disease causing the FUO (34).

REFERENCES

1. Keating MJ III, Klimek JJ, Levine DS, et al. Effect of aging on the clinical significance of fever in ambulatory adult patients. J Am Geriatr Soc 1984; 32:282–287.
2. Wasserman M, Levinstein M, Keller E, et al. Utility of fever, white blood cell, and differential count in predicting bacterial infections in the elderly. J Am Geriatr Soc 1989; 37:534–543.
3. Mourad O, Palda V, Detsky AS. A comprehensive evidence-based approach to fever of unknown origin. Arch Intern Med 2003; 163(5):545–551.
4. de Kleijn E, Vandenbroucke JP, van der Meer J. Fever of unknown origin (FUO): I. A prospective multicenter study of 167 patients with FUO, using fixed epidemiologic entry criteria. Medicine (Baltimore) 1997; 76(6):392–400.
5. Norman DC. Fever and fever of unknown origin in the elderly. Clin Infect Dis 2000 July; 31(1):148–151.
6. Jones SR. Fever in the elderly. In: Machowiak P ed. Fever: Basic Mechanisms and Management. New York: Raven Press, 1991:233–241.
7. Norman DC, Yoshikawa TT. Fever in the elderly. In Cunha BA, ed. Fever: Infectious Disease Clinics of North America. Philadelphia: W.B. Saunders Company, 1996:93–101.
8. Bryant RE, Hood AF, Hood CE, et al. Factors affecting mortality of gram-negative rod bacteremia. Arch Intern Med 1971; 127:120–127.
9. Gleckman R, Hibert D. Afebrile bacteremia: A phenomenon in geriatric patients. JAMA 1981; 1478–1481.
10. Terpenning MS, Buggy BO, Kauffman CA. Infective endocarditis: Clinical features in young and elderly patients. Am J Med 1987; 83:626–634.
11. Werner GS, Schulz R, Fuchs JB, et al. Infective endocarditis in the elderly in the era of transesophageal echocardiography: Clinical features and prognosis compared with younger patients. Am J Med 1996; 100:90–97.
12. Dhawan VK. Infective endocarditis in elderly patients. Clin Infect Dis 2002; 34:806–812.
13. Finklestein MS, Petkun WM, Freedman ML, et al. Pneumococcal bacteremia in adults: Age dependent differences in presentation and in outcome. J Am Geriatr Soc 1983; 31:19–27.
14. Marrie TJ, Haldane EV, Faulkner RS, et al. Community-acquired pneumonia requiring hospitalization: Is it different in the elderly? J Am Geriatr Soc 1985; 33:671–680.

15. Fernandez-Sabe N, Carratala J, Roson B, et al. Community-acquired pneumonia in very elderly patients: Causative organisms, clinical characteristics and outcomes. Medicine (Baltimore) 2003; 82(3):159–169.
16. Metlay J, Schulz R, Li YH, et al. Influence of age on symptoms at presentation in patients with community-acquired pneumonia. Arch Intern Med 1997; 157(13):1453–1459.
17. Korzeniewska-Kosela M, Krysl J, Muller N, et al. Tuberculosis in young adults and the elderly: A prospective comparison. Chest 1994 July; 106(1):28–33.
18. Gorse GJ, Thrupp LD, Nudleman KL, et al. Bacterial meningitis in the elderly. Arch Intern Med 1984; 144:1603–1607.
19. Castle SC, Yeh M, Toledo S, et al. Lowering the temperature criterion improves detection of infections nursing home residents. Aging Immunol Infect Dis 1993; 4:67–76.
20. Castle SC, Yeh M, Norman DC, et al. Fever response in the elderly: Are the older truly colder? J Am Geriatr Soc 1991; 39:853–857.
21. Esposito AL, Gleckman RA. Fever of unknown origin in the elderly. J Am Geriatr Soc 1978; 26:498–505.
22. Berland B, Gleckrnan RA. Fever of unknown origin in the elderly: A sequential approach to diagnosis. Postgrad Med 1992; 92:197–210.
23. Knockaert DC, Vanneste LJ, Bobbaers HJ. Fever of unknown origin in elderly patients. J Am Geriatr Soc 1993; 41:1187–1192.
24. Smith KY, Bradley SF, Kauffman CA. Fever of unknown origin in the elderly: Lymphoma presenting as vertebral compression fractures. J Am Geriatr Soc 1994; 42:88–92.
25. de Kleijn E, van der Meer J. Fever of unknown origin (FUO): Report on 53 patients in a Dutch university hospital. Nether J Med 1995; 47:54–60.
26. Chin C, Lee S, Chen Y, Wann, et al. Mycobacteriosis in patients with fever of unknown origin. J Microbiol Immunol Infect 2003; 36:248–253.
27. Norman DC, Yoshikawa TT. Intra-abdominal infection: Diagnosis and treatment in the elderly patient. Gerontology 1984; 30:327–338.
28. Potts FE, Vukov LF. Utility of fever and leukocytosis in acute surgical abdomens in octogenarians and beyond. J Gerontology (A Bial SCT Med Sci) 1999; 54A(2):M55–M58.
29. Tal S, Guller V, Gurevich A, et al. Fever of unknown origin in the elderly. J Intern Med 2002; 295–304.
30. Amin K, Kauffman C. Fever of unknown origin. Postgrad Med 2003; 114(3):69–76.
31. Arnow PM, Flaherty JP. Fever of unknown origin. Review article. Lancet 1997; 350: 575–580.
32. de Kleijn E, van Lier J, van der Meer J. Fever of unknown origin (FUO): II. Diagnostic procedures in a prospective multicenter study of 167 patients. Medicine (Baltimore) 1997; 76(6):401–414.
33. Kjaer A, Lebech AM, Eigtved A, et al. Fever of unknown origin: Prospective comparison of diagnostic value of ^{18}F-FDG PET and ^{111}In-granulocyte scintigraphy. Eur J Nucl Med Mol Imaging 2004; 31(5):622–626.
34. Knockaert DC, Dujardin KS, Bobbars HJ. Long-term follow-up of patients with undiagnosed fever of unknown origin. Arch Intern Med 1996; 156(6):618–620.

12 Postoperative Fever of Unknown Origin

Tonya Jagneaux, Fred A. Lopez, and Charles V. Sanders

Department of Medicine, Louisiana State University Health Sciences Center, New Orleans, Louisiana, U.S.A.

OVERVIEW

The original definition of fever of unknown origin (FUO), proposed by Petersdorf and Beeson, includes fever 100.4°F ($\geq$38.3°C) on several occasions, with a duration of fever for at least three weeks and an uncertain diagnosis after one week of study in the hospital (1). This definition has been revised due to physicians' current capacity to perform thorough outpatient evaluations for this syndrome. Individuals without a focus for fever $\geq$3 weeks, who have undergone one week of either inpatient or outpatient evaluation specifically to address the fever, are considered to have FUO (2).

The incidence of postoperative fever can range from 13% to 73%, depending upon the patient population and type of surgery performed (3). Routine causes of postoperative fever include both infectious and noninfectious etiologies and, with proper investigation, are usually identified without significant difficulty. The majority of fevers without an identifiable focus resolve without sequelae. The development of postoperative fever that persists $\geq$3 weeks, with a minimum of one week of inpatient evaluation or three outpatient visits specifically to investigate the cause of the fever, meets the criteria for FUO. There is a paucity of data regarding the occurrence of true FUO following surgery. Although the list of common causes of FUO should be considered in treating the patient presenting with this conundrum, the history of recent surgery makes certain disease processes more likely in the differential diagnosis.

Although only minimal data are currently available to characterize differences, there is a theoretical possibility that patients who have developed FUO after ambulatory/outpatient surgery will have a different differential diagnosis than patients who remain hospitalized during recovery. Moreover, the possibility still exists that diseases causing FUO are entirely unrelated to the surgical history. Consequently, a comprehensive workup should be tailored to the patient and should not exclude evaluation of nonsurgical diseases routinely known to result in FUO; such an evaluation should be focused on performing a comprehensive history, physical exam, and diagnostic studies that are guided by the surgical site and type of procedure that has occurred. The focus of this review will be on the evaluation of postoperative patients who develop FUO.

CLINICAL FEATURES
History
An evaluation of FUO in the postoperative patient should include a comprehensive history of the patient's medical condition prior to the operation. This approach serves to account for any specific diagnosis that may present as fever but

may be unrelated to the surgical procedure itself. The condition for which surgery was required should also be investigated as a potential etiology for fever. This is particularly relevant for patients with a history of malignancy or autoimmune disease, as these entities are frequently the cause of FUO, in general patient populations. Talking to the surgeon who performed the operation is another vital component of taking the patient's history, since such a discussion may reveal irregularities in the operative procedure, operative findings, or immediate postoperative/recovery period. The effects of potential immunosuppression due to steroids or adjunctive treatment, such as chemotherapy, should also be considered because they could result in the reactivation of formerly acquired diseases. Although transplant patients are more at risk for these diseases due to the degree of their postoperative immunosuppression, the postoperative reactivation of tuberculosis and malaria after hip surgery and neurosurgery, respectively, has also been evidenced (4,5). In addition, in treating any case of FUO, the physician should review the patient's medication list to determine whether the fever may be drug associated.

With regard to the surgical procedure itself, placement of any type of prosthetic device, graft, or foreign body always increases the likelihood of infection at that particular site. An investigation of perioperative instrumentation should be thorough as this can lead to complications that result in infection and/or inflammation. Intravenous access may result in a hematoma, phlebitis, and/or deep-vein thrombosis (DVT). The use of epidural catheters to deliver anesthesia and/or pain control has been reported to cause epidural abscesses (6). Additionally, the medical record should be reviewed for blood product transfusion(s), because exposure to allogenic blood products carries risk of transfusion-related transmission of infectious agents such as hepatitis, cytomegalovirus (CMV), and Epstein-Barr virus (EBV). The type of surgery and degree of manipulation of tissues and vasculature can also help stratify the risk for DVT, particularly if the postoperative period includes prolonged immobility or suboptimal DVT prophylaxis.

Physical Findings

A thorough physical examination should be performed to assess for signs of disease(s) that could cause FUO. This should begin with an accurate documentation of the occurrence of the fever itself. The pattern of temperature elevation correlates poorly with any particular disease process; however, disorders such as factitious fever can be ruled out with proper measurement of temperature. In the case of factitious fever, measuring the temperature of freshly voided urine will accurately determine the patient's body temperature (7).

The site of the recent surgery should be examined for any evidence of inflammation or suppuration, fluctuation, or induration that would indicate infection and/or hematoma. Examination of the skin may reveal a morbilliform rash consistent with drug hypersensitivity. Stigmata such as Janeway lesions, Osler's nodes, splinter hemorrhages, and petechiae may be suggestive of a diagnosis of infective endocarditis. Sites of recent catheter placement should be examined for indurated cords or erythema indicative of clot or phlebitis. Sites of needle injections should also be evaluated for hematoma formation. Close examination of dentition may reveal dental trauma as a result of endotracheal intubation, potentially resulting in dental abscess formation. Auscultation of the lungs may reveal asymmetric breath sounds that result from pleural fluid due to pulmonary embolus (PE) or postpericardiotomy syndrome. A thorough cardiac exam should be performed to evaluate for murmurs as a potential clue for infective endocarditis. Costovertebral angle (CVA) tenderness may reveal retroperitoneal or perinephric abscess formation as a result of genitourinary instrumentation or injury. The lower extremities should be evaluated for asymmetry and inflammation that would suggest either cellulitus from reduced lymphatic/venous drainage after surgical disruption or the possibility of DVT. The neurologic exam should focus on any meningeal signs and/or new deficits that could result from embolic phenomena after bacteremia or on contamination and/or malfunction of neurosurgical hardware or shunts.

Laboratory/Diagnostic Tests

There is no standard approach to initial diagnostic testing in the evaluation of FUO. Multiple reviews consistently list various tests that are considered to be the minimum of those that should be performed in the investigation of FUO. A routine complete blood count (CBC) with differential assessment, routine blood chemistry including liver enzymes, and urinalysis with microscopy are indicated following a comprehensive history and physical. Blood and urine cultures should also be performed (8). Ideally, the former should include three aerobic and anaerobic cultures performed within a 24- to 48-hour period with 20 mL of blood for each culture. Adsorbent resins for antibiotics and dilution of blood in broth media (1:10) will increase recovery of organisms from patients recently on antibiotic therapy (9). Chest radiography and, in most circumstances, abdominal-computed tomography (CT) are indicated in the absence of localizing signs or symptoms. Although nonspecific, elevated erythrocyte sedimentation rate(s) (ESR) and C-reactive protein level(s) support the presence of inflammatory processes. Any abnormalities identified in the history and physical should subsequently be pursued with additional specific testing.

DIFFERENTIAL DIAGNOSIS
General Postoperative Patients
Infection from Perioperative Instrumentation

Perioperative use of intravenous catheters may result in infection and transient bacteremia, particularly if the catheterization time exceeds five to seven days (10). Patients who present with a history of intravascular catheterization and FUO should be evaluated for endocarditis and/or complications of transient bacteremia. The risk for endocarditis is even more significant for patients with pre-existing cardiac abnormalities, such as valvular heart disease. Focal neurologic signs indicating embolic phenomena also support this diagnosis. Glomerulonephritis and embolic-induced infarcts of other organs, including spleen, lung, and kidney also occur. Splenic or renal abscess(es) may represent late sequelae of vascular access-induced bacteremia. The patient's medical record should be carefully reviewed, particularly regarding the location and duration of vascular catheter use in the perioperative period, and any complications with insertion (hematoma) or discontinuation should be fully investigated.

The increasing use of epidural catheters for pain control and analgesia has resulted in an increase of associated epidural abscesses. The true incidence of catheter-related epidural abscess may be underestimated due to underreporting, but it is believed to be higher than the occurrence of spontaneous epidural

TABLE 1 Risk Factors for Venous Thromboembolism

Increased age	Prolonged immobility
Stroke	Paralysis
Previous venous thromboembolic disease	Cancer
Surgery of abdomen, pelvis, lower extremities	Trauma—particularly hip, pelvis, lower extremity
Obesity	Varicose veins
Cardiac dysfunction	Indwelling central venous catheter
Inflammatory bowel disease	Nephrotic syndrome
Pregnancy/postpartum	Estrogen use

Source: From Ref. 11.

abscess. Symptoms of epidural abscess commonly include fever, back pain, and neurologic deficits. However, early in the course of the disease, neurologic deficits are absent, and back pain may occasionally be unimpressive or attributed to pre-existing disease. The time between catheter insertion and development of symptoms can range from one to 60 days. Regardless of prior patient history of back pain, this diagnosis should be considered for patients with a history of epidural catheter placement, particularly if back discomfort is present (6).

Venous Thromboembolic Disease

Well-known risk factors for venous thromboembolic disease (VTE) include immobility and recent surgery; additional risk factors are listed in Table 1. Because most postoperative patients have an elevated baseline for risk factors (Table 2), an initial investigation for VTE is warranted in every case of FUO unless other diagnoses are strongly suggested. The signs and symptoms of DVT include lower extremity edema, pain, and fever. When venous thromboembolic disease is suspected, important components of the history include a thorough review of the adequacy of prophylaxis used in the perioperative setting, any history of upper extremity DVT or central venous catheterization in the upper extremity that could increase the risk for upper extremity DVT, and the duration of central venous catheterization at any site. An inquiry regarding signs or symptoms of PE (chest pain, dyspnea, and

TABLE 2 Venous Thromboembolism Level of Risk in Surgical Patients[a]

VTE level of risk	
Low	Minor surgery in patients <40 yr, with no additional risk factors
Moderate	Minor surgery in patients with additional risk factors; nonmajor surgery in patients aged 40–60 yr with no additional risk factors; major surgery in patients, <40 yr with no additional risk factors
High	Nonmajor surgery in patients >60 yr or with additional risk factors; major surgery in patients >40 yr or with additional risk factors
Highest	Major surgery in patients >40 yr plus prior VTE, cancer, or molecular hypercoagulable state; hip or knee arthroplasty, hip fracture, surgery; major trauma; spinal cord injury

[a]A thorough description of minor, nonmajor, and major surgery categories is covered in the original source referenced.
Abbreviation: VTE, venous thromboembolic disease.
Source: From Ref. 11.

hemoptysis) is also necessary as the process of evaluation will differ based upon the extent of the disease.

In the absence of signs and symptoms of pulmonary embolism, compression ultrasonography of the lower extremities is routinely the initial diagnostic test. In a study investigating the sole use of venous duplex imaging in a general population of patients identified as having FUO, VTE was diagnosed in 6% of the 89 patients studied. This percentage is likely an underestimate of patients with FUO in the postoperative setting and may also reflect missed diagnoses of DVT, given the poor sensitivity of ultrasound in asymptomatic individuals (12). The addition of D-dimer to ultrasound testing may be helpful in low-risk patients. A negative D-dimer (enzyme-linked immunosorbent assay method) with a negative ultrasound of the lower extremities is sufficient to rule out VTE in low-risk patients. Patients who are at high risk for DVT but who have only fever as a symptom are less likely to have a positive ultrasound. In this circumstance, D-dimer cannot reliably be used to rule out DVT. Contrast venography has been shown to be a specific test in this situation. However, due to its invasive nature, contrast venography is rarely used to screen for DVT (13). Magnetic resonance direct thrombus imaging (MRDT) of the lower extremities offers an alternative to contrast venography in the diagnostic workup of DVT. MRDT imaging offers the advantage of maintaining sensitivity for clots located below the knee and allows visualization of pelvic veins, a potentially useful imaging modality for patients who have undergone pelvic/urologic surgery or orthopedic intervention (14). The test performance characteristics of MRDT have not been extensively studied in asymptomatic patients; therefore, contrast venography may be required in select high-risk patients to rule out DVT effectively.

In patients with symptoms and signs suggestive of PE, diagnostic testing may begin with thoracic imaging studies. Ventilation/perfusion (V/Q) scans are most helpful in patients with a normal chest X ray and no pre-existing cardiopulmonary disease. A normal V/Q scan will essentially rule out the diagnosis of PE; however, nondiagnostic exams necessitate further testing of the patient. A high-probability exam in the setting of a moderate- to high-risk clinical probability of PE establishes the diagnosis. Contrasted spiral CT is routinely the first test ordered to evaluate for PE. With advancing technology, multidetector scanners are able to identify smaller and subsegmental clot(s), thereby increasing the sensitivity of this test. Chest CT also offers the advantage of an imaging evaluation for other competing diagnoses. However, chest CT exams that are negative for PE do not rule out the diagnosis in high-risk patients. Certainly, negative compression-ultrasonography and a negative D-dimer combined with negative chest CT comprise strong evidence against the diagnosis of PE. However, in certain circumstances, pulmonary angiography is required to establish or refute the diagnosis (15).

Transfusion-Related Viral Infections

The risk of acquiring transfusion-related viral infections has been reduced substantially due to sophisticated testing that allows detection of viruses even in the early periods of donor infectivity. However, the risk is not completely absent, particularly for Hepatitis B, Hepatitis C, and CMV (16). The possibility of a transfusion-related viral infection should always be considered in patients who received blood products during the perioperative period. CMV can cause "postperfusion syndrome" in cardiopulmonary bypass graft (CABG) patients. This syndrome is due to primary CMV infection and causes many of the same symptoms as mononucleosis, including fever, malaise, hepatosplenomegaly, and lymphadenopathy. CMV IgM, a four-fold rise in CMV titers, and CMV antigen testing may be helpful in support-ing a diagnosis of acute CMV infection (17).

Miscellaneous Causes

Drug fever can occur at any time during the postoperative period and stem from virtually any type of medication. Even medications that the patient had been taking prior to surgery are potential etiologic agents of drug fever. Characteristic rashes and eosinophilia may be absent. Discontinuation of the drug may provide the only diagnostic indication that the medication was indeed the source of FUO (18). Sinusitis has been implicated as an FUO in postoperative patients, particularly in patients who have had prolonged endotracheal and/or nasogastric intubation. Facial tenderness, edema, and purulent nasal discharge support the diagnosis but may be absent. Evaluation consists of dedicated sinus CT and nasal endoscopy. CT is very sensitive but not specific due to the frequency of radiographic abnorm-alities, such as mucosal thickening and fluid pooling that follow nasopharyngeal instrumentation. Nasal endoscopy offers the advantages of direct visualization, biopsy, and culture in supporting the diagnosis (19).

Factitious fever is a potential cause of FUO in any patient population. Individ-uals will occasionally manipulate or fabricate their own temperature measure-ments, or even ingest drugs, to induce hyperthermia. Factitious fever should be considered when very high, brief episodes of fever are recorded and when corre-sponding signs and symptoms of warm skin and tachycardia are absent during febrile episodes. Some patients will also inject contaminated substances to induce true infection and fever. Characteristic profiles of patients with factitious fever include females with medical backgrounds (2).

Diagnoses Specific to Surgical Subtypes

Neurosurgery: Cerebrospinal Shunt Infection

Patients having undergone neurosurgical placement of a ventriculostomy or ventri-culoperitoneal shunt who develop fever should be evaluated for cerebrospinal fluid (CSF) shunt infection and meningitis. In a recent study, the incidence of shunt infec-tion in a group of 2112 patients was 2.1%, and the range for shunt infection has been reported to be between 2% and 22% (20). The most common features associated with infection included fever, hydrocephalus, depressed consciousness, and seizure activity. Abdominal discomfort was commonly noted in pediatric patients. Neuro-logic abnormalities may be less obvious in patients with underlying neurologic dys-function that preceded shunt placement. Additionally, patients receiving antibiotics at the onset of fever are in danger of having their shunt infection overlooked; prior antibiotic therapy may cause cultures to be negative and symptoms to be attenu-ated. Fever that occurs in patients with these devices should prompt neuroimaging and CSF analysis. Typical organisms include skin-, nasopharyngeal-, and auditory canal-associated flora, and the potential exists for resistant nosocomial organisms if the patient has recently been hospitalized. Treatment includes pathogen-directed antibiotic therapy and usually requires shunt removal (20).

Cardiothoracic Surgery

Postpericardiotomy Syndrome

Postpericardiotomy syndrome results from injury that occurs with trauma to the pericardium and/or myocardium, including the pericardiotomy required during

CABG procedures. It is characterized by development of pericarditis, pericardial and/or pleural effusion, fever, leukocytosis, and an elevated ESR. This syndrome can develop one week to several weeks after bypass surgery. The concurrent chest pain may often be ascribed to recurrence of angina or poststernotomy pain. Even after treatment with nonsteroidal anti-inflammatory drugs, postpericardiotomy syndrome can continue to recur up to six months later (17).

Prosthetic Valve Infection
Patients with prosthetic cardiac valves who develop fever should always be assessed for prosthetic-valve infective endocarditis (PVE). It becomes essential, given the treatment implications and potential for morbidity and mortality, either to establish the diagnosis of infective endocarditis (IE) or to identify and treat an alternative diagnosis for persistent fever in this patient population. The rate of PVE is highest in the first three months following placement, and the risk subsequently declines six months postimplantation. The cumulative risk is estimated to be 1.0% to 1.4% at 12 months and 3.0% to 5.7% at 60 months (21). Early infection occurring within two months can often be traced to acquisition of the offending pathogen either at the time of surgery or in the immediate postoperative period, when invasive hemodynamic monitoring equipment and vascular access devices are in place (21). The most common cause of PVE occurring within 12 months of implantation is coagulase-negative *Staphylococcus* sp. (Table 3) (22). It is therefore imperative to employ appropriate methods for acquiring blood cultures. False-positive cultures due to improper technique may lead to inappropriate treatment, and false-negative cultures due to too few cultures or too little blood volume can delay appropriate therapy. While 90% of blood cultures in the setting of PVE are positive, culture-negative endocarditis can occur, particularly after prosthetic valves have undergone endothelialization. Culture and serology for common causes of culture-negative endocarditis should be included in the evaluation of the persistently febrile patient with a prosthetic valve. It is recommended that the acridine orange test, a fluorescent stain able to identify live bacteria, be performed on an aliquot from the blood culture to increase diagnostic sensitivity (23). In the absence of positive culture, specific criteria that would establish the diagnosis of endocarditis should also be sought. An established diagnosis of endocarditis and

TABLE 3 Microbiologic Features of Prosthetic Valve Endocarditis—Approximate Percentage of Cases Listed

Pathogen	Early <60 days	Intermediate 60–120 days	Late >12 mo
Streptococcus sp.	1	7–10	30–33
Staphylococcus aureus	20–24	10–15	15–20
Coagulase-negative *Staphylococci*	30–35	30–35	10–12
Enterococcus sp.	5–10	10–15	8–12
Gram-negative bacilli	10–15	2–4	4–7
Fungi	5–10	10–15	1
Culture-negative and HACEK organisms	3–7	3–7	3–8
Diphtheroids	5–7	2–5	2–3
Polymicrobial	2–4	4–7	3–7

Abbreviation: HACEK, *Hemophilus* sp., *Actinobacillus actinomycetemcomitans, Cardiobacterium hominis, Eikenella corrodens, Kingella kingae.*
Source: From Ref. 22.

persistent fever in patients with prosthetic valves has serious implications in the form of surgical therapy. Patients with infective endocarditis and persistent fever despite appropriate therapy meet the criteria for valve replacement (21).

The Duke criteria are used to establish or reject a diagnosis in patients with suspected endocarditis (24). There are two major criteria for diagnosis, the first of which is positive blood cultures with organisms typical of infective endocarditis or persistent bacteremia. The second major criterion includes new regurgitant murmur, endocardial involvement, a positive echocardiogram for an oscillating mass, evidence of abscess, or evidence of prosthetic valve dehiscence. Minor criteria include a predisposing cardiac condition or intravenous drug use; fever 100.4°F (≥38°C); vascular phenomena such as arterial emboli, pulmonary infarcts, and Janeway lesions; immunologic phenomena such as Osler's nodes, Roth's spots, and glomerulonephritis; echocardiogram consistent with endocarditis but not meeting major criteria; and positive blood culture not meeting major criteria or positive serology/molecular tests for a compatible microbe (24). Definite endocarditis is defined as positive histology or culture from vegetation or the demonstration of two major criteria, one major and three minor criteria, or five minor criteria. The diagnosis of infective endocarditis is rejected if a firm alternative diagnosis is established or if there is resolution after four days or less of antimicrobial treatment (24).

Modification to the Duke criteria in the setting of PVE has been suggested by Llamas and Eykyn (25). In a prospective study of 118 cases of pathologically proven infective endocarditis, 18 cases of PVE were identified. The addition of several minor criteria improved the diagnostic sensitivity from 50% to 89% without a decrease in specificity. These additional minor criteria included newly diagnosed clubbing, splenomegaly, splinter hemorrhages and petechiae, an elevated ESR, elevated C-reactive protein, the presence of central nonfeeding lines or peripheral lines, and microscopic hematuria. To enhance diagnostic sensitivity in the evaluation for endocarditis, patients with fever following prosthetic valve implantation should be evaluated for these findings in addition to the previously described Duke criteria (25).

Surgical indications to remove prosthetic heart valves in the setting of endocarditis include the development of severe congestive heart failure, demonstration of an unstable prosthesis, paravalvular extension or abscess formation, persistent bacteremia despite adequate antimicrobial therapy, relapse after optimal therapy, and large mobile vegetations (>1 cm). Two indications for valve removal are specific for prosthetic valves; these include infection with fungi, *Pseudomonas aeruginosa*, *Staphylococcus aureus*, or Enterococci in the absence of bactericidal therapy or unexplained persistent fever with evidence for culture-negative PVE (26).

Mediastinitis

The incidence of poststernotomy mediastinitis has been reported to be <1%; however, the mortality associated with this complication can range from 14% to 47% (27). The time interval for the onset of poststernotomy mediastinitis can range from three days to up to one year following surgery, with the majority of cases occurring within two weeks of surgery (28). The typical symptoms and signs of post-CABG mediastinitis include wound pain, purulent discharge, and sternal instability in addition to fever and leukocytosis. On occasion, fever and leukocytosis may be the only clinical findings, while pain and tenderness are attributed to postoperative pain. Risk factors for post-CABG mediastinitis include obesity, bilateral, internal, mammary artery grafts in diabetics, prolonged operative time, and repeated blood transfusions in the perioperative period (27). Blood cultures are indicated to rule out bacteremia, and chest CT is helpful in establishing the diagnosis.

Vascular Surgery: Prosthetic Vascular Graft Infection and Postimplantation Syndrome

Studies examining the incidence of aortic graft infection(s) report rates of 0.5% to 2% at five years (29). Early infection is associated with infection acquired at the time of implantation, whereas late infection may be related to a procedure involving graft revision, enteric erosion, or transient bacteremia from an unrelated process. Signs of graft infection maybe subtle and nonspecific; however, delays in diagnosis maybe catastrophic, resulting in rapid deterioration due to sepsis or hemorrhage. Typical findings in patients with aortic graft infection include pain, gastrointestinal bleeding, a nonhealing wound, and persistent fever. Nonspecific laboratory findings include an elevated ESR and leukocytosis. The mortality associated with infected prosthetic aortic grafts ranges from 25% to 70% (29). Graft infection must be distinguished from postimplantation syndrome, a syndrome of fever, leukocytosis, and perigraft air that is normally seen within 10 days of surgery. Given the time frame, postimplantation syndrome is less likely to meet the criteria for an FUO and would only be considered after other etiologies of infectious complications have been eliminated. With observation, this syndrome resolves over time (30).

Abdominal/Pelvic Surgery

Intra-abdominal and Retroperitoneal Hematoma

Hematoma formation following intra-abdominal surgery is a potential cause of FUO. Bleeding into the peritoneal cavity or retroperitoneal space may result in a hematoma. Hematomas associated with vascular interventions, in which hematoma formation occurs within the wall of an arterial aneurysm or dissection, are prone to catastrophic hemorrhage. In these cases, chest, abdominal, or back pain may precede the development of fever and anemia (18). CT is helpful in identifying fluid collections characteristic of hematomas. In the febrile patient, differentiating hematoma formation from abscess formation remains challenging despite sophisticated imaging techniques. Fine needle aspiration and culture are routinely required to make this distinction and establish the diagnosis.

Intra-abdominal and Retroperitoneal Abscess

Patients who have undergone abdominal surgery have the potential to develop intra-abdominal abscess(es) due to instrumentation or as a complication associated with implantation of a foreign body. Retroperitoneal abscess may also develop following abdominal surgery or genitourinary tract manipulation. Perinephric abscesses have been reported following both abdominal surgery and urologic surgery. Infecting organisms in such circumstances include skin flora arriving by hematogenous route and via postoperative external drains (31). Following cholecystectomy, retroperitoneal abscess occurs due to gallstones dropped into the peritoneal cavity, unbeknownst to the surgeon at the time of the operation (32, 33). The typical symptoms of intra-abdominal abscess include fever, nausea, vomiting, abdominal pain, and diarrhea. Retroperitoneal abscesses present in a similar fashion, but pain may localize to the costovertebral angle or flank on the affected side (34).

With the availability of CTs, intra-abdominal abscess is less frequently reported as a cause of FUO (35). However, in postoperative patients, postsurgical changes may interfere with the diagnostic accuracy of imaging studies. Additionally, associated symptoms may be overlooked or attributed to routine surgical incision pain. Elderly patients are particularly at risk for missed diagnoses of intra-abdominal infection due to their atypical presentation(s) without nausea, vomiting, diarrhea, or pain (36). Therefore, in patients with FUO after recent abdominal surgery, a nondiagnostic abdominal CT should prompt further evaluation for intra-abdominal abscess, which may involve sampling of any abnormal fluid collection, nuclear medicine imaging, and/or potentially positron emission tomography (PET) imaging.

Portal Vein Thrombosis
Portal vein thrombosis (PVT) in the postoperative period has been described in patients having undergone splenectomy. Typical signs and symptoms include fever and abdominal pain. The true incidence of PVT may be underestimated, and many cases may be asymptomatic. In a study of patients undergoing laparoscopic splenectomy, 12 of 22 (55%) patients had a diagnosis of PVT. The diagnosis was identified with surveillance CT performed between postoperative days 3 through 23. (37). The majority of patients were asymptomatic and fever was the most common symptom reported, followed by abdominal pain. Previous studies have reported rates of less than 10% for portal system vein thrombosis after similar procedures. At this time, routine surveillance studies are not performed to screen for PVT. Given the possibility of a higher incidence of PVT than was previously predicted, this diagnosis should be considered when encountering FUO in patients with recent splenectomy (37).

Obstetric/Gynecological Surgery
Septic Puerperal Ovarian Vein Thrombosis
Septic puerperal ovarian vein thrombosis (SPVOT) is a rare complication following either vaginal or cesarean delivery. The disease occurs in approximately 0.02% to 0.18% of all pregnancies, with most cases occurring within one to two weeks of delivery (38) although presentation has been delayed as late as 70 days. Symptoms and signs include fever, leukocytosis, lower-quadrant abdominal pain, and a tender lower abdominal mass with predilection for the right side. The pain may, however, be nonspecific and not associated with a palpable mass, leading to a prolonged duration of evaluation and treatment for other conditions resembling this diagnosis. Disease mimics for which treatment and evaluation are usually initiated prior to diagnosis include pyelonephritis, peritonitis, appendicitis, endometritis, pelvic abscess, and adnexal torsion. Because ultrasound and CT are used when investigating these disease entities, SPVOT is likely to be discovered. However, due to the often difficult physical exam in obese patients and the bowel gas patterns that complicate ultrasound imaging, the typical findings can often be missed. CT offers the additional advantage of evaluating for competing diagnoses in this scenario. However, due to poor contrast filling and visualization, the typical findings associated with SPVT syndrome may also be missed with CT. One study examining the test performance characteristics of CT in evaluating SPVT reported a sensitivity, specificity, and accuracy of 77.8%, 62.5%, and 68.0%, respectively (38). With the appropriate clinical scenario and no competing diagnosis identified, magnetic

resonance imaging (MRI) has been shown to be highly sensitive (100%), specific (100%), and accurate (100%) in identifying or refuting the diagnosis (38).

Ureteral Injury

Ureteral injury may occur during laparoscopic gynecologic surgery and may go unrecognized at the time of operation. The development of symptoms may occur in the early postoperative period, but recognition of this injury has been reported up to 33 days postoperatively. Signs and symptoms include fever, flank pain, abdominal distension, and peritoneal signs. The extent of the injury determines the time to presentation and severity of symptoms. Delayed detection of ureteral injury can result in urinary obstruction and fistula formation. Risk factors for ureteral injury include endometriosis, adhesions, and laparoscopic approach for removal of large uterine myomas. Diagnosis of ureteral injury can be made with pyelography and excretory urograms. Treatment involves drainage if extensive urine-associated ascites is present, ureteral repair, and usually ureteral stenting due to stricture formation (39).

Orthopedic Surgery: Prosthetic Device Infection

The incidence of prosthetic joint infection ranges from 1% to 2%, depending upon the joint involved. Infections presenting within three months of surgery generally have signs referable to the joint involved. Infections that occur outside of the three-month interval may have few localizing signs and symptoms of joint infection, and fever may be the only manifestation. In patients with prosthetic joints and FUO, specific inquiry about recent procedures such as dental work, endoscopy, or cystoscopy should be included in the history. These procedures may lead to transient bacteremia, resulting in seeding of the joint. Radiographic imaging may reveal loosening and joint displacement. CT and magnetic resonance imaging are less helpful in evaluation due to artifact from the prosthesis. Arthrography is useful to demonstrate loosening and/or cystic changes consistent with infection. Nuclear medicine imaging may also support the diagnosis, but the specificity of increased isotope uptake for infection is reduced during the first year after joint implantation. Bone scintigraphy should be combined with leukocyte- or antibody-labeled imaging to increase the specificity for infection during this time interval (40).

DIAGNOSTIC APPROACH

An approach to the evaluation of postoperative FUO includes categorizing and stratifying the risk of potential etiologies based upon clues from the initial history and physical exam. The broad categories of differential diagnoses include recurrence or persistence of the underlying disease requiring surgical therapy, iatrogenic infection due to the procedure or supportive care, thromboembolic disease, drug-related side effects and factitious disorders. A potential focus or number of foci should be identified from the initial history and risk profile of the associated procedure to guide the evaluation of FUO in the postoperative patient. A simplified approach, based upon the signs, symptoms, and recent surgical history, is given in Table 4.

TABLE 4 Diagnostic Methods

Focus	Labs	Microbiology	Imaging	Intervention
Abdominal symptoms/ signs	CBC, complete chemistry, UA	Blood cultures (3 sets), urine culture	Contrasted abdominal CT, nuclear scan, PET	Sample fluid collections or abnormal areas of uptake
Risk of venous thromboembolism, septic phlebitis	CBC, D-dimer	Blood cultures (3 sets)	Ultrasound, contrasted chest CT, MRDT, MRA	Anticoagulation with LMWH or Uf heparin followed by VKA
Risk of endocarditis	ESR, CBC, complete chemistry, rheumatoid factor, UA with microscopy	Blood cultures (3–5 sets), serology for culture-negative IE	TTE, TEE; consider additional imaging for metastatic foci	Institute antimicrobial therapy immediately following cultures
CSF shunt present	CSF analysis, CBC, complete chemistry, UA	CSF culture, blood cultures (3 sets)	Neuroimaging for foci or hydrocephalus	Antimicrobial therapy, consider shunt removal
Recent cardiopulmonary bypass graft	CBC, complete chemistry, UA	Blood cultures (3 sets)	Contrasted chest CT, nuclear scan	Antimicrobial therapy for mediastinitis, surgical debridement
Recent vascular graft	CBC, complete chemistry, UA	Blood cultures (3 sets)	Ultrasound, computed tomography	Antimicrobial therapy; consider graft removal
History of blood products transfused	Serology for hepatitis, CMV, West Nile virus, EBV			
History of prosthetic joint placement	CBC, ESR, CRP	Blood cultures (2 sets)	Radiographs, technetium bone scan, labeled leukocyte and/or labeled antibody scan	Antimicrobial therapy, surgical debridement, joint replacement

Abbreviations: CBC, complete blood count; CMV, cytomegalovirus; CRP, C-reactive protein; CSF, cerebrospinal fluid; CT, computed tomography; EBV, Epstein Barr virus; ESR, erythrocyte sedimentation rate; IE, infective endocarditis; LMWH, low molecular weight heparin; MRA, magnetic resonance angiograpy; MRDT, magnetic resonance direct thrombus imaging; PET, positron emission tomography; TEE, transesophageal echocardiography; TTE, transthoracic echocardiography; UA, urine analysis; VKA, vitamin K antogonists. VTE, venous thromboembolic disease.

Laboratory Tests
Nonspecific
Elevations in leukocyte counts, ESR, and C-reactive protein (CRP) are nonspecific markers of inflammation. An elevation of ESR without a concurrent elevation in CRP may reflect a false positive, indicating that there is inflammation when none is truly present. Serum CRP reflects a broader range of abnormalities and will change more rapidly than ESR with concurrent fluctuations in inflammation. It has been demonstrated that patients with a value of CRP >100 mg/L have bacterial infections 80% to 85% of the time (41). Repeat testing of CRP may be useful to monitor response to therapy or the inflammatory trend. Neither test, alone or in combination, can differentiate infectious from noninfectious processes. Additionally, ESR and/or CRP should not be used in isolation to determine the need for antimicrobial therapy. Other nonspecific laboratory abnormalities that may provide clues to FUO etiologies include eosinophilia as a result of medications, atypical lymphocytosis and elevated serum transaminases due to transfusion-related viruses, and positive rheumatoid factor as a result of subacute bacterial endocarditis (42).

Specific Laboratory Testing
Cultures of normally sterile fluids, such as blood, CSF, and urine, should be obtained based upon any clinical abnormalities revealed during the history and physical. Patients with CSF shunts should undergo CSF fluid sampling to rule out infection, even in the absence of symptoms. Any abnormal collections of fluid, including pleural, peritoneal, or synovial fluid, should also be sampled for culture and routine diagnostic studies to evaluate for other inflammatory conditions. Patients who have received blood products should undergo testing for transfusion-transmitted viruses, including Hepatitis B, Hepatitis C, CMV, EBV, and human immunodeficiency virus (HIV). For patients suspected of having VTE, a negative D-dimer (ELISA) test combined with negative lower extremity ultrasound in patients with a low clinical probability for venous thromboembolic disease can be sufficient to rule out this diagnosis.

Imaging Studies
Initial imaging studies in the postoperative patient include, at minimum, a chest radiograph and an abdominal CT scan. Although routine lower extremity Doppler ultrasound may not be cost effective in patients with FUO in general, lower extremity Doppler ultrasound is a reasonable test to perform in the diagnostic workup of this postoperative patient population (12). As previously noted, the risk of DVT is increased in the surgical patient population, and without an alternate underlying focus, these patients should be screened for DVT with lower extremity Doppler ultrasound for DVT. For patients who have undergone pelvic surgery, more sophisticated imaging of the pelvic veins and ovarian veins may be required. In these cases, contrasted CT and magnetic resonance angiography will be more conclusive (38).

The use of ultrasound for identifying intra-abdominal pathology is typically not helpful and has been largely replaced by CT. Communication with the reading radiologist regarding the type of surgery and any nonspecific clues that have been revealed by history or laboratory testing may also be helpful in identifying a focus. Any abnormalities, such as fluid collections or evidence of inflammation, should be pursued further with additional testing, such as biopsy and/or aspirate culture.

In addition to CT, nuclear medicine imaging may help identify a focus to investigate further in FUO. In an evidenced-based review of diagnostic testing in FUO, technetium-based nuclear scans were recommended as imaging studies of choice in comparison to other types of tracers. Technetium scans have high specificity (93–94%) but low sensitivity (40–75%). Indium-111-labeled leukocyte scans, which have 78% to 86% specificity and 45% to 60% sensitivity as performance characteristics (8), were also recommended for imaging, particularly for localizing infectious processes.

Fluorodeoxyglucose-positron emission tomography (FDG-PET) is becoming increasingly reliable in the evaluation of FUO and may surpass nuclear scans as a method of choice for identifying inflammation. FDG-PET is routinely used in localizing malignancy due to increased uptake of glucose by neoplastic cells. Inflammation and infection also demonstrate increased uptake and are a frequent source of false positives when evaluating for malignancy. Due to this characteristic, FDG-PET can be very useful in identifying inflammatory foci in an otherwise asymptomatic patient. The advantages of using FDG-PET are its high sensitivity, high negative predictive value, and higher resolution imaging compared to nuclear medicine studies. The disadvantages to PET scanning at this time include cost and limited use in patients with poorly controlled diabetes mellitus (43).

THERAPY

Therapy is directed at the underlying cause of fever. Given the circumstances, infection leads the list of etiologies in the workup of postoperative FUO. Appropriate cultures from all potential sources should be obtained prior to the initiation of empiric antibiotic therapy. Therapeutic trials of antibiotics and/or corticosteroids are not recommended unless definitive evidence suggests a diagnosis, the patient is immunosuppressed, or the patient demonstrates rapid deterioration requiring broad-spectrum antimicrobial therapy. Even in these circumstances, efforts to obtain cultures from possible foci should be undertaken to maximize yield. Empiric therapy outside of these circumstances serves only to delay the diagnosis or confuse the clinical picture (44).

Specific Therapies
Antibiotic Regimens
A thorough review of antimicrobial therapy indicated in all infectious etiologies of FUO in the postoperative setting is beyond the scope of this chapter. However, the empiric treatment of two conditions, PVE and postneurosurgical meningitis, are worth mentioning. Recommended empiric therapy for suspected PVE consists of vancomycin, gentamycin, and rifampin (45). Empiric therapy should be converted to specific therapy once a microbiologic agent is identified. Early identification of surgical criteria and surgical consultation are essential to successful therapy (21).

Patients with meningitis who have undergone neurosurgery and/or cerebrospinal shunt placement are at risk for infection with a different spectrum of bacteria compared to community-acquired meningitis. In addition to routine pathogens, these patients have a predisposition for infection with *S. aureus*; coagulase-negative Staphylcocci; aerobic gram-negative bacilli, including *P. aeruginosa*; and *Propionibacterium acnes*. Therefore, empiric therapy in postneurosurgical patients suspected of meningitis should include vancomycin plus either cefepime, ceftazidime, or meropenem. For patients with a CSF shunt and suspected staphylococcal infection, the addition of rifampin to one of the listed regimens is also recommended. Every effort should be made to perform shunt removal in patients who develop meningitis specifically from a shunt, as opposed to bacterial seeding. Additionally, external drainage should be employed to facilitate continued treatment of hydrocephalus and more rapid resolution of ventriculitis. Intraventricular instillation of antimicrobial therapy has been used in addition to conventional regimens for patients who cannot undergo surgical treatment. There are no antimicrobials that are approved by the Food and Drug Administration for delivery by intraventricular route, nor are there specific indications to implement such therapy. A review by Tunkel et al. covering the management of bacterial meningitis provides specific antimicrobials and dosing regimens for intraventricular administration for select patients (46).

Anticoagulation
If a strong suspicion for venous thromboembolic disease develops during the evaluation and confirmatory testing has not yet occurred, anticoagulation should not be withheld. This is particularly true for patients with reduced cardiopulmonary reserve due to pre-existing heart and/or lung disease. Unfractionated heparin or low-molecular-weight heparin are indicated for the initiation of treatment, followed by administration of vitamin K antagonists (coumadin) once a therapeutic partial thromboplastin time is reached (1.5–2.0 times normal). Once therapy is initiated, diagnostic testing that confirms the diagnosis or rules it out with sufficient certainty is needed to guide continued administration or discontinuation of anticoagulation (47).

Surgical Therapy
Identification of fluid collections or devitalized tissue in the postoperative patient with FUO requires intervention. Percutaneous drainage can be both diagnostic and therapeutic for collections of fluid identified during diagnostic imaging, whereas devitalized tissue requires surgical removal. With rare exception, infected hardware and prosthesis require surgical removal for definitive therapy. Exceptions to this rule include early infection (<3 months after surgery) in orthopedic prosthetic hardware in which there is a stable graft and acute onset with symptoms lasting <3 weeks. Even in this regard, treatment failure occurs with medical therapy alone, and careful observation is required (40).

REFERENCES

1. Petersdorf RG, Beeson PB. Fever of unexplained origin: report on 100 cases. Medicine 1961; 40:1–30.
2. Arnow PM, Flaherty JP. Fever of unknown origin. Lancet 1997; 350(9077):575–580.
3. Perlino CA. Postoperative fever. Med Clin North Am 2001; 85(5):1141–1149.
4. Spinner RJ, Sexton DJ, Goldner RD, et al. Periprosthetic infections due to Myobacterium tuberculosis in patients with no prior history of tuberculosis. J Arthroplasty 1996; 11(2):217–222.
5. Chadee DD, Tilluchdharry CC, Maharaj P, et al. Reactivation of plasmodium malariae infection in a Trinidadian man after neurosurgery. N Engl J Med 2000; 342(25):1924.
6. Kindler CH, Seeberger, MD, Staender SE. Epidural abscess complicating epidural anesthesia and analgesia: an analysis of the literature. Acta Anaesthesiol Scand 1998; 42:614–620.

7. Cunha B. Fever of unknown origin. Educational Review Manual in Infectious Disease. New York: Castle Connolly, 2003.
8. Mourad O, Palda V, Detsky AS. A comprehensive evidence-based approach to fever of unknown origin. Arch Intern Med 2003; 163:545–551.
9. Houpikian P, Raoult D. Diagnostic methods: current best practices and guidelines for identification of difficult-to-culture pathogens in infective endocarditis. Cardiol Clin 2003; 21(2):207–217.
10. McGee DC, Gould MK. Preventing complications of central venous catheterization. N Engl J Med 2003; 348(12):1123–1133.
11. Geerts WH, Heit JA, Clagett JP, et al. Preventing venous thromboembolism. Chest 2001; 119(suppl 1):132S–175S.
12. AbuRahma AF, Saiedy S, Robinson PA, et al. Role of venous duplex imaging of the lower extremities in patients with fever of unknown origin. Surgery 1997; 121(4):366–371.
13. Elliott CG. The diagnostic approach to deep venous thrombosis. Semin Respir Crit Care Med 2000; 21(6):511–519.
14. Fraser DG, Moody AR, Morgan PS, et al. Diagnosis of lower-limb deep venous thrombosis: a prospective blinded study of magnetic resonance direct thrombus imaging. Ann Intern Med 2002; 136(2):89–98.
15. Tapson VF, Carroll BA, Davidson BL, et al. The diagnostic approach to acute venous thromboembolism. Clinical Practice Guideline. American Thoracic Society. Am J Respir Crit Care Med 1999; 160(3):1043–1066.
16. Goodnough, LT. Risks of blood transfusion. Crit Care Med 2003; 31(suppl 12):S678–S686.
17. Prince SE, Cunha BA. Postpericardiotomy syndrome. Heart and Lung 1997; 26(2):165–168.
18. Armstrong W, Kazanjian P, Fever of unknown origin in the general population and in HIV-infected persons. In: Cohen and Powderly, eds. Infectious Diseases, 2nd ed. New York: Elsevier, 2004: 871–878.
19. Kortbus MJ, Lee KC. Sinusitis and fever of unknown origin. Otolaryngol Clin North Am 2004; 37(2):339–346.
20. Wang KW, Chang WN, Shih TY, et al. Infection of cerebrospinal fluid shunts: causative pathogens, clinical features, and outcomes. Jpn J Infect Dis 2004; 57(2):44–48.
21. Karchmer AW, Longworth DL. Infections of intracardiac devices. Cardiol Clin 2003; 21(2):253–271.
22. Mylonakis E, Calderwood SB. Infective endocarditis in adults. N Engl J Med 2001; 345(18):1318–1330.
23. Bayer AS, Bolger AF, Taubert KA, et al. Diagnosis and management of infective endocarditis and its complications. Circulation 1998; 98(25):2936–2948.
24. Durack DT, Lukes AS, Bright DK. New criteria for diagnosis of infective endocarditis: utilization of specific echocardiographic findings. Am J Med 1994; 96(3):200–209.
25. Lamas CC, Eykyn SJ. Suggested modifications to the Duke criteria for the clinical diagnosis of native valve and prosthetic valve endocarditis: analysis of 118 pathologically proven cases. Clin Inf Dis 1997; 25(3):713–719.
26. Karchmer AW. Infections of prosthetic valves and intravascular devices. In: Mandell GL, Bennett JE, Dolin R, eds. Principles and Practice of Infectious Disease. New York: Churchill Livingstone, 2000: 903–917.
27. El Oakley RM, Wright JE. Postoperative mediastinitis: classification and management. Ann Thorac Surg 1996; 61(3):1030–1036.
28. Farinas MC, Gald Peralta F, Bernal JM, et al. Suppurative mediastinitis after open-heart surgery: a case-control study covering a seven-year period in Santander, Spain. Clin Infect Dis 1995; 20(2):272–279.
29. Ten Raa S, Van Sambeek MR, Hagenaars T, et al. Management of aortic graft infection. J Cardiovasc Surg 2002; 43(2):209–215.
30. Velazquez OC, Carpenter JP, Baum RA, et al. Perigraft air, fever, and leukocytosis after endovascular repair of abdominal aortic aneurysms. Am J Surg 1999; 178(3):185–189.
31. Sanchez-Ortiz R, Madsen LT, Swanson DA, et al. Closed suction or penrose drainage after partial nephrectomy: does it matter? J Urol 2004; 171(1):244–246.

32. Dashkovsky I, Cozacov JC. Spillage of stones from the gallbladder during laparascopic cholecystectomy and complication of a retroperitoneal abscess mimicking gluteal abscess in elderly patients. Surg Endosc 2002; 16:714–717.

33. Ramia JM, Mansilla A, Villar K, et al. Retroperitoneal actinomycosis due to dropped gallstones. Surg Endosc 2004; 18:345–349.

34. Golden GT, Roberts TL, Donato AT. Prolonged postoperative fever caused by a perinephric abscess: diagnosis by "Mathe's sign." Am Surg 1974; 40(5):302–304.

35. Tal S, Guller V, Gurevich A, et al. Fever of unknown origin in the elderly. J Intern Med 2002; 252(4):295–304.

36. Cooper GS, Shlaes DM, Salata RA. Intraabdominal infection: differences in presentation and outcome between younger patients and the elderly. Clin Infect Dis 1994 19(1): 146–148.

37. Ikeda M, Sekimoto M, Takiguchi S, et al. High incidence of thrombosis of the portal venous system after laparoscopic splenectomy: a prospective study with contrast-enhanced CT scan. Ann Surg 2005; 241(2):208–216.

38. Kubik-Huch RA, Hebisch G, Huch R, et al. Role of duplex color Doppler ultrasound, computed tomography, and MR angiography in the diagnosis of septic puerperal ovarian vein thrombosis. Abdom Imaging 1999; 24(1):85–91.

39. Oh BR, Kwon DD, Park KS, et al. Late presentation of ureteral injury after laparoscopic surgery. Obstet Gynecol 2000; 95(3):337–339.

40. Zimmerli W, Ochsner PE. Management of infection associated with prosthetic joints. Infection 2003; 31(2):99–108.

41. Gabay C, Kushner I. Mechanisms of disease: acute-phase proteins and other systemic responses to inflammation. N Engl J Med 1999; 340(6):448–454.

42. Cunha BA, Fever of unknown origin. Infect Dis Clin North Am 1996; 10(1):111–127.

43. Zhuang H, Yu JQ, Alavi A. Applications of fluorodeoxyglucose-PET imaging in the detection of infection and inflammation and other benign disorders. Radiol Clin N Am 2005; 43:121–134.

44. Mackowiak PA, Durach DT. Fever of unknown origin. In: Mandell GL, Bennett JE, Dolin R, eds. Principles and Practice of Infectious Disease. 5th ed. Philadelphia: Churchill Livingstone, 2000:623–633.

45. Gilbert DN, Moellering RC, Eliopoulos GM, et al., eds. The Sanford Guide to Antimicrobial Therapy. 35th ed. Hyde Park, Vermont: Antimicrobial Therapy, 2005:19.

46. Tunkel AR, Hartnam BJ, Kaplan SL, et al. Practice guidelines for the management of bacterial meningitis. Clin Inf Dis 2004, 39(9):1267–1284.

47. Buller HR, Agnelli G, Hull RD, et al. Antithrombotic therapy for venous thromboembolic disease. The Seventh ACCP Conference on Antithrombotic and Thrombolytic Therapy. Chest 2004; 126(suppl 3):401S–428S.

Recurrent Fever of Unknown Origin

Daniel C. Knockaert

Department of General Internal Medicine, Gasthuisberg University Hospital, Leuven, Belgium

DEFINITION

Fever of unknown origin (FUO) is generally considered a major diagnostic challenge because many diseases may cause this well-defined, rather rare, clinical syndrome. The diagnostic criteria of classic FUO were delineated in the landmark article of R. Petersdorf and P. Beeson in 1961 and subsequently modified by D. Durack and A. Street in 1991 (1,2). Recurrent FUO is probably the most perplexing and intriguing presentation that can be defined as a subtype of FUO, meeting the classic criteria of FUO and characterized by at least two episodes of fever with fever-free intervals of at least two weeks and seeming remission of the underlying illness (3). We realize that the proposed duration of the fever-free interval is somewhat arbitrary, but, in cases of rare clinical syndromes, adherence to standardized definitions is needed to permit comparison of groups of patients over time and in countries and between different hospital settings. This symptom-free period may vary from weeks to years, and we suggest this fever-free interval of at least two weeks for several reasons. First, this time window allows exclusion from the category of recurrent FUO those diseases that recur due to interruption or tapering of an inadequate empiric therapy. Typical examples are incompletely treated endocarditis (too short- and/or too low-dosed antibiotic therapy) and noninfectious inflammatory disorders treated with nonsteroidal anti-inflammatory agents or corticosteroids. Second, as long as fever persists, patients presenting with prolonged fever remain prepared to undergo the whole battery of less or more costly, invasive tests in order to reach a final diagnosis and get appropriate treatment. However, when fever subsides spontaneously, they become reluctant for further investigations in a few days, a week to 10 days, in our experience. Third, physicians who are familiar with the good prognosis of unexplained FUO stop the investigations when fever and symptoms subside and propose a watchful, waiting outpatient follow-up (4).

We prefer the term recurrent or episodic FUO to the term periodic fever, because the latter term is sometimes used for familial Mediterranean fever (FMF), a common cause of recurrent fever also designated as "maladie périodique," a periodic disease, in the French literature. Periodic fever has also been considered as a distinct clinical entity since the 1940s, mainly by the work of H Reimann (5,6). It was included in a broader group of disorders of unknown origin, named periodic disease and characterized by symptoms that recur with a sometimes remarkable periodicity. Particular attention was paid to a specific periodicity of 21 days, being a multiple of the biblical holy number of 7, or multiples of these numbers. When fever was the prominent symptom, without other signs or symptoms, the periodic disease was called periodic fever and analysis of the temperature chart was the key diagnostic factor (6). This entity remained popular from the 1950s through the early 1970s, but this is no longer the case. The sole periodic disease in adults with a rather fixed interval, about 21 days, is cyclic neutropenia (7). PHAPA (periodic fever, aphtous stomatitis, pharyngitis, adenitis) or Marshall syndrome is a pediatric disease with an individually predictable, sometimes clock-work periodicity. The interval is mostly about 28 days at the peak of the disease activity, but the interval may lengthen gradually before eventual, seemingly spon-taneous remission. Persistence through adulthood is very rare (8).

EPIDEMIOLOGY

Recurrent FUO represented 22.6% of the cases in our first cohort of 199 patients with FUO (9); 33.5% of 167 cases in the study of De Kleyn et al. (10); 18.6% in one French study (11); and 36% of 290 cases with prolonged fever recently studied in our center (12). It should be kept in mind that all these data are from ter-tiary care centers and these centers can expect to see more patients with recurrent FUO due to referral bias of these difficult cases.

A recurrent fever pattern has been found to be the strongest independent pre-dictor of the diagnosis in FUO in several large studies. The overall chance of finding the cause of recurrent FUO is no more than 50%. We were able to establish a final diagnosis in only 49% of 45 patients with recurrent FUO versus 82% final diagnoses in 154 cases with continuous fever (9). De Kleyn et al. reported similar figures, a final diagnosis in 50% of 56 recurrent FUO versus a final diagnosis in 80% of 111 patients with continuous fever, although the required interval between two epi-sodes was only 48 hours (10). In our second series, a diagnosis could be established in 52% of 105 cases with recurrent FUO versus 74% of 185 cases with continuous FUO (12).

Recurrent FUO remains a frustrating experience for both patients and inves-tigators because many cases continue to evade a final diagnosis despite repeated assessment. Recurrent FUO represents a subgroup of patients with very prolonged disease duration, and it is known that the chance of reaching a diagnosis in cases with fever lasting >6 months is relatively low. In the large series of 347 patients with FUO lasting >6 months referred to the National Institutes of Health, United States of America from 1961 to 1977, a cause could be identified in only 54% of the cases (13). In a less well-defined population of 85 patients with recurrent fever for >6 months, 40% remained unexplained (14).

CAUSES

Recurrent FUO may be caused by relapse of a partially treated disorder, by a disease with a known course of spontaneous remission and relapses, or by repeated exposure to pyrogens, whether micro-organisms or other substances. Typical examples of this last category are extrinsic allergic alveolitis or hypersensitivity pneumonitis caused by inhalational allergens (e.g., pigeon breeder's disease) and drug fever due to repeated intake of medications (e.g., nitrofurantoin for urinary tract infection). Diseases with a typical, fluctuating course are Still's disease, relap-sing polychondritis, Behçet's disease, mastocytosis, and the familial autoinflamma-tory syndromes such as FMF and others.

The causes of recurrent FUO can be classified into four major categories: infec-tions, tumors, noninfectious inflammatory diseases, and others or miscellaneous.

The "Big 3" namely, infections, tumors, and NIIDs account roughly for only 20% of the causes. The miscellaneous group accounts for 30% and 50% remain unexplained. In a review of the literature of FUO from 1961 to 1991, we were able to identify 55 different conditions that met the criteria of recurrent FUO among 179 reported causes of FUO. Of these 55 diseases, 33 belonged to the miscellaneous category (3). In a renewed search, up to April 2005, we could identify 70 different disorders as causes of recurrent FUOs, and 40 belonged to the miscellaneous category. Numerous case reports of so-called recurrent FUO can be found in the literature, but most of them do not meet our proposed criteria or represent cases of partially treated infectious or inflammatory conditions. We do not consider this overview of the literature as exhaustive and are well aware of the possible, unexpected recurrent course of more than 200 diseases reported as causes of classic FUO. A recurrent course with spontaneous remissions is indeed an unexpected one, yet well-documented for diseases such as giant cell arteritis and tuberculosis (15,16).

Infections

Only a limited number of infections cause recurrent FUO (Table 1). Typical bacterial causes are prostatitis, cholangitis, and otitis media/mastoiditis. Cholangitis may occasionally be a late manifestation of Caroli's disease, a congenital segmental saccular dilatation of the large intrahepatic bile ducts. The mechanism of fever is intermittent seeding of bacteria from these silent foci with spontaneous resolution of the fever.

Partially treated, deep-seated abscesses, endocarditis, septic jugular or subclavian vein thrombosis, and osteomyelitis may present as so-called recurrent FUO. The mechanism here is temporary suppression, but not cure, of infection in patients who received antibiotic trials. In our experience, dental and sinus abnormalities are frequently found in FUO patients, but they are rarely the cause of FUO, whether classic or recurrent (9).

Some unusual bacterial infections should be kept in mind. Brucellosis may cause a pattern of so-called undulating fever, characterized by episodes of higher temperature and of less elevated temperature but, seldom, normal temperature.

TABLE 1   Infections Reported as Causes of Recurrent FUO

Chronic prostatitis
Recurrent cholangitis (Caroli's disease)
Otitis media/mastoiditis
Brucellosis
Dental abscess
Sinusitis
Yersinia enterocolitica
Rat bite fever (*Spirillum minor, Streptobacillus moniliformis*)
Melioidosis
Q-fever
Relapsing fever (*Borrelia* sp.)
Trypanosomiasis
Whipple disease
Epstein Barr virus infection
Toxoplasmosis

Persistent Yersinia infection has been reported as a cause of recurrent FUO, but the final proof of persistent infection is difficult to yield and specificity of specialized serologic tests may be a matter of debate (3). Leptospirosis may present in a biphasic pattern, but the interval between two phases is too short to meet the criteria of recurrent FUO. Melioidosis is a typical granulomatous, bacterial infection caused by *Burkholderia pseudomallei*, endemic in Southeast Asia, that may cause repeated bouts of fever during years. It may become symptomatic years after a stay in the endemic area (17).

Relapsing fever, caused by either flee- or tick-transmitted Borrelia species, mostly causes a distinct, recurrent fever pattern, with short fever-free intervals. It is limited to well-described geographic areas, and travel history must be the clue (18).

The same holds true for malaria, particularly the nonfalciparum species such as *Plasmodium vivax* and *Plasmodium ovale*, which can cause relapsing, repetitive disease in patients who not receive liver-stage prophylaxis.

Viral infections nearly never cause recurrent FUO but might be a trigger for the so-called macrophage activation syndrome or hematophagocytic lymphohistiocytosis, a nonmalignant, yet potentially fatal, immune dysregulation syndrome (19). All members of the herpes virus group are notorious causes of FUO in HIV-associated, nosocomial, and neutropenic FUO. Herpes simplex and herpes zoster reactivate also in immunocompetent individuals but not as unexplained fever. An unusual 13-year history of recurrent, persistent Epstein-Barr virus infection has been reported in a child without immune deficiency (20). Human herpes virus 6 and human herpes virus 8 are suspected to play a role in some of the atypical histiocytic or lymphocytic proliferative disorders such as Rosai-Dorfman syndrome and Castleman's disease, respectively (21,22).

Tumors

All tumors may probably cause recurrent fever based upon the mechanism of tumor necrosis, but this is especially the case in rather large tumors (Table 2). In the past, cancer of the liver and the kidneys were typical examples, but, nowadays, even the criteria of classic FUO are mostly no longer met, because these tumors are readily detected by ultrasonography and computed tomography (CT) scan (9,23).

Particular attention should be paid to lymphoma, and not only Hodgkin's lymphoma, which may present as recurrent FUO, well-known in the literature as Pel-Ebstein fever (24). Spontaneous remission of fever and even regression of enlarged lymph nodes is a surprise for most physicians involved in the care of these patients.

Colon carcinoma remains a classic neoplastic cause of recurrent FUO. The repeated bouts of fever are due either to recurrent infection in the ulcerated area or to tumor necrosis.

TABLE 2   Neoplastic Diseases Reported as Causes of Recurrent FUO

Hodgkin's lymphoma
Non-Hodgkin's lymphoma
Malignant histiocytosis
Angioimmunoblastic lymphadenopathy
Craniopharyngioma
Schnitzler syndrome
Artrial myxoma
Hepatocellular carcinoma

Schnitzler syndrome is a very rare disease but should be known by FUO experts because intermittent fever is a cardinal feature. Other typical features are chronic urticaria, bone pain, and bone densification on X rays and monoclonal IgM gammopathy. It has a slow, chronic course without remissions and truly malignant lymphoplasmocytic transformation has been documented in 20% of the cases (25).

Cardiac myxoma is a benign tumor of endocardial origin that may cause fever by silent distal embolization and by production of interleukin-6 by the tumor itself (3,26).

Noninfectious Inflammatory Diseases

This third category represents a whole array of diseases designated as rheumatic diseases, vasculitides, multisystem diseases, connective tissue diseases, collagen vascular diseases, autoimmune diseases, and so on. The term noninfectious inflammatory diseases (NIID), as suggested by De Kleyn et al. from the Nijmegen group, Netherlands, solves this semantic problem (10). Most of these entities are rather rare diseases with which most physicians are not so familiar. Several of them have an indolent course over years before the diagnosis is established because diagnosis is based upon a number of criteria that must be fulfilled. Many patients get empiric treatment with nonsteroidal anti-inflammatory drugs (NSAIDs) or corticosteroids and experience relapse of disease activity when the treatment is tapered. These cases do not meet the criteria of recurrent FUO, because they have a fluctuating course due to a disease that is suppressed by treatment. However, a seemingly spontaneous remission of the inflammatory process, with relapse months or even years later, is even typical for a number of diseases of this group, such as Still's disease, Behçet's disease, and relapsing polychondritis, but very unusual for others, for example, giant cell arteritis (16) and ankylosing spondylitis (3).

Still's disease is by far the most common NIID, with a really classic course of recurrent FUO with asymptomatic intervals that may last more than one year. However, we plead for diagnostic stringency and strict adherence to the criteria of Still's disease, which, in our opinion, are too sensitive and not specific enough (27). There is no single, true specific diagnostic test nor specific feature, and, in our experience, many physicians too readily consider this diagnosis in case of recurrent FUO, even in a first episode of fever accompanied with myalgia, arthralgia, and a rash. It is a disease to consider only in patients < 35 or 40 years of age, although numerous case reports of so-called Still's disease in older patients can be found in the literature. We only establish the diagnosis as definite after exclusion of other diseases and a prolonged follow-up or the presence of several of the most typical features, such as very high fever, sore throat without pharyngitis, a typical evanescent, macular, salmon-colored rash, diffuse lymphadenopathy, pleuritis or pericarditis, markedly elevated erythrocyte sedimentation rate (ESR) or C-reactive protein (CRP) value, neutrophil leukocytosis $>15.10^9$ cells/L and highly elevated ferritin levels (28).

Behçet's disease is another NIID with a tendency of recurrence and spontaneous remission. Its prevalence is high along the ancient Silk Road (the eastern Mediterranean littoral, particularly Turkey, over the Middle East to Japan) but very low in the United States and the Western countries (29). Recurrent aphtous stomatitis, genital ulcerations, and uveitis are the typical manifestations, which, when present as a triad, allow immediate diagnosis. Thrombophlebitis is common, and

TABLE 3 Miscellaneous Conditions Reported as Causes of Recurrent FUO[a]

Addison's disease
Aorta-enteric fistula
Brewer's yeast ingestion
Castleman's disease
Cirrhosis (68)
Cholesterol embolism
Chronic fatigue syndrome (2)
Crohn's disease
Cryopyrin-associated periodic syndromes
   Muckle-Well's disease (urticaria, deafness, and ayloidosis)
   Familial cold autoinflammatory syndrome (familial cold urticaria)
   Neonatal onset multisystem inflammatory disease or
      chronic infantile neurologic, cutaneous and articular syndrome
Cyclic neutropenia
Erdheim-Chester disease (58)
Drug fever
Fabry disease
Factitious fever
Familial Mediterranean fever
Periodic fever, aphtous stomatitis, pharyngitis (cervical) adenitis
Gaucher's disease
Gout
Granulomatous hepatitis
Habitual hyperthermia
Hemolytic anemia (69)
HIDS (hyper IgD syndrome)
Hypersensitivity pneumonitis
Hypothalamic hypopituitarism
Hypertriglyceridemia
Idiopathic granulomatosis
Inflammatory pseudotumor of lymph nodes
Lung embolism
Mastocytosis (70)
Metal fume fever
Milk protein allergy
Poikilothermia
Polymer fume fever
Pseudogout
Ratke's cleft cyst
Rosai-Dorfman syndrome (21)
Seizures
TNF-receptor-1-associated periodic syndrome (familial Hibernian fever)

[a]For references, see Ref. 3 unless references given between parentheses.
Abbreviation: TNF, tumor necrosis factor.

aneurysm of the peripheral arteries and pulmonary arteries is a dreaded complication. It is a well-known cause of recurrent FUO in ethnic groups at risk for that disease (30).

     Relapsing polychondritis has also a fluctuating course, as suggested by the name of the disease, and this rare diagnosis is easily missed in the early phase. It is characterized by bouts of fever and inflammation of one or more of the cartilaginous structures of the body (nose, external, and inner ear, larynx and trachea, joints), the sclera, and the heart valves (31).

Miscellaneous

The miscellaneous category is the most important one, both in number and types of diseases. It is said that FUO is more frequently caused by an unusual presentation of common, well-known diseases than by rare, exotic diseases but this is not the case with recurrent FUO. In this subtype of FUO, major attention should be paid to the list of miscellaneous disorders that contains diseases with exotic names many physicians never have heard of (Table 3).

Drug-related fever due to intermittent intake of drugs and factitious fever are classic but frequently forgotten causes (3,32,33).

Factitious fever is more prevalent in young females, allied with health professions but it has also been described in elderly patients (3). It was the cause in 9% of 343 cases with very prolonged FUO evaluated at the National Institutes of Health, United States (33). Factitious fever must be suspected in case of unusual fever patterns with very high or very brief spikes, loss of diurnal variation, rapid defervesence without diaphoresis, lack of tachycardia or so-called pulse-temperature differential, absence of signs of inflammation, and good appearance despite an impressive history. Polymicrobial bacteremia, the presence of a mixed bacterial flora in blood cultures, suggests self-inoculation of saliva or fecal or other material when the search for the classic sources of mixed bacteremia such as the gastrointestinal or genitourinary tract and soft tissues remains negative (33).

Habitual hyperthermia was a very popular entity in the 1950s, and it was the reason for R. Petersdorf to introduce the cut-off value of 101°F (38.3°C) as a criterion of FUO (1). Habitual hyperthermia displays some overlap with chronic fatigue syndrome and fibromyalgia (2). The main complaint is fever, particularly after physical or intellectual exertion and in most cases also fatigue, but not as debilitating as in chronic fatigue syndrome. Patients sometimes remember an acute infection, mostly of the upper airways, as first manifestation, and they know that their body temperature was normal before that acute event. In these cases, habitual hyperthermia cannot be considered a normal variant with exaggeration of the diurnal rhythm. Physical examination is normal, except an increased body temperature, particularly at evening and after exertion. Laboratory tests and radiographs are all normal and spontaneous resolution mostly ensues, but sometimes after one or two years. Reassurance about the innocent nature of the elevated body temperature is more appropriate than an FUO investigation.

Crohn's disease was an unexpected cause in four of our initially reported 45 patients. The lack of abdominal complaints and normal bowel habits were the reason why bowel investigations were not done in the initial evaluation (3).

It is easily understood that hypersensitivity pneumonitis, also known as extrinsic allergic alveolitis, may cause episodic FUO when exposure to inhaled allergens is intermittent or when symptoms subside spontaneously during hospital admission. Exposure may occur at home (e.g., pet birds, indoor molds, contaminated humidifiers) or it may be linked to certain occupations and hobbies (farmers, mushroom workers, bakers, woodworkers, bird breeders, etc.). Diagnosis will easily be established when respiratory symptoms dominate the clinical presentation, yet missed when systemic symptoms such as fever overshadow other manifestations. The same reasoning holds true for lung embolism, an overlooked cause of episodic FUO (3).

Several hereditary periodic fever syndromes are now grouped as familial autoinflammatory syndromes (35,36). FMF is the most common worldwide and best known. During the last decades, new but much rarer syndromes have been described, mostly in families from or originating from northern and western Europe (Table 4). At first glance, these syndromes look similar with lifelong, spontaneously resolving periods of fever, inflammation, rash, and abdominal and musculoskeletal symptoms. Specific clinical characteristics can be found, but genetic analysis has yielded the final proof of the true identity of these initially clinically defined syndromes. The advent of molecular genetic tools, indeed, brought a real breakthrough in the diagnostic approach of recurrent FUO in certain ethnic groups. The term autoinflammatory, rather than autoimmune, has been proposed to define these disorders, because autoantibodies or antigen-specific T cells do not play a role in the pathogenesis (36).

FMF is a typical episodic disease, autosomal recessive. It is by far and large the most common hereditary periodic fever syndrome worldwide and highly prevalent in Jews, Turks, Arabs, Armenians, and other people of Mediterranean littoral origin (35,37). Its most prominent feature is short (one to three days), spontaneously resolving attacks of fever, mostly starting before the age of 20 years. Fever, malaise, and inflammation may be accompanied by signs and symptoms of serositis, particularly abdominal but also pleural and pericardial, arthritis frequently confined to one large joint, and, less frequently, an erysipelas-like rash of the distal lower limbs (37,38). The frequency of attacks varies considerably and diagnosis is, in our experience, frequently missed during childhood in the case of low-frequency attacks. These episodes are then considered as transitory viral infections. The genetic basis is a mutation of the MEFV gene on the short arm of chromosome 16 that encodes for a protein, named pyrin or marenostrin. That particular protein is predominantly expressed in neutrophils and in monocytes. It has a so-called PYD domain shared with other proteins that play a role in inflammation and apoptosis. Numerous mutations of the MEFV gene have already been identified and the list continues to grow (36,37). AA-type amyloidosis is a dreaded complication with a variable prevalence in different genetic populations. Colchicine is the first-line treatment and essential in the prevention of amyloidosis.

Hyper IgD syndrome (HIDS), an autosomal recessive disorder has been described in the Netherlands in 1984 by Van der meer et al. The majority of the cases, collected in an international registry (www.HIDS.NET), originate from western Europe and particularly the Netherlands and France (39). The genetic basis is mutation in the gene encoding for mevalonate kinase, an enzyme of the isoprenoid pathway with cholesterol, ubiquinone, and other substances as endproducts (40). This gene is located on the long arm of chromosome 12. It is not known how this metabolic defect leads to inflammation, and the relation to the characteristically elevated IgD level is unclear. Most patients develop fever episodes in the first year of life, and abdominal symptoms and (cervical) lymphadenopathy are nearly always present. The attacks last a little bit longer than in FMF, three to five days or more. Rash, arthritis, and oral and genital aphthous ulcers are not so uncommon. No effective treatment is available, but provisional data from a trial with simvastatin, an hydroxy-methylgluteryal coenzyme A (HMG-CoA) reductase inhibitor, are encouraging (41).

Muckle-Wells syndrome, familial cold autoinflammatory syndrome (FCAS), and neonatal-onset multisystemic inflammatory disease (NOMID), also known as chronic infantile neurologic, cutaneous, and articular syndrome (CINCA), are three clinically defined, autosomal dominantly inherited syndromes, caused by mutations of the same gene (36,42–45). This CIAS$_1$ gene (cold-induced autoinflammatory syndrome 1), also named NALP3 and PYFAP gene, is located on the long

TABLE 4 Features of Familial Autoinflammatory Syndromes

	FMF	HIDS	TRAPS	CAPS[a]
Age of onset	Variable <20–30 years	Mostly <1 year	Variable; mostly infancy or childhood	Infancy or childhood
Mode of inheritance (autosomal)	Recessive	Recessive	Dominant	Dominant
Chromosome	16 p	12 q	12 p	1 q
Duration of attacks	1–4 days	3–7 days	1–3 weeks	1–2 days
Abdominal pain	+++	++	+	+
Diarrhea	–	+	–	–
Chest pain	+	–	+	–
Skin involvement	Rare, erysipelas-like (below the knee)	++ Macules, papules	++ Erysipelas-like (upper limbs)	++ Urticaria
Arthritis// arthralgia-myalgia	++//+	+/–//++	+//++	++//++
Lymphadenopathy	–	+ Cervical, inguinal, axillar, abdominal	+/– Cervical, inguinal, axillar	–
Splenomegaly	+/–	+	–	+
Risk for AA-type amyloidosis	+	Very rare	Rare	+
Distinguishing feature	Testicular pain (prepubertal)	Elevated IgD levels	Conjunctivitis, periorbital edema, testicular pain	Conjunctivitis Triggered by cold exposure[b] Deafness later in life[c]
Effective treatment	Colchicine	None, simvastatin?	Etanercept (corticosteroids)	IL-1 RA(anakinra)

[a]CAPS encompasses familial cold autoinflammatory syndrome, Muckle-Wells syndrome, and neonatal onset multisystemic inflammatoty syndrome (NOMID) or chronic infantile neurologic, cuataneous and articular syndrome (CINCA).
[b]familial cold urticaria syndrome.
[c]Muckle-Wells syndrome.
Abbreviations: CAPS, cryopyrin-associated periodic syndrome); FMF, familial Mediterranean fever; HIDS, hyperimmunoglobulin D and periodic fever syndrome; TRAPS, tumor necrosis factor receptor-1-associated periodic syndrome.

arm of chromosome 1. It encodes for cryopyrin, a protein that, like pyrin or mare-nostrin, is predominantly expressed in neutrophils and monocytes. Its N-terminal domain, called PYD, is similar to that of pyrin and it has a role in inflammation by activating caspase 1, an IL1-converting enzyme, and NF-κB, resulting in release of the proinflammatory cytokines IL6 and IL8 (44,45).

These three syndromes, originally described as distinct clinical entities and now grouped as CAPS (cryopyrin-associated periodic syndromes) reflect actually a spectrum of illnesses, ranging from the most severe, NOMID or CINCA, to Muckle-Wells syndrome and FCAS, the mildest forms (44). The latter, also described as familial cold urticaria, is characterized by very short bouts of fever, joint inflammation, and urticaria-like rash, typically induced by exposure to mild cold (cool breezes of air-conditioned rooms, for instance). The temperature required to provoke symptoms is no lower than 22°C and the interval between exposure and attack is frequently <1 hour. Conjunctivitis is a typical symptom for that syndrome, and the attacks resolve spontaneously within 24 to 48 hours. Muckle-Wells syndrome has been described in 1962 as "urticaria, deafness, and amyloidosis" in an English family. The typical distinguishing feature here is progressive neural deafness, occurring later in life. The correlation between cold exposure and onset of symptoms is said to be absent (42,45) but this is contradicted by a recent study (44). NOMID or CINCA, the most severe of CAPS, is a pediatric disease, characterized by very early onset, severe joint malformation, hearing loss, chronic aseptic meningitis, and mental retardation.

The new insights in the pathogenesis of these rare disorders have already resulted in a new therapeutic approach, anakinra (recombinant IL-1 receptor antagonist), shown to be effective in Muckle-Wells syndrome and in FCAS (42,44).

TNF-receptor-1- associated periodic syndrome (TRAPS) is an autosomal dominant disorder originally described in 1982 as "familial Hibernian fever" in an Irish family (46). The genetic basis is mutations in the gene of TNF-receptor type 1, located on the short arm of chromosome 12, probably resulting in defective shedding of the receptor (47,48). The age of onset of symptoms is variable and attacks last several weeks. Centrifugal migratory erysipelas-like painful skin lesions on distal upper limbs, but also on torso, unilateral periorbital oedema, and testicular pain are the distinguishing features. Amyloidosis occurs rather commonly. Etanercept, a recombinant soluble TNF receptor, is a logical therapeutic approach and found to be an effective treatment (47,49).

Gaucher's disease and Fabry disease, lysosomal storage diseases, are also hereditary diseases that occasionally present as episodic FUO (3,50–52). Cases may remain undiagnosed until adulthood in the absence of a family member in whom the diagnosis has already been established.

Another group of little known, rare disorders that arise as rather classic causes of recurrent FUO, can be grouped as nonspecific reactive, autoimmune, or infection-triggered lymphoproliferative or histiocytic disorders mostly presenting as pseudotumor or lymphadenopathy. This group encompasses Castleman's disease (20,53), Kikuchi-Fujimoto disease (54,55), Rosai-Dorfman syndrome (21), inflammatory pseudotumor of lymph nodes (56,57) and Erdheim-Chester disease (ECD) (58,59). Several other diseases resemble, at first glance, these entities but they should no longer be included in this group for the following reasons. Angio immunoblastic lymphadenopathy and Schnitzler syndrome are considered neoplastic hematological disorders (Table 2) (25,60). Large granular lymphocyte lymphocytosis is also a malignant, not a reactive, lymphoid proliferation in most cases (61,62). The macrophage-activation syndrome, formerly described as hematophagocytic lymphohistiocytosis, may cause episodic fever but the course is mostly fulminant, requiring early aggressive empiric treatment with corticosteroids and immunosuppressive drugs (19,63–65). PHAPA is a pediatric disease that may occur in adolescents, but onset in adults has not been reported to our knowledge (8,66).

Castleman's disease is a lymphoproliferative disorder that presents with two clinical subtypes, a localized or unicentric and a multicentric form. Histologically, three variants can be discerned: hyaline vascular, plasma cell, and a mixed type. These differences are important both for clinical presentation, and prognosis and treatment. Fever and constitutional symptoms are rarely present in the hyaline vascular type in contrast to the other histological variants. Increased IL-6 production, possibly linked to human herpes virus 8 infection might play a role in the inflammatory response. The localized type can be cured by surgical resection, whereas the multicentric form mostly requires treatment with corticosteroids and occasionally chemotherapy (20,53).

Kikuchi-Fujimoto disease mainly affects young females; it is common in Japan and other Asian countries, but it is reported from all over the world. It is a histiocytic necrotizing lymphadenitis, typically located in the cervical lymph nodes. Cat scratch disease is the main differential diagnosis, which can be established by appropriate serology and by the presence of a granulomatous type of inflammation. Kikuchi-Fujimoto disease is easily recognized by clinicians and pathologists familiar with this benign self-limiting disease but it continues to be reported as cause of FUO (54) and recurrent FUO (55).

Inflammatory pseudotumor of lymph nodes resembles histologically plasma cell granuloma, also called inflammatory pseudotumor (56,57). This latter entity is a benign mesenchymal proliferation, found in various extranodal sites throughout the body. It is predominantly reported in children and young adults, frequently without fever. Inflammatory pseudotumor of lymph nodes presents as lymphadenopathy and as episodic FUO, particularly when located in hidden sites such as the mediastinum, the mesentery, or retroperitoneum (3,57,67). The histological picture consists of a mixture of lymphocytic, plasmocytic, histiocytic, and myofibroblastic cells (57). Surgical resection, mostly performed for diagnostic reasons, frequently leads to cure. Corticosteroids suppress fever and inflammation and even nonsteroidal anti-inflammatory drugs suffice in some cases (56).

Erdheim-Chester disease (ECD) resembles Langerhans-cell histiocytosis (LCH) but the typical characteristics of Langerhans dendritic cells, a positive stain for S-100 proteïn, and Birbeck granules or X bodies, are lacking. Moreover, ECD causes osteosclerosis of long bones, easily pointed to by bone scintigraphy, whereas LCH causes lytic bone lesions on standard radiographs (58,59). The lack of plasma cells and presence of many foamy histiocytes allow the differential diagnosis with retroperitoneal fibrosis in case of perirenal localization.

All these reactive disorders present as lymphadenopathy or as extranodal mass, a pseudotumor, frequently ill-delineated on classic imaging techniques. In our experience, they are Gallium and fluoro-deoxyglucose avid and, hence, easily detected in hidden areas such as the mediastinum and abdomen by appropriate total body radioisotope scanning method (56,67). The definite diagnosis is based on characteristic histological features but less experienced pathologists frequently miss the diagnosis and they classify the findings as nonspecific reactive abnormalities (56,57).

In Table 3, we summarize the difficult-to-classify cases of recurrent FUO that came to our attention by careful analysis of the literature on FUO since 1961. Most of these disorders have been tabulated in our initial study (3) but for a number of them, the existence as a separate entity has been questioned in the meantime. Etiocholanolone fever and periodic fever are no longer considered as disease, and, in our opinion, granulomatous hepatitis is not a disease but a distinct histological reaction caused by a broad array of infectious, neoplastic, and other conditions (68). A number of these rare disorders have been better delineated, particularly the hereditary periodic-fever syndromes, and renamed. Some authors tend to classify Crohn's disease in the NIID group, but we prefer to reserve the term NIID for the classic collagen vascular diseases.

Central nervous system abnormalities with lesions in the thermoregulation zone of the brain stem mostly cause poikilothermia with episodes of hypothermia and, very rarely, episodes of hyperthermia (69).

DIAGNOSTIC STRATEGY

The diagnostic strategy in case of recurrent FUO is different from continuous FUO for several reasons. Although the approach to the patient should be individualized, some general principles must be kept in mind and followed.

First, the spectrum of causative disorders is different, and the risk of life-threatening infections or fulminant neoplastic disorders is low, particularly in cases with duration of more than a half year (3,4). Second, starting an investigation in an asymptomatic phase is not indicated except for a routine laboratory battery, including complete blood count, liver tests, urinalysis, radiograph of the chest, and abdominal ultrasonography. Third, lack of laboratory signs of inflammation during a symptomatic phase points to either habitual hyperthermia, factitious fever, or seizures, the latter being a very rare cause of recurrent FUO, well-described in a number of older case reports (3). Fourth, an underlying disease will be found in no more than 50% of the cases, and ordering multiple diagnostic tests in patients at low risk for the tested conditions increases considerably the chance of false-positive results (4,10–12).

Fifth, most patients remain in good health despite repeated episodes of fever even for many years without a diagnosis (3,4). Patients with recurrent FUO are therefore rarely inclined for another in-depth, in-hospital diagnostic round. They mostly accept a watchful, waiting strategy in an outpatient setting that permits the underlying disease to reveal itself during follow-up. Sixth, the initial diagnosis in case of recurrent FUO is sometimes a probable one, established by excluding other diseases, by the response to specific therapy, or by studying the course of the disease.

Particular attention should be paid to the ethnic origin and family history, to possible intermittent drug intake (e.g., quinine for occasional nocturnal leg cramps), to travel history, and to occupation and hobbies, with possible exposure to inhalational antigens causing hypersensitivity pneumonitis, such as pigeon breeder's disease, farmer's lung, and so on.

A complete, repeated physical examination with particular attention to the skin, looking for the typical Still's disease rash, should be performed. In case of suspicion of factitious fever, temperature measurement should be supervised, and, in case of doubt, simultaneous body and urine temperature can solve the problem (70).

Blood and other cultures should only be taken during a symptomatic phase, and few serologic and immunologic tests are required in addition to the standard laboratory battery of the FUO patient (68). Undirected serologic and immunologic tests have very poor predictive value in a setting of low prevalence of the screened disorders. Even for tests with high specificity, the rate of false-positive results remains high. Chest radiograph and abdominal ultrasonography belong to the initial workup of patients with prolonged fever (68).

Abdominal and chest spiral CT should be performed in all cases, with both oral and intravenous contrast, mainly to search for neoplastic and nonspecific histiocytic or lymphoproliferative disorders. Additional appropriate CT modalities are required in case of suspicion of lung embolism or hypersensitivity pneumonitis. Colonoscopy belongs to the initial workup because colon cancer or Crohn's disease are two classic causes of recurrent FUO (3). Up to now, magnetic resonance imaging (MRI) is only used to identify specific features of lesions detected by other techniques.

In case of recurrent fever for more than one year, additional tests should be guided by clues that point to the classic, very prolonged recurrent FUOs such as Still's disease, the hereditary periodic fever syndromes, and the atypical histiocytic and lymphoproliferative diseases. Low white blood cell count suggests cyclic neutropenia, large granular lymphocyte lymphocytosis, and macrophage activation syndrome, and bone marrow biopsy is an essential procedure in these cases (7,19,62). Serum ferritin concentrations >10.000 µg/L are typical for the active phase of Still's disease and also macrophage activation syndrome (27,64). In other conditions such as acute liver necrosis, hemochromatosis, and some malignancies, the values rarely exceed 3000 µg/L. Genetic testing allows confirmation of FMF in more than 90% of the cases (37,38). These tests are indicated for atypical cases of FMF, and they are widely available, in contrast to tests for the other hereditary periodic fever syndromes (35).

After this standard assessment, we prefer a wait-and-see strategy or a whole body FDG-PET scintigraphy in a symptomatic phase, mainly in search of neoplastic, atypical reactive lymphoproliferative and histiocytic disorders, and inflammatory bowel disease. We prefer FDG-PET to Gallium because FDG-PET takes less time and it allows a better assessment of the abdomen. It seldom yields the diagnosis, but allows to detect focal abnormalities, which can be pursued with directed radiologic, ultrasonographic, MRI, endoscopic, and surgical procedures (67,68).

Periodic reassessment with complete physical examination is indicated but repeating the standard assessment makes little sense. Renewed investigation should be directed by new clues. Elevated alkaline phosphatase value is an indication for ordering a bone scintigraphy that may yield the first clue to mastocytosis, Schnitzler's disease, or ECD, all causes of bone densification on standard bone radiographs (25,59,74). Increased LDH (lactic dehydrogenase) should raise suspicion not only of a neoplastic disease but also of a hemolytic crisis and pulmonary embolism. Measurement of lung diffusion capacity may be useful in selected cases, pointing toward hypersensitivity pneumonitis or lung embolism. Venous thromboembolism must be actively searched for in patients with predisposing factors but D-dimer levels are nearly always increased in case of inflammation and hence probably worthless.

Invasive procedures such as liver biopsy and exploratory laparotomy may only be helpful when other features point to abdominal disease. Slight liver abnormalities are so common in FUO patients that this sole finding does not warrant liver biopsy (68).

THERAPEUTIC TRIALS

Therapeutic trials make little sense and have very poor, if any, diagnostic value in case of recurrent FUO because spontaneous resolution of fever is common. Moreover, defervescence following institution of a therapy, designed to treat a specific disorder, may not be considered as proof of the diagnosis.

NSAIDs are more effective than paracetamol as symptomatic treatment pending a definite diagnosis. However, according to our experience, attention should be paid to liver toxicity of NSAIDs in this clinical setting and, particularly, in case of possible Still's disease. The antipyretic effect of naproxen is not specific for neoplastic fever and the so-called naproxen test lacks differential diagnostic value in unselected patients with a prolonged febrile illness (71). Sometimes corticosteroids may be required for symptomatic reasons. These therapeutic trials should be interrupted as soon as the illness subsides, but a small percentage of patients require a continuous low dose of corticosteroids (e.g., 4 to 6 mg prednisolone per day) for suppression of fever and debilitating symptoms of inflammation (3,4). In the 21st century, there is no longer room for empiric treatment with heparins in the case of suspicion of venous thromboembolism as cause of recurrent FUO. Appropriate imaging techniques, particularly, CT scan, allow to exclude thromboembolic disease in these cases of prolonged illness.

REFERENCES

1. Petersdorf RB, Beeson PB. Fever of unexplained origin: report on 100 cases. Medicine 1961; 40:1–30.
2. Durack DT, Street AC. Fever of unknown origin—reexamined and redefined. Curr Clin Top Inf Dis 1991; 11:35–51.
3. Knockaert DC, Vanneste LJ, Bobbaers HJ. Recurrent or episodic fever of unknown origin. Review of 45 cases and survey of the literature. Medicine 1993; 72(3):184–196.
4. Knockaert DC, Dujardin KS, Bobbaers HJ. Long-term follow-up of patients with undiagnosed fever of unknown origin. Arch Intern Med 1996; 156(6):618–620.
5. Reimann HA. Periodic disease. Medicine 1951; 30:219–245.
6. Reimann HA, Mc Closkey RV. Periodic fever. Diagnostic and therapeutic problems. JAMA 1974; 228(13):1662–1664.
7. Dale DC, Bolyard AA, Aprikyan A. Cyclic neutropenia. Semin Hematol 2002; 39(2):89–94.
8. Thomas KT, Feder HM, Lawton AR, Edwards KM. Periodic fever syndrome in children. J Pediatr 1999; 135(1):15–21.
9. Knockaert DC, Vanneste LJ, Vanneste SB, et al. Fever of unknown origin in the 1980s. Arch Intern Med 1992; 152(1):51–54.
10. De Kleijn EMH, Vandenbroucke JP, Van Der Meer JWM, and the Netherlands FUO Study Group. Fever of unknown origin (FUO). Medicine 1997; 76(6):392–400.
11. Vidal E, Liozon E, Loustaud-Ratti V. Prise en charge d'une fièvre intermittente chez l'adulte. Rev Prat 2002; 52(2):167–171.
12. Vanderschueren S, Knockaert D, Adriaenssens T, et al. From prolonged febrile illness to fever of unknown origin. Arch Intern Med 2003; 163(9):1033–1041.
13. Aduan RP, Fauci AS, Dale DC, et al. Prolonged fever of unknown origin (FUO): a prospective study of 347 patients. Clin Res 1978; 26:558A.
14. Winckelmann G, Lütke A, Löhner J. Uber 6 Monate besthendes rezidivierendes Fieber ungeklärter Ursache. Bericht über 85 Patienten. Deutsche Medizinische Wochenschrift 1982; 107(26):1003–1007.
15. Collazos J, Guerra E, Mayo J, Martínez E. Tuberculosis as a cause of recurrent fever of unknown origin. J Infect 2000; 41(3):269–272.
16. Rho JP, Montori VM, Bauer BA. 74-year-old women with intermittent fever, headache and stroke. Mayo Clin Proc 1998; 73(1):73–76.

17. Case records of the Massachusetts general hospital. Case 40-1992. N Engl J Med 1992; 327(15):1081–1087.
18. Dworkin MS, Schwan TG, Anderson DE. Tick-Borne relapsing fever in North America. Med Clin North Am 2002; 86(2):417–433.
19. Grom AA. Macrophage activation syndrome and reactive hemophagocytic lymphohistiocytosis: the same entitites? Curr Opin Rheumatol 2003; 15(5):587–590.
20. Herrada J, Cabanillas F, Rice L, Manning J, Pugh W. The clinical behavior of localized and multicentric Castleman Disease. Ann Intern Med 1998; 128(8):657–662.
21. Sakai Y, Atsumi T, Itoh T, Koike T. Uveitis, pancarditis, haemophagocytosis, and abdominal masses. Lancet 2003; 361(9360):834.
22. Lekstrom-Himes JA, Dale JK, Kingma DW, et al. Periodic illness associated with Epstein-Barr virus infection. Clin Infect Dis 1996; 22(1):22–27.
23. Scully RE, Mark EJ, McNeely WF, McNeely BU. Case records of the Massachusetts general hospital. Case 2-1996. N Engl J Med 1996; 334(3):176–182.
24. Kaufmann Y, Many A, Rechavi G, et al. Brief report: Lymphoma with recurrent cycles of spontaneous remission and relapse—possible role of apoptosis. N Engl J Med 1995; 332(8):507–510.
25. Lipsker D, Veran Y, Grunenberger F, et al. The Schnitzler syndrome. Four new cases and review of the literature. Medicine 2001; 80(1):37–44.
26. Pinede L, Duhaut P, Loire R. Clinical presentation of left atrial cardiac myxoma: a series of 112 consecutive cases. Medecine 2001; 80(3):159–172.
27. Fautrel B, Zing E, Golmard JL, et al. Proposal for a new set of classification criteria for adult-onset Still disease. Medicine 2002; 81(3):194–200.
28. Mert A, Ozaras R, Tabak F. Fever of unknown origin: a review of 20 patients with adult-onset Still's disease. Clin Rheumatol 2003; 22(2):89–93.
29. Sakane T, Takeno M, Suzuki N, Inaba G. Behcet's disease. N Engl J Med 1999; 341(17):1284–1291.
30. Saltoglu N, Tasova Y, Midikli D, Aksu H, Sanli A, Dündar I. Fever of unknown origin in Turkey: evaluation of 87 cases during a nine-year-period of study. J Infect 2004; 48(1): 81–85.
31. Trentham DE, Le CH. Relapsing polychondritis. Ann Int Med 1998; 129(2):114–122.
32. Johnson DH, Cunha BA. Drug fever. Infect Dis Clin North Am 1996; 10(1):85–91.
33. Aduan RA, Fauci AS, Dale DC, et al. Factitious fever and self-induced infection. A report of 32 cases and review of the literature. Ann Intern Med 1979; 90(2):230–242.
34. Winckelmann G, Maass G, Schmidt H, Löhner J. Vegetative Hyperthermie: Thermoregulationsstörung oder Variante der Norm? Dtsch Med Wochenschr 1986; 111(42):1590–1594.
35. Drenth JPH, van der Meer JWM. Hereditary periodic fever. N Engl J Med 2001; 345(24):1748–1757.
36. Hull KM, Shoham N, Chae JJ, Aksentijevich I, Kastner DL. The expanding spectrum of systemic autoinflammatory disorders and their rheumatic manifestations. Curr Opin Rheumatol 2003; 15(1):61–69.
37. Samuels J, Aksentijevich I, Torosyan Y, et al. Familial Mediterranean fever at the millenium. Clinical Spectrum, ancient mutations, and a survey of 100 American referrals to the National Institutes of Health. Medicine 1998; 77(4):268–297.
38. Ben-Chetrit E, Levy M. Familial Mediterranean fever. Lancet 1998; 351(9103):659–664.
39. Drenth JPH, Haagsma CJ, van der Meer JWM, and the International Hyper-IgD study group. Hyperimmunoglobulinemia D and periodic fever syndrome. The clinical spectrum in a series of 50 patients. Medicine 1994; 73(3):133–144.
40. Simon A, Cuisset L, Vincent MF, et al. Molecular analysis of the mevalonate kinase gene in a cohort of patients with the hyper-IgD and periodic fever syndrome: its application as a diagnostic tool. Ann Intern Med 2001; 135(5):338–343.
41. Simon A, Drewe E, van der Meer JWM, et al. Simvastatin treatment for inflammatory attacks of the hyperimmunoglobulinemia D and periodic fever syndrome. Clin Pharmacol Ther 2004; 75(5):476–483.
42. Hawkins PN, Lachmann HJ, Aganna E, Mc Dermott MF. Spectrum of clinical features in Muckle-Wells syndrome and response to Anakinra. Arthritis Rheum 2004; 50(2): 607–612.

43. Johnstone RF, Dolen WK, Hoffman HM. A large kindred with familial cold autoinflammatory syndrome. Ann Allergy Asthma Immunol 2003; 90(2):233–237.
44. Hoffman HM, Rosengren S, Boyle DL, et al. Prevention of cold-associated acute inflammation in familial cold autoinflammatory syndrome by interleukin-1 receptor antagonist. Lancet 2004; 364(9447):1779–1785.
45. Dodé C, Le Dû N, Cuisset L, et al. New mutations of CIAS1 that are responsible for Muckle-Wells syndrome and familial cold urticaria: a novel mutation underlies both syndromes. Am J Hum Genet 2002; 70(6):1498–1506.
46. Williamson LM, Hull D, Mehta R, Reeves WG, Robinson BHB, Toghill PJ. Familial Hivernian fever. Q J Med 1982; 51(204):469–480.
47. Hull KM, Drewe E, Aksentijevich I, et al. The TNF receptor-associated periodic syndrome (TRAPS). Emerging concepts of an autoinflammatory disorder. Medicine 2002; 81(5):349–368.
48. Dodé C, André M, Bienvenu T, et al. The enlarging clinical, genetic, and population spectrum of tumor necrosis factor receptor-associated periodic syndrome. Arhritis Rheum 2002; 46(8):2181–2188.
49. Simon A, Van Deuren M, Tighe PJ, van der Meer JWM, Drenth JPH. Genetic analysis as a valuable key to diagnosis and treatment of periodic fever. Arch Intern Med 2001; 161(20):2491–2493.
50. Yosipovitch Z, Katz K. Bone crisis in Gaucher disease—an update. Isr J Med Sci 1990; 26(10):593–595.
51. Brady RO, Schiffmann R. Clinical features of and recent advances in therapy for Fabry disease. JAMA 2000; 284(21):2771–2775.
52. Desnick RJ, Brady R, Barranger J, et al. Fabry disease, an under-recognized multisystemic disorder: expert recommendations for diagnosis, management, and enzyme replacement therapy. Ann Intern Med 2003; 138(4):338–346.
53. Lachmann HJ, Gilbertson JA, Gillmore JD, Hawkins PN, Pepys MB. Unicentric Castleman's disease complicated by systemic AA amyloidosis: a curable disease. Q J Med 2002; 95(4):211–218.
54. Parappil A, Rifaath A, Doi SAR, Pathan E, Surrun SK. Pyrexia of unknown origin: Kikuchi-Fujimoto disease. Clin Infect Dis 2004; 39(1):138–143.
55. Rezai K, Kuchipudi S, Chundi V, Ariga R, Loew J, Sha BE. Kikuchi-Fujimoto disease: hydroxychloroquine as a treatment. Clin Infect Dis 2004; 39(12):e124–e126.
56. Knockaert DC, Schuermans A, Vlayen, et al. Fever of unknown origin due to inflammatory pseudotumour of lymph nodes. Acta Clin Belg 1998; 53(6):367–370.
57. Moran CA, Suster S, Abbondanzo SL. Inflammatory pseudotumor of lymph nodes: a study of 25 cases with emphasis on morphological heterogeneity. Hum Pathol 1997; 28(3):332–338.
58. Oliveira L, Moraes MF, Oliveira P, et al. A train driver with painful legs. Lancet 1999; 353(9169):2034.
59. Veyssier-Belot C, Cacoub P, Caparros-Lefebvre D, et al. Erdheim-Chester disease. Clinical and radiological characteristics of 59 cases. Medicine 1996; 75(3):157–169.
60. Dogan A, Attygalle AD, Kyriakou C. Angioimmunoblastic T-cell lymphoma. Br J Haematol 2003; 121(5):681–691.
61. Scott CS, Richards SJ, Sivakumaran M, et al. Transient and persistent expansions of large granular lymphocytes (LGL) and NK-associated (Nka) cells: the Yorkshire Leukaemia Group Study. Br J Haematol 1993; 83(3):504–515.
62. Lamy Th, Loughran Jr. Clinical features of large granular lymphocyte leukaemia. Semin Hematol 2003; 40(3):185–195.
63. Reiner AP, Spivak J. Hematophagic histiocytosis. A report of 23 patients and a review of the literature. Medicine 1988; 67(6):369–388.
64. Imashuku S. Differential diagnosis of hemophagocytic syndrome: underlying disorders and selection of the most effective treatment. Int J Hematol 1997; 66(2):135–151.
65. Ramanan AV, Schneider R. Macrophage activation syndrome. What's in a name! J Rheumatol 2003; 30(12):2513–2516.
66. Long SS. Syndrome of periodic fever, aphthous stomatitis, pharyngitis, and adenitis (PFAPA). What it isn't. What is it? J Pediatr 1999; 135(1):1–5.

67. Blockmans D, Knockaert D, Maes A, et al. Clinical Value of [18F]fluoro-deoxyglucose positron emission tomography for patients with fever of unknown origin. Clin Infect Dis 2001; 32(2):191–196.
68. Knockaert DC, Vanderschueren S, Blockmans D. Fever of unknown origin in adults: 40 years on. J Intern Med 2003; 253(3):263–275.
69. MacKenzie MA, Hermus RM, Wollersheim HC, et al. Poikilothermia in man: pathophysiology and clinical implication. Medicine 1991; 70(4):257–268.
70. Murray HW, Tuazon CU, Guerrero IC, et al. Urinary temperature. A clue to early diagnosis of factitious fever. N Engl J Med 1977; 296(1):23–24.
71. Vanderschueren S, Knockaert DC, Peetermans WE, Bobbaers HJ. Lack of value of the naproxen test in the differential diagnosis of prolonged febrile illnesses. Am J Med 2003; 115(7):572–575.
72. Singh N, Yu VL, Wagener MM, et al. Cirrhotic fever in the 1990s: a prospective study with clinical implications. Clin Infect Dis 1997; 24(6):1135–1138.
73. Roth M, Blum U, Hellerich V. Rezidivierende hyperbilirubinämie und Fieber. Med Klin 1993; 88(12):699–700.
74. Lopez-Gomez M, Garcia JDM, Jimenez-Alonso J, et al. Systemic mast cell disease as a cause of fever of unknown origin. Eur J Intern Med 1993; 4(2):171–175.

Nonspecific Tests in the Diagnosis of Fever of Unknown Origin

Burke A. Cunha

Infectious Disease Division, Winthrop-University Hospital, Mineola, New York, U.S.A.

OVERVIEW

Fevers of unknown origin (FUOs) are caused by a limited number of infectious and noninfectious disorders. The diagnosis of the various etiologies of infectious and noninfectious FUOs depends on demonstrating the pathogen, which may involve culture or tissue biopsy. The definitive diagnostic tests for FUO are discussed elsewhere in this book. This chapter reviews the diagnostic significance of nonspecific tests in the diagnosis of FUO. Nonspecific laboratory tests are important because they may suggest an otherwise unsuspected diagnosis or increase/decrease the diagnostic probability of a particular disorder. Nonspecific laboratory tests should not be used in place of definitive tests but rather provide clinical clues to diagnostic possibilities. Such abnormal test results should suggest a further diagnostic workup to include specific testing to make a definitive diagnosis (1–11).

IMAGING TESTS IN THE DIAGNOSIS OF FUO

The two most important imaging tests in the diagnosis of FUO are radionucleotide scanning tests and computed tomography and magnetic resonance imaging (CT/ MRI) scans. The radionucleotide scans of most diagnostic usefulness in patients with FUO include the bone scan, the indium scan, or the gallium scan (1,2).

The indium scan requires that blood be taken from the patient and tagged with a radioisotope and given back to the patient. The radioisotope in the white blood cells (WBCs) concentrates in areas of inflammation, infection, or malignancy. A focal pickup on the indium scan localizes the pathology of the FUO to a particular organ or organ system. Because each disorder has a particular pattern of organ involvement, localization by indium scan to a particular organ helps narrow differential diagnostic possibilities. Further imaging tests or tissue biopsy may be done to determine the nature and extent of the focal uptake determined by the indium scan. Indium scans have a high false negativity in patients with osteomyelitis. Excluding vertebral osteomyelitis, patients with osteomyelitis are not usually diagnostic problems, because their infectious process is readily recognizable before meeting the definition of FUO (11–13).

Gallium scanning involves the injection of a radioisotope that concentrates in areas of inflammation, infection, or neoplasm. Gallium scan is the preferred radionucleotide scan in patients with FUO. Total body indium scan should be requested to determine the focality of the infectious or noninfectious process. As with indium scans, gallium scans are useful in determining the pattern of organ involvement responsible for the FUO process. As with the indium scan, further imaging with CT or MRI scans will further delineate the extent and nature of the pathology.

Gallium scans, as with indium scans, should be used in concert with CT/MRI scanning to provide the basis for further diagnostic testing, which usually requires biopsy for definitive tissue diagnosis (14,15).

Computed Tomography/Magnetic Resonance Imaging

If there are symptoms or signs referable to the chest, abdomen, or pelvis, then CT/MRI scanning of these anatomical areas should be part of the FUO workup. CT/MRI scanning also has a role in FUO cases where the diagnosis is obscure and there are no localizing findings. CT/MRI scanning of the chest, abdomen, and pelvis may provide important positive or negative diagnostic information. As mentioned previously, CT/MRI scanning is usually used in concert with indium or gallium scanning. The indium/gallium scans localize the abnormality, and the CT/MRI scans provide higher resolution and detail in areas of increased uptake on the indium/gallium scan. Otherwise unsuspected findings on the CT/MRI scans in FUO patients include occult abscesses, retroperitoneal adenopathy, hepatic/splenic masses, splenomegaly, hepatic, pancreatic, renal neoplasms, and so on. After localization and characterization by CT/MRI scanning, biopsy of some lesions may be warranted. Tissue biopsy by CT guidance in difficult-to-reach areas may be helpful. With today's imaging techniques, including PET scans, exploratory laparotomy is rarely necessary in patients with intra-abdominal signs or symptoms (11,16–18).

NONSPECIFIC LABORATORY TESTS
The Complete Blood Count

The complete blood count (CBC) is often helpful in pointing to the etiology of prolonged fevers in FUO patients. The peripheral WBC count is the least helpful diagnostic parameter in the CBC in patients with FUO. FUO patients rarely have a marked leukocytosis, and the WBC count is often unremarkable. Leukopenia, if present, may be drug induced, secondary to viral infection or collagen vascular disease, or may be part of a myelophthisis bone marrow problem. Many patients with FUO are elderly and not uncommonly have the anemia of chronic disease. The anemia of chronic disease by itself is unhelpful, because elderly patients often have a variety of chronic disorders that are responsible for the anemia of chronic disease. The platelet count in the CBC is the most helpful of the CBC parameters in terms of delineating the diagnosis of the FUO. Thrombocytopenia may be on a viral, drug, or neoplastic basis. Thrombocytosis suggests a chronic, inflammatory, or infectious process as well as the possibility of a myelodysplastic syndrome or malignancy. In internal medicine in general, and in infectious disease in particular, nonspecific diagnostic clues take on added diagnostic specificity in the context of associated findings. For example, if the patient with an FUO has both leukopenia and thrombocytopenia, the most likely diagnostic possibilities include a medication-related problem, a viral infection, for example, cytomegalovirus (CMV), or a neoplastic process. More helpful diagnostically is the differential WBC count in FUO patients (19,20).

The WBC differential count can be helpful particularly if abnormal. Normal WBC counts with a normal differential have little diagnostic value. More important than leukocytosis, leukopenia, thrombocytosis, or thrombocytopenia are abnormalities in the WBC count. Parameters with particular diagnostic importance are eosinophilia, lymphocytosis/lymphocytopenia, atypical lymphocytosis, and basophilia.

While abnormalities of these WBC elements are not always present, they are very helpful in narrowing diagnostic possibilities when they are present. As with other nonspecific diagnostic tests, their diagnostic specificity is enhanced when combined with other abnormalities. Eosinophilia in a patient with FUO suggests the possibility of vasculitis, for example, periarteritis nodosa (PAN), or a drug reaction. Lymphocytosis is present with many chronic inflammatory and infectious diseases, but lymphopenia is a more specific finding. Relative lymphopenia in a patient with FUO suggests the possibility of malignancy or viral infection. The presence of atypical lymphocytes suggests the presence of viral infection, certain parasitic disorders, for example, toxoplasmosis, or a drug reaction. Basophils are an uncommon finding in patients with FUO; however when present, basophilia indicates a myeloproliferative disorder or a malignancy (20–30).

Liver Function Tests
Although there are no tests of liver function, liver function tests (LFTs) usually refer to the serum transaminases, that is, serum glutamic-oxaloacetic transaminase (SGOT) or serum glutamic pyruvate transaminase (SGPT), as well as the serum alkaline phosphatase. Mild elevations in serum transaminases in FUO patients may suggest a viral process, for example, CMV or drug-induced hepatitis. Increases in alkaline phosphatase may suggest an obstructive process in the hepatobiliary system, or may suggest a bone metastasis or temporal arteritis (20,31,32).

Serum Protein Electrophoresis
The serum protein electrophoresis (SPEP) is useful in confirming the diagnosis of multiple myeloma or Waldenström's macroglobulinemia, which are rare causes of FUO. SPEP is also important in detecting elevations in the alpha 1 and alpha 2 globulin fraction, which may suggest lymphoma or adult Still's disease. The SPEP should be part of the FUO diagnostic workup when collagen vascular diseases or neoplasms are in the differential diagnosis (20–25).

Serum Ferritin Levels
Serum ferritin levels are an underappreciated indicator of a variety of disorders that may present as an FUO. Ferritin is an acute phase reactant when elevated slightly and early in the course of an illness. Patients with FUO, by definition, have been ill for a month or more with fever. Therefore, patients presenting with FUO and elevated ferritin levels should not be ascribed to acute phase elevations. In patients with FUO, diagnostically useful elevated serum ferritin levels have two characteristics. The serum ferritin levels in the rheumatic diseases and neoplastic diseases are persistently and highly elevated. A patient with an FUO and otherwise unexplained highly elevated ferritin levels should prompt diagnostic testing for a neoplasm. If the patient does not have a neoplasm, the case presentation should be reviewed, looking for the features of adult Still's disease (20,33–37).

Erythrocyte Sedimentation Rate
The erythrocyte sedimentation rate (ESR) is an invaluable test in the differential diagnosis of infectious diseases. The ESR is highly sensitive but not very specific. The key to its usefulness lies in its high sensitivity and interpreting it in the context of other clinical or laboratory abnormalities. As with other laboratory

TABLE 1 Fever of Unknown Origin: Laboratory Clues

Leukopenia	Atypical lymphocytosis	ESR ($>$100 mm/hr)
Miliary TB	EBV	Adult JRA
Brucellosis	CMV	PMR/TA
SLE	Brucellosis	Hypernephroma
Lymphomas	Toxoplasmosis	SBE
Preleukemias	Drug fever	Drug fever
Typhoid fever	Thrombocytosis	Carcinomas
Kikuchi's disease	MPD	Lymphomas
Monocytosis	TB	MPD
TB	Carcinomas	Abscesses
PAN	Lymphomas	Subacute osteomyelitis
TA	Sarcoidosis	LORA
CMV	Vasculitis	Hyper IgD syndrome
Sarcoidosis	Temporal arteritis	SPEP
Brucellosis	Subacute osteomyelitis	Polyclonal gammopathy
SBE	Hypernephroma	Atrial myxoma
SLE	Thrombocytopenia	Alcoholic cirrhosis
Lymphomas	Leukemias	Sarcoidosis
Carcinomas	Lymphomas	PAN
Regional enteritis	MPD	HIV
(Crohn's disease)	EBV infectious mono	Takayasu's arteritis
MPD	Drug fever	$\uparrow$ α_1/α_2 globulins
Eosinophilia	Vasculitis	Lymphoma
Trichinosis	SLE	SLE
Lymphomas	Rheumatoid factor	Monoclonals spike
Drug fever	SBE	Multiple myeloma
Addison's disease	Chronic active hepatitis	Increased serum transaminases
PAN	Malaria	EBV mononucleosis
Hypersensitivity vasculitis	Hypersensitivity	CMV
Hypernephroma	vasculitis	Q fever
MPD	LORA	Drug fever
Basophilia	Alkaline phosphatase	Leptospirosis
Carcinomas	Hepatoma	Toxoplasmosis
Lymphomas	Miliary TB	Brucellosis
Preleukemia (AML)	Lymphomas	Kikuchi's disease
MPD	EBV	Abnormal renal tests
Lymphocytosis	CMV	SBE
TB	Adult JRA	Renal TB
EBV	Subacute thyroiditis	PAN
CMV	TA	Leptospirosis
Toxoplasmosis	Hypernephromas	Brucellosis
Non-Hodgkin's lymphoma	PAN	Lymphomas
Lymphopenia	Liver metastases	SLE
Whipple's disease	Granulomatous hepatitis	Hypernephroma
Miliary TB	Serum ferritin levels	Myeloproliferative Disorders
SLE	Malignancies	Malignancies
Lymphomas	SLE	SLE
Multiple myeloma	TA	TA
	LORA	LORA
	Adult JRA	Adult JRA

Abbreviations: AML, acute myelogenous leukemia; CMV, cytomegalovirus; EBV, Epstein-Barr virus; ESR, erythrocyte sedimentation rate; HIV, human immunodeficiency virus; JRA, juvenile rheumatoid arthritis; LORA, late onset rheumatoid arthritis; MPD, myeloproliferative disorders; PAN, periarteritis nodosa; PMR, polymyalgia rheumatica; SBE, subacute bacterial endocarditis; SLE, systemic lupus erythematosus; SPEP, serum protein electrophoresis; TA, temporal arteritis; TB, tuberculosis.

tests, elevations of the ESR have different diagnostic specificity depending upon the degree of ESR elevation. Elevations of the ESR >100 mm/hour narrow differential diagnostic possibilities to six clinical categories. An ESR >100 is found in relatively few disorders, that is, endocarditis, osteomyelitis, drug fevers, abscesses, collagen vascular diseases, and malignancies. All of these disorders that may be associated with an ESR >100 may present as an FUO. However, it is relatively straightforward to narrow this list even further by history, physical examination, and selected laboratory tests, for example, osteomyelitis is easily ruled out with a plain film or CT/MRI of the bone likely to be involved. Endocarditis can be ruled out with negative blood cultures, and a negative echocardiogram for cardiac vegetation. Abscess can be ruled out with a CT/MRI of the appropriate anatomical region. Drug fever is accompanied by its characteristic signs, and the patient must be on a sensitizing medication. A highly elevated ESR does not differentiate among the rheumatologic causes of FUO or the neoplastic causes of FUO. Other tests are necessary to make the definitive collagen vascular disease- or neoplastic-specific diagnosis.

The ESR, if not elevated, has no exclusionary diagnostic value. The diagnostic possibilities of an elevated sedimentation rate depend upon the degree of elevation and the company it keeps. The ESR is found in concert with other history, physical, and laboratory findings, which make certain diagnostic possibilities more or less likely. Various disorders have certain ranges of sedimentation rate elevation, which are helpful diagnostically, for example, even in advanced tuberculosis, the ESR is rarely elevated >70 mm/hour. Lower intra-abdominal infections, for example, pelvic inflammatory disease (PID), appendicitis, and diverticulitis are associated with higher ESR ranges (50–80 mm/hr) than upper abdominal disorders, that is, cholecystitis and gastritis, where the ESR does not usually exceed 50 mm/hour. The ESR is also helpful at extremes of either very high or very low values. An ESR that is within the normal range has no significance, but an ESR approaching zero, that is, 1 mm/hour–3 mm/hour would suggest the possibility of trichinosis in a patient with an FUO and myositis (20,38). (Table 1)

NONSPECIFIC LABORATORY TESTS IN THE DIAGNOSTIC APPROACH

Nonspecific laboratory tests are nonspecific when considered alone or in a clinical vacuum. The diagnostic utility of nonspecific tests lies in their ability to suggest an otherwise unthought of diagnostic possibility. Nonspecific tests also can increase or decrease the likelihood of a particular diagnostic consideration. The diagnostic specificity of nonspecific tests is enhanced if multiple nonspecific abnormalities are present, for example, highly elevated ESR plus a serum ferritin has much more diagnostic specificity than either an isolated elevation of the ESR or serum ferritin level. While nonspecific laboratory tests are rarely nondiagnostic in and of themselves, they often represent important and easily overlooked diagnostic clues to an otherwise obscure diagnosis. In every patient with an otherwise unexplained FUO, this battery of nonspecific laboratory tests should be ordered (19,20).

REFERENCES

1. Petersdorf RG, Beeson PB. Fever of unexplained origin: report on 100 cases. Medicine (Baltimore) 1961; 40:1–30.
2. Louria DB. Fever of unknown etiology. Del Med J 1971; 43:343–348.

3. Weinstein L. Clinically benign fever of unknown origin: a personal retrospective. Rev Infect Dis 1985;7:692–699.
4. Murray HW, ed. FUO: fever of undetermined origin. Mount Kisco, New York: Futura Publishing, 1983.
5. Kauffman CA, Jones PG. Diagnosing fever of unknown origin in older patients. Geriatrics 1984; 39:46–51.
6. Kazanjian PH. Fever of unknown origin. Review of 86 patients treated in community hospital. Clin Infect Dis 1992; 15:968–973.
7. Knockaert DC, Vanneste LJ, Vannester SB, et al. Fever of unknown origin in the 1980s: an update of the diagnostic spectrum. Arch Intern Med 1992; 152:51–55.
8. Knockaert DC, Vanneste LJ, Bobbears HJ. Fever of unknown origin in elderly patients. J Am Geriatr Soc 1993; 41:1187–1192.
9. Cunha BA. Fever of unknown origin. Infect Dis Clin North Am 1996; 10:111–128.
10. Cunha BA. Fever of unknown origin. In: Gorbach SL, Bartlett JG, Blacklow NE, eds. Infectious Diseases. 3rd ed. Philadelphia: Lippincott Williams and Wilkins, 2004: 1568–1577.
11. Brusch JL, Weinstein L. Fever of unknown origin. Med Clin North Am 1988; 72: 1247–1261.
12. Peters AM. Nuclear medicine imaging in fever of unknown origin. Q J Nucl Med 1999; 43:61–73.
13. Datz FL, Anderson CE, Ahluwalia R, et al. The efficacy of indium-111 polyclonal IgG for the detection of infection and inflammation. J Nucl Med 1994; 35:74–83.
14. Hilson AJW, Maisey MN. Gallium-67 scanning in pyrexia of unknown origin. Br Med J 1979; 2:1130–1131.
15. Knockaert DC, Mortelmans LA, De Roo MC, et al. Clinical value of gallium-67 scintigraphy in evaluation of fever of unknown origin. Clin Infect Dis 1994; 18: 601–605.
16. Quinn MJ, Sheedy PF II, Stephen DH, et al. Computed tomography of the abdomen in evaluation of patients with fever of unknown origin. Radiology 1980; 136:407–411.
17. Rowland MD, Del Bene VE. Use of body computed tomography to evaluate fever of unknown origin. J Infect Dis 1987; 156:408–409.
18. Blockmans D, Knockaert D, Maes A, et al. Clinical value of [(18)F] fluorodeoxyglucose positron emission tomography or patients with fever of unknown origin. Clin Infect Dis 2001; 32:191–196.
19. Sen P, Louria DB. Noninvasive and diagnostic procedures and laboratory methods. In: Murray HW, ed. FUO: Fever of Undetermined Origin. Mount Kisco, New York:Futura Publishing, 1983:159–190.
20. Cunha BA. Diagnostic significance of nonspecific laboratory abnormalities in infectious diseases. In: Gorbach SL, Bartlett JG, Blacklow NE, eds. Infectious Diseases, 3rd ed. Philadelphia: Lippincott Williams and Wilkins, 2004:158–165.
21. Ravel R. Clinical Laboratory Medicine. 6th ed. New York: Mosby, 1995.
22. Henry JB. Clinical Diagnosis and Management by Laboratory Methods 19th ed. Philadelphia: WB Saunders, 1996.
23. Sacher RS, McPherson RA, Campos JM. Widmann's Clinical Interpretation of Laboratory Tests. 11th ed. Philadelphia: FA Davis, 2000.
24. Tilton RC, Balows A, Hohnadel DC, et al., eds. Clinical Laboratory Medicine. St. Louis: Mosby, 1992:1–1207.
25. Wallach J. Interpretation of Diagnostic Tests. 7th ed. Philadelphia: Lippincott Williams and Wilkins, 2000.
26. Tietz NW, ed. Clinical Guide to Laboratory Tests, 4th ed. Philadelphia: WB Saunders, 2006.
27. Shafiq M, Cunha BA. Diagnostic significance of lymphopenia. Infect Dis Pract 1999; 23:81–82.
28. Sullivan CL, Cunha BA. The significance of eosinophilia in infectious disease. Hosp Pract 1989; 25:21–27.
29. Cunha BA. The diagnostic significance of thrombocytosis and thrombocytopenia in infectious disease. Infect Dis Pract 1995; 19, 68.
30. Cunha BA. Fever in malignant disorders. Infect Dis Pract 2004; 28:335–336.

31. Bailey EM, Klein NC, Cunha BA. Kikuchi's disease with liver dysfunction presenting as fever of unknown origin. Lancet 1989; 2:986.
32. Johnson DH, Cunha BA. Drug fever. Infect Dis Clin North Am 1996; 10:85–91.
33. Krol V, Cunha BA. Diagnostic significance of serum ferritin levels in infectious and noninfectious diseases. Infect Dis Pract 2003; 27:196–197.
34. Beyan E, Beyan C, Demirezer A, et al. The relationship between ferritin levels and disease activity in systemic lupus erythematosus. Scand J Rheumatol 2003; 32:225–228.
35. Cunha BA. Fever of unknown origin caused by adult juvenile rheumatoid arthritis: the diagnostic significance of double quotidian fevers and elevated serum ferritin levels. Heart Lung 2004; 33:417–421.
36. Schwarz-Eywill M, Helig B, Bauer H, et al. Evaluation of serum ferritin as a marker for adult Still's disease activity. Ann Rheum Dis 1992; 51: 683–685.
37. Cunha BA, Parchuri S, Mohan S. Fever of unknown origin: temporal arteritis presenting with persistent cough and elevated serum ferritin levels. Heart Lung 2006; 35:112–116.
38. Cunha BA. The diagnostic significance of erythrocyte sedimentation rate. Intern Med 1992; 13:48–51.

Specific Tests in the Diagnosis of Fever of Unknown Origin

Aaron R. Kosmin and Bennett Lorber

Section of Infectious Diseases, Department of Medicine, Temple University School of Medicine, Philadelphia, Pennsylvania, U.S.A.

INTRODUCTION

Investigating a fever of unknown origin (FUO) is challenging. Even after completing a sound clinical evaluation and developing a differential diagnosis, obstacles remain. Every potential etiology has its associated diagnostic quirks. Selecting the right test at the right time impacts the accuracy of a fever investigation. This chapter provides a practical summary of diagnostic tests for specific causes of FUO. The diagnostic entities considered in this chapter are listed in Table 1.

This chapter will focus on testing that must be requested with a specific diagnosis in mind. We will assume that routine evaluations have already been completed, including a history and physical, chest X ray, complete blood count (CBC), comprehensive metabolic panel, urinalysis, and routine cultures of blood and urine. Unlike detecting hypernatremia on a serum chemistry panel from a confused elderly patient, a test for a specific entity causing FUO often must be ordered with a diagnosis in mind. The clinician's differential diagnosis may need to be relayed directly to the laboratory personnel doing the test, particularly in the case of microbiology specimens, in order to insure that the most appropriate processing is performed. We have attempted to provide the content for these discussions in this chapter. Although we have tried to be thorough, this discussion is not intended to be exhaustive. Moreover, diagnostic imaging modalities are discussed in the next chapter.

This chapter has been organized by etiologic categories. We will first discuss bacterial causes of FUO, focusing in particular on special culturing or testing conditions required to identify certain bacteria. Next, the diagnostic challenges for mycobacterial diseases will be investigated. Then histoplasmosis, a fungal infection that may present as a FUO yet not be detected using routine cultures, will be explored. We will continue by exploring some viral causes of FUO. Parasitic infections will constitute the last infectious category of FUO etiologies to be explored. Finally, some noninfectious etiologies will be discussed.

BACTERIAL CAUSES OF FUO
Gram-Positive Organisms
Nocardia *Species and Other Related Actinomycetales*
Actinomycetales is an order of bacteria that includes aerobic and filamentous, often branching, gram-positive human pathogens that may not be isolated using routine laboratory cultures. *Nocardia*, *Mycobacterium*, and *Corynebacterium* are well-known members of this order, but the following genera have also been implicated in human infections: *Actinomadura*, *Dermatophilus*, *Gordona*, *Nocardiopsis*, *Rhodococcus*,

(Text continues on p. 163.)

TABLE 1 Recommended Diagnostic Tests for Specific FUO Etiologies

Organism or syndrome	Test(s)	Comments
Bacteria		
Gram-positive bacteria		
Nocardia spp.	Microscopy culture	Long incubation time needed
		Modified AFB-positive
Tropheryma whipplei	PCR of infected tissues or body fluids	Extra-duodenal PAS staining not diagnostic
Actinomyces spp.	Microscopy culture	Use anaerobic media
		Modified AFB-negative
Gram-negative bacteria		
Salmonellae spp. (Enteric fever)	Culture of blood, stool and urine	If routine cultures negative, may culture bone marrow or rose spots
Bartonella spp.	Serology	Prolonged incubation on solid media may increase culture yield
	Peripheral smear (*B. bacilliformis* only)	
Brucella spp.	Serology	*B. canis* not detected using routine serology
HACEK group	Blood culture	Incubate for two weeks
Legionella spp.	Urine antigen	Urine antitgen only detects infections caused by *L. pneumophila* serogroup 1
Neisseria meningitidis	Culture of blood	Consider blind subculture onto chocolate agar and incubation in humid environment with increased carbon dioxide
Streptobacillus moniliformis	Microscopy of peripheral blood	Use specialized enriched media with increased carbon dioxide
	Culture of blood	
Intracellular bacteria		
Chamydophila (*Chlamydia* spp.)	Serology	IgG seroconversion most accurate. IgA may indicate chronic, active infection
Mycoplasma pneumoniae	Serology	Negative IgM does not exclude active infection
Rickettsial illnesses		
Coxiella burnetii	Serology	Phase I antigen seroconversion associated with chronic infection
	Microscopy of infected tissues	
Ehrlichiosis	Microscopy of Buffy coat	Serology only available for HME
	Serology	
Spirochetes		
Leptospira interrogans	Serology	IgG seroconversion is standard. IgM specific but not sensitive
Borellia spp.	Microscopy of blood	Yield greatest during febrile episodes
Mycobacteria		
Mycobacterium tuberculosis	Culture	Liquid media reduces detection time

(Continued)

TABLE 1 Recommended Diagnostic Tests for Specific FUO Etiologies (*Continued*)

Organism or syndrome	Test(s)	Comments
Disseminated MAI	Culture of blood for AFB	High yield with two separate AFB blood cultures
Fungi		
Histoplasma capsulatum	Urine antigen	Antigen can be used to detect relapses
Viruses		
EBV	Serology	Negative EBNA necessary to attribute febrile illness to EBV
Cytomegalovirus	Virus detection in blood or pathologic specimens	Shell vial culture is old standard. Several molecular techniques being studied
HIV seroconversion	Serology and P24 antigen Viral load if P24 negative	P24 highly specific. Viral load highly sensitive
Parasites		
Plasmodium spp.	Expert inspection of peripheral blood smears	Rapid organism detection tests available that require little expertise but not as accurate
Babesia spp.	Microscopy of blood	Serology available but seroconversion may be delayed and it cross-reacts with *P. falciparum*
Leishmania spp.	Microscopy of buffy coat and serology Biopsy, if above negative	Patients with impaired cellular immunity more likely to have false negative serology. Patients in endemic areas (non-travelers) more likely to have false positive serology
Toxoplasma gondii	Pathology Serology	Serology unreliable in patients with impaired cell-mediated immunity
Schistosoma spp. (Katayama fever)	Microscopic inspection of stool and urine Serology	Serology reliable only in sojourners because of high seropositivity in patients from endemic areas
Noninfectious causes of FUO		
Temporal arteritis	Biopsy of temporal artery	Discontinuous lesions can cause false negatives
Wegener's granulomatosis	Pathology $+/-$ Anti-PR-3 (c-ANCA)	Necrotizing granulomas of small to medium blood vessels
Churg-Strauss syndrome	Pathology plus eosinophilia and/or atopy Anti-MPO (p-ANCA)	Granulomatous inflammation of smaller vessels with eosinophils
Microscopic polyangiitis	Pathology Anti-MPO	Small vessels, necrotizing vasculitis
Periarteritis	Angiography Pathology if mononeuritis multiplex	Low prevalence of anti-MPO. Significant minority associated with Hepatitis B

(*Continued*)

TABLE 1 Recommended Diagnostic Tests for Specific FUO Etiologies (*Continued*)

Organism or syndrome	Test(s)	Comments
Rheumatoid arthritis	Anti-cyclic citrullinated peptide antibody	More specific than rheumatoid factor. Still not sensitive enough to rule out RA
Systemic lupus erythematosus	ANA $\geq$ 1:160	Highly sensitive, but at best 90% specific. Peripheral or nucleolar patterns more specific for rheumatologic disease
Kikuchi-Fujimoto disease	Lymph node biopsy, preferably excisional	Experienced pathologist needed to exclude infectious etiologies and SLE
Adult-onset Still's disease	Ferritin often dramatically elevated	Diagnosis based on clinical criteria
Inflammatory bowel disease	Endoscopy with biopsy and exclusion of infections Autoantibodies may help diagnose indeterminate colitis	ASCA associated with Crohn's disease, while p-ANCA (not anti-MPO) associated with ulcerative colitis
Behçet's disease	Pathergy skin test Mucocutaneous biopsy	Diagnosis is clinical
Familial Mediterranean fever	Genetic testing for known *MEFV* gene mutations	Diagnosis is clinical when gene test negative
Hyper-IgD syndrome	Test for elevated IgD twice over at least a month Gene testing for mevalonate kinase gene if IgD normal	Despite name, not all patients have increased IgD
TNF receptor-associated periodic syndrome	Genetic testing for known *TNFRSF1A* gene mutations	Family history often negative because of incomplete penetrance and spontaneous mutations
Malignant causes of FUO		
Primary illness due to malignancy	Pathology	Must exclude infection
FUO in patients with known malignancy	Consider naproxen challenge once infections excluded	Tumor fever still a diagnosis of exclusion. Accuracy of naproxen challenge in modern health care setting not established
Endocrine causes of FUO		
Adrenal insufficiency	Cosyntropin stimulation test using 250 μg IM/IV	Any cortisol level $\geq$18 μg/dL makes AI unlikely
Thyrotoxicosis	TSH with Free T4 and T3	Free thyroid hormones more accurate and easier to interpret than total levels
Pheochromocytoma	24-hour urine collection for catecholamines, VMA and metanephrines Plasma free metanephrines	False positives may occur with certain medications, renal failure or severe systemic illness

Abbreviations: AFB, acid-fast bacilli; ANA, anti-nuclear antibodies; AI, adrenal insufficiency; Anti-MPO, anti-myeloperoxidase; Anti-PR-3, anti-proteinase 3; ASCA, anti-*Saccharomyces cerevisiae* antibodies; c-ANCA, cytoplasmic-antineutrophil cytoplasmic antibodies; CMV, cytomegalo virus; EBNA, Epstein-Barr nuclear antibody; EBV, Epstein-Barr virus; FUO, fever of unknown origin; HME, human monocytic ehrlichiosis; Ig, immunoglobulin; TS-aclcl: HACEK, *Hemophilus sp.*, *Actinobacillus actinomycetemcomitans*, *Cardiobacterium hominis*, *Eikenella corrodens*, *Kingella kingae*; MAI, *Mycobacterium avium* intracellulare; p-ANCA, perinuclear-antineutrophil cytoplasmic antibodies; PAS, periodic acid-Schiff PCR, polymerase chain reaction; stain; RA, rheumatoid arthritis; SLE, systemic lupus erythematosus; TSH, thyroid-stimulating hormone; VMA, vanillylmandelic acid.

Streptomyces, Tropheryma, and *Tsukamurella* (1–3). These organisms are difficult to isolate because of their slow growth rate. However, with the notable exception of *Tropheryma whipplei,* these organisms can be isolated in routine laboratories.

These pathogens can cause febrile infections involving the lymph nodes, liver, brain, lungs or nearly any organ. If a tissue biopsy is performed during the evaluation of a FUO, an attempt to isolate these bacteria should be made. This is most important when evaluating FUO in a patient with impaired cell-mediated immunity, as *Nocardia* spp. and other aerobic Actinomycetales are important potential pathogens (4–9). Specimens can be transported to the lab on routine or fungal media. The specimen should not be refrigerated, as this can reduce the viability of some species. A Gram stain and a modified acid-fast stain should be performed to make a presumptive diagnosis and guide further isolation techniques. These organisms range from weakly gram-positive to vividly so. *Nocardia* spp. may be suggested in the right context if delicate, branching, beaded, weakly gram-positive organisms are seen. Many of these genera, excluding *Mycobacterium,* are weakly acid-fast. This property refers to the "fastness" of carbolfuchsin dye to the bacteria if milder decolorizers, such as 1% sulfuric acid, are used for shorter durations than in traditional acid-fast stains (1).

Actinomycetales will grow on most media; however, they are often isolated in the mycology division of the laboratory. Fungal cultures are routinely held for at least three weeks, affording time for detection of slow growing micro-organisms. Most aerobic Actinomycetales will not be isolated in the mycobacterial lab because they do not survive the decontamination phase of specimen processing for acid-fast bacilli (AFB). Holding traditional bacterial media for at least three weeks may be sufficient to isolate the organism. Alternatively, particularly for *Nocardia,* a buffered charcoal-yeast extract (BCYE) agar with antibiotics that suppress normal flora increases the yield (10). Molecular techniques for the diagnosis of nocardiosis are being researched (11–14) but are not yet ready for widespread use.

Tropheryma whipplei (Whipple's Disease)

Tropheryma whipplei, the cause of Whipple's Disease, cannot be cultivated in routine laboratories (15–17). This organism is traditionally associated with lipodystrophy of the small bowel causing diarrhea but often also causes a systemic disorder (18–19). It can involve the central nervous system, eyes, joints, (20) lungs, and heart (21,22). *Tropheryma whipplei* should be included in the differential diagnosis for culture negative endocarditis (21, 23–25). Duodenal biopsy characteristically reveals periodic acid-Schiff (PAS)-positive inclusions in large macrophages infiltrating the lamina propria. However, PAS stains of extraduodenal tissue are not considered diagnostic. Electron microscopic evaluation of tissues may help, but this technique is not often readily available.

Polymerase chain reaction (PCR) and immunohistochemistry tests have been developed to detect *T. whipplei* (26–27) in small bowel (28), synovial fluid (20), lymph node, cardiac valves, vitreous humor, cerebrospinal fluid (CSF), (29–30) feces (31), bone marrow (32), or peripheral blood (31,33). These tests are still being standardized, and because of the potential for contamination, they may result in false positives (26,34). They should only be considered diagnostic, therefore, when other clinical or laboratory features of Whipple's disease are present. Associated laboratory features include evidence of malabsorption (with resultant malnutrition), lymphopenia, eosoinophilia, and IgM and IgA hypo-gammuglobulinemia.

Actinomyces *Species (Actinomycosis)*

Actinomycosis is usually caused by anaerobic or facultatively anaerobic filamen-tous gram-positive bacteria that belong to the genus *Actinomyces*. These organisms can cause indolent, progressive infections in hosts with normal immunity (35). They tend to violate tissue planes and anatomic barriers, and thus may be misdiagnosed as malignancies (36–40). Because most species are quite sensitive to multiple anti-biotics, it is important to obtain specimens prior to the use of any empiric therapy.

The key to diagnosis is to obtain sufficient material for laboratory evaluation with the help of a surgeon or an interventional radiologist (41–43). The yield from transbronchial biopsy has been questioned (44,45), and thus a negative broncho-scopic evaluation should not preclude further study. *Actinomyces* spp. colonize the oral cavity and genital tract (46); so mere isolation of this potential pathogen does not establish a cause for a FUO. However, isolation of these bacteria is suffi-cient for diagnosis if the specimen is obtained from a sterile body site or if there is a compatible clinical syndrome.

Culture material in the form of tissue or purulent fluid should be transported to the laboratory quickly, ideally in anaerobic transport media. The presence of sulfur granules in the specimen increases the yield. Swab cultures should be avoided, as they foster small sample size and limit viability. Although many organ-isms causing actinomycosis are facultative anaerobes, they are best isolated on special media under anaerobic conditions (47). These bacteria grow slowly; one to four weeks may be required to detect growth. Selective media may increase the yield if rapidly growing organisms are also present (48).

Microscopic evaluation of clinical specimens can help establish the diagnosis of actinomycosis. In fact, especially after exposure to antibiotics, a simple Gram stain may be more sensitive than culture for detecting these bacteria. Attempts should be made to localize and examine sulfur granules in specimens. Sulfur gran-ules occur only in vivo and represent tightly grouped microorganisms with sur-rounding inflammatory cells. The bacteria can be visualized at the periphery of the granule(47) and often appear as branching filamentous gram-positive bacteria. They must be distinguished from other bacteria and fungi. Of note, hematoxylin and eosin (H&E) stain, a routine stain used in histopathology, will not detect the organisms (35,38). Gram, silver, or Giemsa stains are required. *Actinomyces* spp. are unable to hold carbolfuchsin dye even when using modified acid-fast stains, thus distinguishing them from *Nocardia* spp. When the diagnosis remains in doubt despite culture and direct microscopy, immunofluorescence stains directed at the more common species can be performed by the pathologist (35,47).

Gram-Negative Organisms

Salmonella *Species (Enteric Fever)*

Enteric fever, in addition to sustained elevation of body temperature, may result in any combination of the following signs or symptoms (49): abdominal pain, head-ache, pulse-temperature dissociation, rash, leukopenia, hepatitis (50), or splenome-galy (51). This syndrome is traditionally caused by gastrointestinal infection with *Salmonella enterica*, subspecies *enterica* serotype typhi (*Salmonella* typhi) (49), but may also be caused by other *Salmonella* spp. Less frequently other pathogens, including *Brucella* spp., *Yersinia* spp., *Campylobacter* spp., and *Francisella tularensis*, cause enteric fever.

Leukopenia in the absence of eosinophilia, although not entirely specific, is suggestive of a bacterial cause of a patient's abdominal pain, especially in regions where invasive parasitic diseases are common. Microscopic examination of the stool may reveal leukocytes with a predominance of mononuclear cells. The mainstay of diagnosis, however, is by culture.

Unfortunately, stool cultures are insensitive for enteric fever, so alternate means are necessary to make the diagnosis in about two-thirds of cases (52,53). Culture of urine and blood should be obtained in every suspected case. Ultimately, urine culture has limited sensitivity, so the diagnosis is most often made via blood cultures. Multiple blood cultures should be taken, as the yield increases with each. In addition, a relatively large volume of blood (10 mL–15 mL) should be used, as the amount of blood inoculated also increases yield (49). The sensitivity of routine blood cultures range from 73% to 97% depending on the volume of blood inoculated, the number of cultures obtained and the prior exposure to antibiotics. Some have suggested that culturing the blood clot after the removal of the serum may increase culture sensitivity (54,55).

If cultures of blood, urine, and stool are not revealing, there are some alternatives. Tissue from rose spots, if present, may be cultured and may be positive in >60% of patients, even after prior antibiotic exposure (52). Culture of bone marrow aspirates is more sensitive than blood culture (53,56) and in one series was positive in 56 of 62 patients even after antibiotic exposure (52).

Salmonella typhi infection used to be diagnosed using the Widal test. This test is designed to detect host antibodies to the surface polysaccharides and flagellar antigens of *S.* typhi (57). Although a four-fold increase in acute and convalescent titers drawn at least two weeks apart is diagnostic, this is not helpful initially. It has been suggested that a single O-antigen antibody titer of at least 1:320 or a single H-antigen antibody titer of at least 1:160 is sufficient to establish a diagnosis without waiting for convalescent sera. Serologic studies, however, are of limited value for the diagnosis of enteric fever. Because the Widal test is species specific, many causes of enteric fever are missed. Despite its design as a species-specific test, cross-reactions with other Enterobacteriaceae have been reported (49). Furthermore, even among the same species, such as *S.* typhi, the breakpoints for antibody positivity should be altered based on the region from which the organism was acquired (57,58). Moreover, false-positive tests have been documented because of other infections, such as malaria (59). Given these limitations, we do not recommend relying on the Widal test to diagnose enteric fever.

Bartonella *Species*

Bacteria in the genus *Bartonella* are increasingly being determined to cause a wide range of febrile syndromes that used to defy explanation. To date, there are at least eight species that cause disease in humans, the most notable of which are *B. henselae* and *B. quintana*. Specific syndromes attributed to *Bartonella* spp. include cat-scratch disease, bacillary angiomatosis, bacillary peliosis hepatitis, culture-negative endocarditis (14), Oroya fever, verruga peruana, and trench fever. Because the signs and symptoms of these illnesses are variable and significantly host dependent, *Bartonella* infection is often included in the differential diagnosis of FUO. This organism can cause very different syndromes in immune-compromised hosts. Patients with impairments in cell-mediated immunity may have systemic illness with fever and less obvious exposure histories. One rule of thumb for FUO in HIV-infected patients is to include bartonellosis in the differential diagnosis whenever one considers disseminated *Mycobacterium avium* intracellulare (MAI) infection.

Bartonella spp. are gram-negative bacilli. Unlike rickettsial organisms, *Bartonella* will grow on regular media, but is seldom isolated using routine lab protocols because it is fastidious and slow growing. Clinical specimens should be processed as soon as possible after collection. If a delay is anticipated, specimens should be frozen until processing is available (60). *Bartonella* grows best on solid or semi-solid media, and thus may not be detected in a thioglycollate broth. The optimum medium is rabbit-heart infusion agar, but blood and chocolate agars will support its growth (60–62). Optimum incubation for most *Bartonella* spp. is between 35°C and 37°C in a humid, carbon dioxide-enriched atmosphere (62). At least seven days, but up to one month, of incubation is required to detect growth. Colony morphology is unique, and can take on either a smooth or verrucous form.

When it comes to isolating *Bartonella* spp. from the blood, routine automated cultures are limited by the use of liquid media, the short incubation period, and the limited amount of detectable metabolic byproducts (60,63–65). In addition, broth media used in automated systems often contain sodium polyanethol sulfonate (SPS), which inhibits the growth of *Bartonella* (61). Adding agents to neutralize SPS may help, but may not be practical in routine labs. Theoretically, lytic blood culture systems may be useful because the hemolysis releases intracellular organisms, whereas the freed hemoglobin neutralizes any SPS (60,61). Still, most routine blood culture media will sustain viable organisms even if they fail to detect growth. Thus blind subculturing to solid media after five to seven days of routine incubation will likely increase the yield (65–67). Although not required for cultivation, cell cultures using endothelial cells may detect growth in as little as 72 hours (68,69). At least one research group has also developed a unique cell-free media designed to detect *Bartonella* spp (70). However, endothelial cell culture and special cell-free culture media for *Bartonella* are not available in most laboratories.

Because of the above detailed difficulties in isolating *Bartonella* spp. in the routine laboratory, alternative techniques are often used to make a diagnosis. These techniques include direct examination of clinical specimens and serology. *Bartonella bacilliformis*, the causative agent in Oroya fever, can be visualized on Giemsa stains of peripheral blood (71). Other species, however, are usually not present in the blood in high enough concentrations to make the peripheral smear useful. H&E stain of pathologic specimens will show inflammation and proliferative changes, but will not demonstrate the bacteria. Instead, silver stain will detect organisms, especially in early lesions (72). Organisms may be difficult to visualize at all in more mature, granulomatous lesions but may still be detected by electron microscopy. Alternatively, immunohistochemistry has been developed (73–78).

Because culture and microscopy have limited sensitivity for bartonellosis; diagnosic testing is often supplemented by serologic testing. Serologic tests have been developed for *B. bacilliformis* (79), *B. quintana*, and *B. henselae* (80). These tests are limited by the cross-reactivity with other species and the lack of a gold standard to help define the predictive value of serology. Additionally, different levels of disease activity and site of organ involvement are associated with variability in the titers. Still, these tests do have clinical utility. In parts of South America where Oroya fever is endemic, immunoblot or indirect fluorescent antibody (IFA) tests help establish a diagnosis (81). Serology in some endemic areas, however, is limited by false positives (71). Indirect fluorescent antibody and enzyme immunoassay (EIA), usually designed to detect IgG, have been developed for *B. henselae* and *B. quintana*. [Note: enzyme immunoassay (EIA) is a newer term referring to the same lab technique as enzyme-linked immunosorbent assay; term EIA is used for the remainder of this chapter.] Serology has been used to diagnose cat-scratch disease and culture-negative endocarditis in the appropriate clinical settings. Also, these tests have been used in HIV-positive patients with FUO. The sensitivity ranges from 85% to 95% and specificity is again limited by cross-reactivity with other *Bartonella* spp. and a low level of background seropositivy in healthy control populations. When the cutoffs are increased to improve specificity, the tradeoff can be significant: the sensitivity in one series using EIA to diagnose cat-scratch disease fell to 75% (82). While imperfect, serologic testing has replaced skin testing as a way to detect host exposure to pathogenic *Bartonella* spp. PCR tests have been developed and are accurate and useful (14,83–85). As they become perfected, molecular tests may be used in the future as the standard by which to calibrate serologic tests. However, such PCR is not yet widely available.

Brucella *Species (Brucellosis)*

The zoonotic infection brucellosis often causes FUO when it affects humans. The signs and symptoms of illness are nonspecific and routine laboratory studies are not diagnostic. *Brucella* spp. are gram-negative coccobacilli that grow aerobically but may require supplementation with carbon dioxide for growth. These species are cultivatable from blood, urine, bone marrow, liver, lymph node, and, occasionally, CSF. However, the yield ranges from 15% to 90% (86) and depends on inoculum, exposure to antibiotics, and laboratory techniques used (87,88). Because brucellosis accounts for many of those infections acquired by specimen handling in the microbiology laboratory (89,90), personnel should be alerted whenever brucellosis is suspected. Lysis centrifugation blood culture technique may be superior to routine blood cultures (87,91). Automated identification systems can be unreliable (92), and so results should be questioned if there is clinical suspicion that a gram-negative isolate is a *Brucella* spp. but has been misidentified.

The diagnosis of brucellosis is often made serologically because, in practice, the yield from culture is poor. IgG and IgM antibodies directed against *Brucella* spp. are most often detected using serum agglutination tests (93,94). IgM antibodies are useful for common causes of brucellosis: *B. abortus* (cows), *B. suis* (pigs), and *B. melitensis* (goats). EIA is more accurate (95) but less widely available. Using any available method, though, rising titers with a compatible syndrome or high titers on presentation are usually sufficient for diagnosis. False positives may occur in patients with prior infections. One major caveat to the use of serology to diagnose brucellosis involves *Brucella canis*: this species is not detected using routine antibody assays (96,97). If the epidemiology suggests that exposure to dogs is the source of illness, then specific serology for *B. canis* must be requested. Finally, molecular methods using PCR to detect *Brucella* DNA in blood samples are being studied (98–102).

Hemophilus, Actinobacillus, Cardiobacterium, Eikenella, *and* Kingella *Species*

The HACEK group (*Hemophilus*, *Actinobacillus*, *Cardiobacterium*, *Eikenella* and *Kingella* species) contains slow growing gram-negative organisms that are classically associated with culture-negative endocarditis. Modern blood culture media with automated continuous monitoring have improved the yield of these organisms while following routine lab protocols (103). However, it is still advisable to allow blood cultures to incubate for two weeks to maximize yield (104,105); one must ask the lab to let the bottles continue incubating before they are discarded in accordance with routine practice (usually after five days).

Legionella *Species (Legionnaires' Disease, Pontiac Fever)*

Legionella spp., usually *pneumophila*, are well known to cause atypical community-acquired pneumonia (106,107). However, these bacteria can cause a wide range of febrile syndromes from Pontiac fever to culture-negative endocarditis (108) to metastatic abscesses. *Legionella* spp. are gram-negative bacilli that grow slowly and are fastidious. Uniquely, the media used to isolate these bacteria use protein as an energy source instead of the usual sugars (109). Culture of sputum, blood or other specimens is best performed on BCYE agar (110). This agar is buffered at a pH of 6.9, which is optimal for *Legionella* growth. The charcoal is used to absorb fatty acids that are toxic to these bacteria. Finally, BCYE agar contains several unique nutrients including ferric pyrophosphate, vitamins, and amino acids. L-cysteine amino acid is always present, as it is an essential growth factor for *Legionella*. The plates are incubated at 37°C for three weeks. Positive cultures from an ill patient are highly specific; however, the sensitivity can be as low as 20% (111,112). The yield depends on the severity of illness (more severe illness is more likely to show culture positive) (113,114), prior exposure to antibiotics, the specific culture medium used (115–117), and the expertise of the laboratory personnel. Finally, growing the organism is the only way to detect infection due to a less common species or serogroup (118,119).

Immunologic testing is often more sensitive and less cumbersome than culture, but will only reliably detect disease caused by *Legionella pneumophila* serogroup 1. The most convenient and widely available of such tests detects *L. pneumophila* antigens in the urine. Similar to routine cultures, the likelihood of test positivity correlates with severity of illness (120,121). Monoclonal antibodies are used in card-based immunoassays for this test. The average sensitivity for *Legionella* infection is between 70% and 80% (reported range 57% to 99%) (106), owing to the less frequent species and serogroups that the test is not designed to detect (122). The sensitivity in patients with impaired cellular immunity is likely to be lower because such patients are at greater risk for acquiring less pathogenic and less common varieties of these bacteria (123).

Serology may be used to make a diagnosis of *Legionella* disease retrospectively. At best, however, these tests have a sensitivity of 75% for legionellosis (124). Acute serology alone lacks accuracy, and thus convalescent sera must be used. Most seroconversions will occur by four weeks, but as many as 20% will occur between weeks five and twelve. Thus, multiple convalescent sera samples are recommended.

Immunoflourescent microscopy or PCR of sputum may be helpful when routine culture or urine antigen are not diagnostic (125,126). However, these tests are neither well standardized nor widely available (127,128).

Neisseria meningitidis

Neisseria meningitidis causes well-known, acute illnesses and thus are not found on most lists of FUO etiologies. However, in patients with complement deficiencies who become infected with atypical, less virulent serotypes, a more subacute or chronic illness may ensue with less specific signs or symptoms (129–131) *Neisseria meningitidis* may defy isolation from the blood by routine laboratory means because the bacteria are fastidious and exquisitely sensitive to many antibiotics (132–134).

These bacteria die if not kept warm, moist, and in neutral to acidic pH; thus specimens should be transported and processed as quickly as possible (135). For optimal isolation, specimens from sterile body sites may be plated onto chocolate agar. Incubation should occur in a humid environment at body temperature, with an atmosphere enriched with carbon dioxide. Routine blood cultures in most centers will detect *N. meningitidis*. However, growth may be delayed because of inhibition by SPS, which is often included in the broth media used in automated blood culture systems. Options for overcoming this limitation include incubating the cultures longer than the standard five days, blind subcultures to nutrient rich media or direct inoculation onto solid media.

The fastidious growth requirements of *N. meningitidis*, along with the need for rapid diagnosis in bacterial meningitis, have spurred the development of molecular-based tests. Anticapsular antibodies in latex agglutination assays are widely used on CSF (136). Although rapid and easy to perform, these tests lack sensitivity and thus are limited in their clinical applicability (137). PCR has been developed, which is most sensitive when a buffy coat is used (138). The sensitivity and specificity depends on the specific assay used but is usually >90% (139,140). Prior antibiotic administration in some series did not impact the accuracy (138,140). At this point, however, such tests are not widely available.

Streptobacillus moniliformis *and* Spirillum minus *(Rat-Bite Fever)*

Rat-bite fever, an uncommon febrile illness, may be caused by *Streptobacillus moniliformis* or, particularly in Asia, *Spirillum minus* (141,142). *Streptobacillus moniliformis* is a microaerophilic gram-negative bacillus that is part of the normal oral flora of rats. It should be suspected whenever a history of rat exposure is obtained from a febrile patient, especially if they have a rash or arthritis. These bacteria can be visualized directly on Gram or Giemsa stains of blood smears. Definitive diagnosis requires culture. Routine blood or broth cultures may fail to identify the organism if they contain SPS (143). When growth in broth does occur, the bacteria appear as white fluffy granules (144). Yield is optimized on heart infusion agar supplemented with horse serum or rabbit blood and yeast extract. Incubation should occur at 36°C in a humid, carbon dioxide enriched environment. Most routine labs will need to consult a reference laboratory. PCR has been developed to detect species specific 16S ribosomal RNA (145,146), but is not widely available for use in humans.

Intracellular Bacteria

Chlamydophila *and* Chlamydia *Species*

These bacteria are obligate intracellular organisms that lack peptidoglycan in the cell wall. They can only be grown using cellular media (147), which is cumbersome, dangerous, and lacks sensitivity. *Chlamydophila psittaci*, *Chlamydophila pneumoniae*, and certain biovars of *Chlamydia trachomatis* can cause atypical febrile illnesses, including culture-negative endocarditis.

If cell culture is attempted, sputum should not be used as a specimen source as it is toxic to the cell lines used for culture. Alternatively, nasopharyngeal wash or swab should be used. However, swabs should not contain calcium alginate, cotton, or wood as these materials interfere with the growth of these bacteria (148). If possible, the swab should be placed in specialized transport media that contains a buffered solution. Special freezing protocols must be followed if the specimen will not be processed for >24 hours (148,149).

Because of the difficulty inherent to cellular culture of these fastidious organisms, molecular or serologic techniques are often the mainstays of diagnosis (150). Serology using complement fixation is the most widely available and standardized method, but does not distinguish among species (151,152). This is because antibodies to a shared lipopolysaccharide antigen are detected. Species-specific IgG, IgM, and IgA antibodies can be detected using IFA (151,152) and are becoming increasingly available in reference laboratories. However, these tests have not been completely standardized and are technically difficult (150). In addition, the result depends on human interpretation of a pattern of immunofluorescence and is somewhat subjective. False positives may occur in the presence of rheumatoid factor, but these antibodies can be neutralized in vitro. Finally, EIA is available, but it lacks species specificity and is not yet standardized (150).

Although a positive IgM titer suggests active infection, the sensitivity of this isotype is limited (153) for two reasons. First, the appearance of IgM may be delayed a few weeks into the course of an illness, and thus may be missed if serology is sent early on. Second, because illnesses caused by *Chlamydophila* spp. often reflect reinfection following remote prior exposure, IgM may not be made for the current illness. Thus, absence of IgM does not exclude chlamydiosis. Testing for IgG is limited by the opposite problem: there is a high prevalence of positive IgG among even healthy adults, reflecting past infection. Thus, acute and convalescent sera must be compared to confidently establish the diagnosis. The rate of rise in the titer depends on whether the patient has a history of prior infection. It ranges from six to eight weeks for primary infection down to one to two weeks for reinfection. Measurements of IgG antibody should be made between three to six weeks apart. IgA antibodies are also being evaluated as a diagnostic tool for chlamydiosis. Because the half-life of IgA is considerably shorter than IgG, positive IgA serology is thought to correlate better with chronic, active infection. How clinically useful this will be remains to be established.

Molecular-based detection techniques are becoming more widely available and could greatly improve diagnosis. Molecular-based detection of organisms in urogenital specimens has been standardized and is now a widely used method for detecting sexually transmitted diseases. Attempts to use PCR for other specimen types that contain *C. psittaci* or *C. pneumoniae* are being studied (127,153–156). Finally, pathologists may use immunohistochemistry to localize disease-specific antigens in tissue or sputum (155,157), but these methods are somewhat subjective and not always practical or available.

Mycoplasma pneumoniae

Mycoplasma pneumoniae is a slow growing bacterium that lacks a cell wall. Thus, it is not visible on routine Gram stain. Besides *Legionella*, *M. pneumoniae* is the only common cause of atypical pneumonia that can grow on cell-free media. For as long as one month into the course of illness, cultures of throat swabs or sputum may be positive, even in the face of antibiotics. Culturing *Mycoplasma* is a specialized process that most labs are not used to doing (158). Transport media similar to viral media are used and they contain peptides, albumin, and antibiotics. Culture is usually done on SP-4 medium that, when positive, yields small spherical colonies with a mulberry-like morphology. Because growth is subtle, chromogens are often exploited to detect *Mycobacteria* spp. The range of time needed to cultivate *M. pneumoniae* ranges from five to 14 days.

Because of the complexity of culturing *M. pneumoniae*, serologic tests are often used clinically. Cold agglutinins are classically associated with this infection (159), but are usually detected only as a consequence of severe disease. These agglutinins are oligoclonal IgM antibodies that react with altered red cell antigens in infected patients (160). These antibodies are often present early in disease, peaking between two and three weeks, and thus may help with diagnosis at the time a patient presents for medical attention. Titers are determined by incubating a patient's serum with type O red blood cells at 4°C. Visible clumping is considered positive. The mixture is then serially diluted to determine the titer. A titer >1:64 is suggestive of *M. pneumoniae* infection (158). A bedside version of this test may be done using 1 mL of the patient's blood in a tube containing an anticoagulant (161). This test is considered positive if cooling the blood to 4°C leads to agglutination that resolves when the blood is rewarmed to body temperature. Bedside positivity has been shown to correlate with a titer of 1:64. The main drawback to cold agglutinins is the lack of specificity. These antibodies are also present in some viral illnesses, including Epstein-Barr Virus (EBV) (162) and cytomegalovirus (CMV) (163), as well as lymphoma.

Several comparable methods have been used to detect IgG or IgM to *M. pneumoniae* (164–166). Testing for both isotypes is complementary. Although a positive IgM is good evidence of active infection, a significant number of adults will mount only an IgG response. Furthermore detectable IgM responses may be delayed by one to two weeks into the course of symptomatic illness (166). IgG seroconversion, on the other hand, is accurate but will usually delay the diagnosis by at least a month (166). False positives occur, most often with the widely available complement fixation tests in the setting of acute systemic inflammation. Although not as widely available, EIA serology for *M. pneumoniae* preserves sensitivity while being more specific than complement fixation (167).

Molecular techniques are available for the detection of *M. pneumoniae* in nasopharyngeal specimens or sputum (168,169). Such tests can be performed rapidly with >90% sensitivity (170). The sensitivity cited varies depending on sample type (171) and whether seroconversion or culture is used as the reference standard (125,168,169,172,173). Specificity is good (98% in one study) (172), but the negative predictive value may be poor in patients with a low pretest probability of disease. Although intriguing, these molecular techniques are not yet ready for widespread clinical use.

Rickettsiales Bacteria

Most illnesses caused by bacteria in the order Rickettsiales have an acute, sometimes fulminant course, and thus are unlikely to be considered as causes of FUO. Rocky Mountain spotted fever, for example, has a high (20%) mortality rate if treatment is not instituted prior to laboratory confirmation. Testing methods include acute and convalescent serology and molecular-based assays (174). *Coxiella burnetii*, however, is well known to cause more prolonged febrile syndromes often without obvious localizing signs or symptoms. Along with *Bartonella* spp or HACEK group organisms, *C. burnetii* should always be in the differential for culture-negative endocarditis (175,176).

Coxiella burnetii (Q Fever)

C. burnetii is a gram-negative intracellular organism that is endemic to livestock. Human infection occurs via aerolization of infectious particles from animal excretions or soil contaminated by animal excreta (177). The organism progresses through two entirely different antigenic phases in vivo, which complicates serologic evaluation of infection. Still, diagnosis is usually made serologically. In general, acute disease causes elevated antibodies to phase II antigens, whereas the more chronic syndromes that cause FUO are associated with seroconversion to phase I antigens. Antibodies are usually screened for using a cutoff titer of 1:50 by IFA. Complement fixation assays are also available. Seroconversion, involving a four-fold rise in IgG directed at phase I antigens, is diagnostic of chronic disease. However, at the time of evaluation, seroconversion may already have taken place, and thus a high initial titer is also diagnostic: IgG ≥ 1:200 for complement fixation (178) and IgG ≥ 1:800 for IFA (179). The detection of abnormal levels of IgM antibodies is variable and of undetermined diagnostic significance.

Coxiella burnetii can also be detected in infected tissues through special culture methods, immunohistochemistry, and PCR. The organism can be cultivated from blood (180), heart valves, and other tissues, but it is hazardous to do so in the general laboratory (177). Biologic materials may be inoculated into fibroblast cell cultures (181). Growth can be detected in as little as a week using shell vial techniques. The organism can also be grown in chick embryos, but in vivo cultures are more hazardous and cumbersome (177).

PCR can detect C. burnetii in blood or tissue (182), but is not widely available. Rapid nested PCR assays have been developed to improve specificity and ease of use and their performance is being evaluated. One such assay was tested in a series of 191 patients with and without endovascular infections caused by C. burnetii and the specificity was outstanding (100%) (182). The sensitivity, however, was as low as 64%. Prolonged storage of the serum samples prior to testing and markedly elevated IgG titers were found to decrease the sensitivity of the test. PCR will be most helpful in diagnosing Q fever infection when, relatively early in the course of the disease, the serology may not yet be diagnostic (183).

Finally, the detection of C. burnetii in pathologic tissue can also establish the diagnosis in a patient with a compatible febrile illness. Methods of detection include electron microscopy, immunohistochemisty (184,185), and special stains (176). Although helpful, these tests require invasive procedures to obtain tissue and also depend on the pathologist's interpretation of test results.

Ehrlichiosis

Ehrlichiosis is caused by bacteria that are tick-borne intracellular pathogens. Two patterns of disease occur: human granulocytic anaplasmosis (HGA) and human monocytic ehrlichiosis (HME) (186). The former is a result of infection with Anaplasma phagocytophilum, the latter Ehrlichia chaffeensis (187). When faced with a patient with a nonspecific febrile syndrome and a history of tick exposure, a high index of suspicion is needed to prompt further testing for these illnesses (188). Ehrlichia chaffeensis has been cultivated in the laboratory (189,190), but such techniques are limited to specialized research centers. Microscopy of peripheral blood, serology, and PCR are means by which to make the diagnosis in clinical practice.

Microscopic examination of a Wright- or Giemsa-stained buffy coat may reveal the intracytoplasmic inclusions known as morulae in neutrophils or mononuclear cells. Sensitivity of microscopy, a highly operator-dependent technique, ranges from 7% to 80% in different case series (188,191,192).

Serology using IFA is available for HME through state health departments (193). A positive result is defined as a titer of at least 1:64 with a four-fold rise between acute and convalescent sera. The need for repeat testing to confirm the diagnosis limits the clinician's ability to use serology for decision making in the acute setting. Another drawback for IFA is that it is organism specific and thus will not help with the diagnosis of HGA.

PCR for both HME and HGA are becoming increasingly available (194–199). In small case series these tests have been highly accurate and afford diagnosis in smear-negative patients at the time of presentation. Once standardized (194), PCR will likely become the diagnostic method of choice for human ehrlichiosis (197).

Spirochetes
Leptospira interrogans *(Leptospirosis)*

Leptospira interrogans and other pathogenic species of this spirochete can cause febrile illnesses during warmer months ranging from flu-like symptoms to Weil's disease, a severe syndrome marked by hyperbilirubinemia, renal failure, and bleeding. With effort these organisms can be grown from CSF, blood, peritoneal fluid, or urine (200). Specimens must be processed as soon as possible, preferably within one hour. Most routine laboratories will need to send the specimen to a reference laboratory for processing. These bacteria grow best in a semisolid albumin-polysorbide media, which should be incubated at 30°C for one to four months. Of note, organisms can be cultured from the urine later in the course of the illness; thus, urine culture may yield a diagnosis two to four weeks after onset of illness.

Direct visualization of *Leptospira* requires dark-field microscopy (201) or special staining techniques, such as immunofluorescence, immunoperoxidase, and silver stains (200). These methods lack sensitivity and also specificity because of the difficulty in distinguishing true organisms from artifact (200,201). A promising strategy that would allow early confirmation of infection is PCR on clinical specimens (202–209). However, these tests are not available in most centers.

Most diagnoses of leptospirosis are made serologically. The reference standard is a microscopic agglutination assay, but this test is cumbersome and done only in specialized facilities (210). Most centers use an indirect hemagglutinin test, which detects total antibody (211). The accuracy of serology depends on the species prevalent in the region where it is used (212–214). Although 90% of patients will seroconvert within 30 days of becoming ill (215), it is customary to obtain acute and convalescent sera to increase the yield of serology. False positives have been associated with other spirochete infections (216), legionellosis, and autoimmune diseases (215). An EIA test directed at IgM is available and, when positive, will make the diagnosis sooner (217,218). However the false-negative rate ranges from 21% to 48% depending on how early in the course of infection EIA for IgM is done (219).

Borrelia hermsii *and* Borrelia recurrentis *(Relapsing Fever)*

Intermittent spirochetemia with *Borrelia* spp. leads to a relapsing fever syndrome. This zoonosis can be tick-borne (*B. hermsii* and others) or louse-borne (*B. recurrentis*). *Borrelia* spp. can be cultured either in vivo or in vitro, but these methods are not generally available (220). Diagnosis is often based on visualization of spirochetes in the peripheral blood during febrile episodes (221). Routine thick and thin smears using Wright or Giemsa stains can be used to detect the organisms. Darkfield microscopy may also be used. The yield of microscopy is at best 70%, so the procedure may need to be repeated to confirm the diagnosis. Yield may be increased by examining the buffy coat instead of whole blood or by using acridine orange-stained smears (222). With central nervous system involvement these organisms may occasionally be detected by direct smear of CSF.

Serological tests are available, but the relapsing nature of the illness, which is based on antigenic variation (223), complicates the use of these tests (220). Serological tests are used more for epidemiologic purposes and are not widely available. False-positive Lyme or syphilis serology may occur with this infection (216). In such cases, Western blot (Lyme) or antitreponemal serology (syphilis) may help interpret the misleading test results. Glycerophosphodiester phosphodiesterase (GlPQ) antigen is a promising target for future development of a clinically useful, relapsing fever-specific serologic test (220,224,225).

MYCOBACTERIAL CAUSES OF FUO
Mycobacterium Tuberculosis Complex (Tuberculosis)
Tuberculosis (TB) can affect any organ system in both normal and immune-compromised hosts worldwide, and thus should always be in the differential for FUO. Skin testing is most helpful to determine the presence of latent disease in asymptomatic patients. Delayed hypersensitivity to purified protein derivative (PPD), has limited predictive power in the setting of a FUO for a myriad of host-dependent factors. Thus, diagnosis of atypical presentations of tuberculosis requires culture confirmation or the direct detection of organisms in clinical specimens by other means.

Pulmonary, Smear Negative
Patients with FUO due to TB may have nonspecific radiographic abnormalities. Although negative sputum smears for AFB are helpful in determining the need for isolation, they do not exclude the diagnosis. Traditional culture systems start by exposing sputum to chemicals to liquefy the specimen and kill other microorganisms (226). Specimens from sterile body sites, however, do not require decontamination. Solid agar, egg-based media, or liquid broth media may be used to cultivate *M. tuberculosis*, a slow grower that can take up to six weeks to grow. Liquid broth media with automated growth detection may shorten the isolation time to two to four weeks. Once growth has been detected, DNA probes are often available to expedite species determination.

Still, waiting weeks for culture to diagnose smear-negative TB is problematic. PCR designed to detect *M. tuberculosis* DNA or RNA have been developed to diagnose smear-negative disease. These tests still are not as sensitive as culture, detecting only about two-thirds of smear negative infections (227–232). Furthermore, PCR for TB is not yet perfected; any PCR diagnosis should be followed by culture confirmation if possible (233).

Extrapulmonary Tuberculosis
Extrapulmonary tuberculosis can involve any tissue or body site, causing persistent fever. In general, examination of tissues is more sensitive than examination of body fluids. This is why, for example, pleural biopsy is preferable to simple thoracentesis

to make a diagnosis of pleural TB (234,235). Genitourinary or central nervous system involvement can be diagnosed indirectly by examination of urine or CSF, and may be preferable in these infections because of the risk associated with biopsy. Extrapulmonary TB is usually diagnosed via histopathology and culture of tissue obtained from biopsy. Pathologic examination should reveal granulomas. If caseous necrosis is present along with AFB on special stains, a diagnosis of TB is likely. Stains for fungi should also be included because they can cause similar findings on histopathology. Even when granulomas are detected with AFB in the absence of fungi, culture confirmation should be attempted whenever possible because other mycobacteria are also pathogenic in humans. Although not as well-studied in extrapulmonary TB, PCR has been tried on nonrespiratory specimens, with promising initial results (229,236,237). The role, if any, for rapid testing in extrapulmonary disease remains to be established.

Interestingly, elevated adenosine deaminase (ADA) activity is often present in fluid specimens taken from patients with TB. ADA levels are measurable in cerebrospinal, bronchial lavage (238), pleural, and pericardial fluids. In one series, for example, ADA activity in pericardial fluid was significantly higher in patients with confirmed or probable TB pericarditis than in malignant or normal controls (239). Using an ADA activity cutoff of 40 U/L in this small study population, the test had a sensitivity of 93% and a specificity of 97%. Sensitivity may be lower in patients with military TB (240) and when applied to CSF samples (241). Moreover, brucellosis can cause elevation in CSF ADA (242). Because determinations of ADA activity are quick and relatively inexpensive, these tests are worth studying in larger patient populations to help guide early empiric therapy for TB. Confirmation of these results and determination of optimal cutoffs are needed prior to widespread use of ADA testing for the diagnosis of TB. As PCR becomes less expensive and more widely available, ADA, a simple biochemical test, will have to compete with rapid molecular-based tests as well as routine clinical evaluation and culture (241).

Miliary Tuberculosis

The term miliary tuberculosis is now used to refer to disseminated hematogenous infection with *M. tuberculosis* (243,244), and thus classic radiographic findings may not be present (240,245). Patients with impaired cellular immunity are at increased risk for miliary tuberculosis (246), and such patients often will present with FUO. These patients rarely (10% of the time) have a positive PPD (245). Diagnosis depends on culturing multiple fluids and tissues because no one type of culture is highly sensitive. Blood cultures in patients with AIDS, for example, have a sensitivity of at best 60% (247,248). Other noninvasive culture sources include sputum, urine, and gastric aspirates. Of note, urine cultures for mycobacteria should not be sent in the general urine culture tubes because they are too small and often contain preservatives, such as boric acid and sodium formate, which prevent the growth of AFB.

Other, more invasive, options include biopsy and culture of lymph nodes, liver, and bone marrow. Liver biopsy has the highest yield (240), but is also more risky than lymph node or bone marrow biopsy. Bone marrow aspirates are most likely to be positive in the setting of pancytopenia (240,249). Diagnosis of progressive disseminated TB as a cause of FUO requires a balance between the aggressive pursuit of a diagnostic specimen and due caution when subjecting a patient to the morbidity of invasive procedures. Till date, there is no suitable gold standard.

Mycobacterium Avium Complex

Disseminated *Mycobacterium avium* intracellulare (MAI) infection is a prevalent cause of FUO in patients with advanced HIV disease, usually in those with a CD4 count $<50/mm^3$. Isolation of MAI from a usually sterile body site in a patient with AIDS and FUO is strong evidence of infection. Positive cultures from a lymph node, liver or spleen, however, may occasionally represent localized disease, and thus should be interpreted with caution. Isolation from a bone marrow aspirate is strong evidence for disseminated disease; this procedure may help establish the diagnosis in the rare cases in which blood cultures are negative (249). MAI can also be detected in sputum, urine, gastric or colonic tissue, or stool. Isolation from one such site can reflect mere colonization. However, disseminated disease becomes more likely as the number of sites from which MAI is isolated increases.

The most reliable way to diagnose disseminated MAI is by performing two separate blood cultures for AFB (248,249). This method will detect systemic infection 99% of the time (250,251). Incubation in liquid media has shortened the interval to detect growth, which often is <2 weeks. Six weeks are still needed, however, to finalize a culture as negative. Once isolated, DNA probes can be used to confirm the organism as MAI. A direct blood smear for AFB has low sensitivity even in advanced disease (249,252). Although a positive smear is suggestive, patients with HIV are at risk for other disseminated AFB infections—for example, TB. PCR tests have been developed to hasten the detection of MAI in blood cultures and may be as accurate as blood cultures (253–255). In the future, as PCR becomes more routine, this test may be preferred to blood cultures.

FUNGAL CAUSES OF FUO
Endemic Fungi

Most endemic mycoses, such as coccidioidomycosis or blastomycosis, occur with localizing signs and symptoms that, when coupled with pertinent exposure histories, suggest the diagnosis. With the notable exception of histoplasmosis, endemic fungal infections are rare causes of FUO.

Histoplasma capsulatum (Histoplasmosis)

Histoplasma capsulatum is a dimorphic fungus that usually causes self-limited infections in normal hosts. However, in patients with impaired cell-mediated immunity, *H. capsulatum* can cause progressive disseminated infection with significant morbidity and mortality (256,257). *Histoplasma capsulatum* can be cultured from sputum, blood, bone marrow (249) or other tissues; however, the yield is variable and dependent on several host factors. Sputum or biopsy specimens can be cultured onto brain-heart infusion agar with chemicals added to select out bacteria and saprophytic fungi (258). Incubation will often yield growth in as little as one week, but the cultures should be observed for at least three weeks. The organism can be isolated from pericardium or pleura, but is seldom cultivated from pleural or pericardial fluid. CSF from patients with central nervous system involvement can yield a positive culture. It is important to note, however, that high volume samples of CSF increase yield because the fungi have a predilection for the basal meninges (257,259).

Blood or bone marrow cultures have a sensitivity approaching 50% (260). Dedicated fungal blood cultures using lysis centrifugation technique increases the yield.

Immunologic testing includes skin testing and serology. In the past, skin testing was done in a manner analogous to PPD testing for TB, but is no longer available commercially. Skin test positivity is poorly correlated with active infection due to the high prevalence of skin test positivity in endemic areas. Moreover, those patients at highest risk for disseminated infection have impaired cell-mediated immunity that may lead to false-negative skin testing (261). Serology is available (261,262), but its role is limited to retrospective confirmation of histoplama infection in acute pulmonary syndromes. Seroconversion often does not occur in patients with disseminated infection (261).

Detection of the organism in blood or other tissues is a highly specific means of diagnosis (261). Dedicated inspection of Giemsa or Wright stained peripheral blood smears will detect the organisms in some patients with disseminated disease. Periodic acid-Schiff or silver stains of pathologic specimens will demonstrate organisms when present, and thus can suggest the diagnosis.

Species-specific polysaccharide antigen can be detected from blood, CSF, or urine using EIA. Urinary antigen detection is widely available and is the most accurate and efficient method available for diagnosis of disseminated histoplasmosis (260,263), with a yield approaching 90%. Moreover, unlike serological tests, urine antigen tests can be used to detect relapses. These tests are very specific; however, cross-reactions can occur with infections caused by *Blastomyces dermatitidis, Paracoccidioides brasiliensis,* or *Penicillium marneffei.* First-generation assays were also susceptible to false positives owing to the presence of heterophile antibodies (264,265). This problem has been largely eliminated in second-generation assays.

VIRAL CAUSES OF FUO
Herpes Viruses
Epstein Barr Virus
Infection with Epstein Barr Virus (EBV) is very common and frequently asymptomatic. Symptomatic disease may be mild and nonspecific, or can cause infectious mononucleosis or even more severe febrile syndromes with atypical features. Although the presence of atypical lymphocytes on a peripheral blood smear is suggestive (266,267), the diagnosis is made serologically. Heterophile antibodies are detected when a patient's serum agglutinates red blood cells from another species. When present in the context of an acute febrile illness, they are suggestive of EBV (268). However, heterophile antibody production may be delayed such that early false negatives often occur. Furthermore, their presence is transient. Thus alternative serologic tests are often relied upon.

Viral capsid antibodies (VCA) are often used. Because clinical disease caused by EBV has a long incubation period, by the time a patient is symptomatic isotype class switching often has already occurred, leading to detectable IgG and undetectable IgM. Thus the presence of IgG can indicate either past infection or an acute, more recent infection. Epstein-Barr nuclear antibody (EBNA), which occurs only after resolution of infection, will help interpret a positive VCA-IgG test (269). Consequently, the pattern of antibodies that would suggest EBV as the cause of FUO is a positive VCA-IgG and a negative EBNA. The presence of heterophile antibodies or VCA-IgM helps support the diagnosis but is unreliable (269–271).

Cytomegalovirus
Active cytomegalovirus (CMV) disease is notoriously difficult to diagnose. Widespread seropositivity by adulthood, intermittent shedding of live virus

even in healthy persons, and unusual serological patterns mar attempts at establishing a diagnosis. CMV can cause a mononucleosis-like syndrome in adolescents or adults and mild nonspecific illness in children. Occasionally CMV can cause severe, persistent disease, most notably in immune-compromised patients.

CMV IgG has little diagnostic value, as up to 60% of the population are seropositive. Counterintuitively, CMV IgM does not correlate well with acute disease and false-positive rates as high as 75% have been documented. Thus routine serology has little if any role in the diagnosis of acute CMV disease (272). A possible exception is retrospective diagnosis using IgG seroconversion.

Instead, the diagnosis of CMV must be made by detecting the virus itself. Convincing evidence may come from the pathologist when characteristic cytopathic changes are detected in affected tissues. Immunohistochemistry may increase the yield from biopsy (273). Alternatively, the virus may be detected from blood, saliva, or urine. Isolation of CMV from the blood, although not perfect (274), does suggest active infection more than periodic shedding in the nasopharynx, for example. Viral cultures, PCR, and antigen detection are methods with varying availability. Most microbiology labs will culture CMV by inoculating clinical specimens into human fibroblast cell lines (273). Detection of virus has been hastened by using monoclonal antibodies to detect early antigens well before cytopathic effects would be detected. These are the so-called "shell vial" assays, which may detect virus in as little as 24 hours.

Alternatively, multiple assays have been developed to directly detect CMV antigens or DNA in clinical specimens. The antigenemia test uses monoclonal antibodies to detect pp64, a viral matrix protein, in peripheral blood polymorphonuclear leukocytes (275). Antigen test results are reported as a ratio between the number of cells positive to the total number of cells evaluated. Multiple PCR tests have been developed that are highly sensitive. Ultrasensitive molecular techniques are compromised by both the prolonged and intermittent presence of CMV in humans, even in the absence of disease. Many of these assays are quantitative, which is necessary because the mere presence of virion components can occur in the absence of disease. Correlation with active disease or development of disease has been studied (276–280). Currently these molecular tests need standardization. Complicating standardization is the likelihood that every type of immune-compromised host will need different cutoffs to attribute a febrile syndrome to CMV. Research is being conducted to determine what breakpoints will be most meaningful (275,278,281–285).

Human Immunodeficiency Virus

Acute seroconversion syndrome has protean manifestations and should be high on the list of FUO for any patient with risk factors for human immunodeficiency virus (HIV) acquisition (286–288). Patients are systemically ill, often with flu-like symptoms including fever, myalgias, and headache (289). Nonspecific rashes, lymphadenopathy, and meningeal inflammation may occur. The syndrome is caused by the host's initial immune response, and usually reflects high grade viremia with an acute drop in T-lymphocytes (288). As the syndrome resolves the CD8 cells increase more rapidly than CD4 cells. Symptomatic illness usually occurs within six weeks of exposure to HIV. Clinical suspicion should prompt further testing, which needs careful interpretation, but will usually establish a diagnosis. Uncommonly, patients with acute HIV infection may develop opportunistic infections; thus, illnesses more often associated with advanced HIV disease should also be considered and tested for when appropriate.

Enzyme Immunoassay with Confirmatory Western Blot
The currently employed third generation EIA test is more sensitive than earlier assays. Cases of seroconversion syndrome that may have been missed by EIA previously will often be detected (288,290). Furthermore, a positive test may indicate prior infection with HIV, thus altering the diagnostic evaluation of a patient with FUO. Negative or indeterminate test results should prompt repeat testing up to six months later (291). Other testing, outlined below, may help make the diagnosis in the meantime.

P24 Antigen and Viral Load
HIV p24 antigen is a Gag protein and may be detected in up to 88% of patients with acute seroconversion syndrome (288,292). This test is highly specific and will help make the diagnosis in seronegative patients. The negative predictive value, however, is unacceptably low given the stakes. So detection of viral RNA is often used because of its high (100%) sensitivity (291). A high level of reported HIV viremia (usually greater that 100,000 copies/mL) indicates acute HIV infection in a seronegative patient. The drawback of using a viral load is the higher risk of a false positive, with the attendant psychological distress and increased cost, when compared with p24 antigen assays (292,293). False positives should be suspected with low levels of reported viremia, usually <10,000 copies/mL. Despite the additional information these assays provide in the acute setting, any patient tested for HIV should have a repeat HIV EIA with confirmatory Western blot done up to six months later.

PARASITIC CAUSES OF FUO
Protozoa
Plasmodium Species (Malaria)
Infection with *Plasmodium* spp. usually causes fever, but the classic patterns of periodicity that would suggest the diagnosis are often absent during the initial course of illness. Malaria must be considered in anyone with FUO and a history of travel to an endemic area, blood transfusion or needle sharing (294). Diagnosis depends on examination of the peripheral blood smear by experienced personnel (295). Thick and thin smears of peripheral blood should be performed and then subjected to Giemsa staining. Thick smears are nearly forty times as concentrated as thin smears and increase the detection rate of parasites. Thick smears, which can also help quantify parasitemia, should be examined at high-power magnification (×400) and under oil immersion for 20 minutes or until 200 high-power fields have been examined. Thin smears, on the other hand, are used differentiate the four human *Plasmodium* species. Mature forms of *Plasmodium falciparum* are sequestered in the microvasculature, and thus are seldom detected in samples of peripheral blood. Therefore, serial blood samples should be examined twice daily to detect the immature forms, which can appear in the blood stream intermittently.

Rapid diagnostic tests for malaria are under development and are helpful when experienced personnel are not available (296–299). These tests may also be used when the diagnosis of falciparum malaria is still suspected despite initially negative light microscopy. One such test, in fact, is designed to detect *P. falciparum*. It uses a monoclonal antibody directed against the histidine-rich protein (HRP) 2 found in this parasite. Unfortunately, some *P. falciparum* strains produce too little HRP-2 to be detected. Still, the test is rapid, easy to perform, and sensitive. Its specificity can be limited by the fact that the antigen remains detectable for up to one month after infection. Also, cross reactivity with rheumatoid factor can cause a false positive test.

Another available rapid test can detect all four species of *Plasmodium* known to infect humans (300,301). It relies on the detection of *Plasmodium* lactate dehydrogenase. This test is as sensitive for *P. falciparum* as the HRP-2 based assay. Although convenient, neither type of rapid diagnostic test is as accurate as serial peripheral blood microscopy by an experienced technician (296,302–305). PCR assays have been studied for the diagnosis of malaria (296,301,306–309); though accurate, these tests are not yet available for widespread use. When used directly on blood smears that are also used for microscopy, care must be taken not to contaminate the slide leading to false-positive PCR (310).

Babesia *Species (Babesiosis)*

This tick-borne illness is caused by numerous *Babesia* spp. that infect human erythrocytes and cause a febrile syndrome marked by hemolysis (311). Usually mild, this illness can mimic malaria in its severity when immune-compromised hosts (311), especially asplenic patients, are infected (312). Direct microscopic examination of Giemsa-stained blood smears is the usual means of diagnosis (295,313). Organisms are most commonly detected in ring forms that are similar in appearance to the ring forms seen in falciparum malaria. Considerable expertise is needed to differentiate the two and the following features of babesiosis may be used: (*i*) absence of hemozoin; (*ii*) lack of schizonts or synchronous states; (*iii*) absence of gametocytes; and (*iv*) presence of merozoite tetrads (so-called Maltese crosses) (312). Using in vivo techniques, the diagnosis of *B. microti* can be made by inoculation of infected blood into hamsters, whereas the diagnosis of *B. divergens* can be made using gerbils. After inoculation into the peritoneum, two to four weeks is required for the peripheral blood smears to turn positive in these animals.

Serologic tests for *B. microti* have been developed (313) but are often not readily available. IFA titers of at least 1:256 are specific for acute infection, but seroconversion may occur later in the course of illness (311,314–316). Somewhat analogous to the diagnostic dilemma of the peripheral smear, IFA tests cross-react with *P. falciparum*. EIA (317), immunohistochemistry (318), and PCR (313,319–320) techniques are in development in the hopes of providing increased accuracy and species-specific diagnosis.

Leishmania donovani *and Other Species (Kala–Azar, Visceral Leishmaniasis)*

Leishmania donovani and other *Leishmania* spp. can cause clinical syndromes ranging from limited skin involvement to disseminated infection of the reticuloendothelial system (321). The latter syndrome is called visceral leishmaniasis and is more likely to occur in hosts with impaired cell-mediated immunity (322,323). However, even normal hosts can develop disseminated disease with *Leishmania* spp. that have increased tropism for visceral tissues. For example, unusually invasive strains of *L. tropica* were found to cause visceral leishmaniasis in Americans who served in the Persian Gulf War (321,324). Patients with FUO occurring within a year of travel to India, Africa, South America, the Mediterranean, or the Middle East should be evaluated for Leishmania infection, especially if they have impaired cell-mediated immunity.

Although the diagnosis can be made clinically in endemic areas, the diagnosis in the United States depends on laboratory confirmation. Methods of diagnosis include visualization of organisms, culture, and serology. Needle aspiration of the spleen, bone marrow, liver, or lymph nodes (325) is often needed to establish a diagnosis. The yield is greatest from the spleen (326,327), but this procedure also has a higher risk of bleeding complications (328). Material obtained can be cultured onto special media available from the CDC (329,330). The cultures should be incubated at room temperature and, when positive, will yield motile promastigotes. Growth may be detected in as little as three days, but it often takes several weeks.

Clinical specimens can also be subjected to Wright or Giemsa staining, which allows detection of amastigotes, an asexual stage of *Leishmania* found in human reticuloendothelial cells (330). Amastigotes appear as small (3–5 μm) organisms with blue cytoplasm and red, eccentrically located nuclei. Organisms may also be detected in buffy coat smears, or atypically infected tissues, such as lung or gastrointestinal mucosa, especially in a patient with impaired cellular immunity (331).

Serologic testing is available using several methods including an EIA and a dipstick test (322,332–335). In the former, specific antileishmanial antibodies are detected. In the latter, reactions between host serum and a recombinant antigen are detected. These tests are highly sensitive in immunocompetent patients and are especially useful in patients who normally live outside of endemic areas. False positives occur in the presence of some other infections, including cutaneous leishmaniasis, leprosy, and Chagas disease. Patients with advanced HIV disease often do not generate significant antileismanial titers, thus serologic testing has low sensitivity in this high-risk population (336–338). To facilitate diagnosis in resource poor locales, serological tests using urine are being developed (339–342). PCR tests have been devised, but are not yet available for routine clinical use (343–348).

A reasonable approach to diagnosis in nonendemic areas would be to inspect smears obtained from a buffy coat and to check serology. If both of these tests are negative, especially in a patient with marked cellular immunodeficiency, needle aspirates of the spleen, liver or bone marrow should be obtained for culture and pathologic examination. Biopsies of other organs, such as the lung, may be positive if directly involved in advanced cases of leishmaniasis.

Toxoplasma gondii *(Toxoplasmosis)*

Toxoplasma gondii, despite its worldwide prevalence, rarely causes febrile illness. This sporozoan parasite is acquired via ingestion of infected meat or through direct or indirect contact with cat feces. Organisms may disseminate widely to many tissues but are usually kept in check by the host's immune system. Patients with impaired cellular immunity are at increased risk for symptomatic acute infection or reactivation disease. We are used to thinking of toxoplasmosis in patients with advanced HIV and brain lesions. However, disseminated toxoplasmosis can be associated with fever and a myriad of signs or symptoms depending on the organ system affected. In humans, *T. gondii* exists in either a tachyzoite or bradyzoite form (349,350). The former replicates rapidly and detection of it in a symptomatic patient suggests active infection.

Diagnosis of infection may be made using various combinations of serology, culture, molecular amplification or histopathology. *T. gondii* can be cultured (350) from tissue or blood in vitro using cell lines used in routine viral cultures; however, this technique is done only at reference laboratories. Growth can be detected using special stains within one week. In vivo culture using mice is more sensitive but is slower and not readily available in most laboratories. Direct microscopic inspection of biopsied tissues may yield a diagnosis (350). The presence of tachyzoites implies active disease. Encysted bradyzoite forms most often reflect latent infection; however, a heavy parasite burden with surrounding host inflammatory response can also suggest active toxoplasmosis. Organisms may be visualized using Wright or Giemsa stains or immunohistochemistry. In immunocompetent patients, characteristic lymph node pathology, even without the direct visualization of organisms, can establish the diagnosis (351,352).

PCR assays have been developed to detect *T. gondii* in clinical specimens. Although highly specific, the sensitivity depends on the type of assay used along with the quantity of parasite present in the fluid tested (353–362). PCR has been used on CSF, whole blood, buffy coats, urine, ocular fluids, respiratory secretions, as well as placental and fetal tissue. Sensitivity of PCR on blood from patients with disseminated disease approaches 90%.

Serology can establish the diagnosis in immunocompetent patients. EIA and IFA assays directed against IgM, IgG, and even IgE or IgA, antibodies, are widely available (362–364). IgG seroconversion, with or without the initial presence of IgM antibodies, establishes the diagnosis of acute infection in a symptomatic patient (365). Patients with impaired cell-mediated immunity, however, usually have reactivation disease, thus seroconversion cannot be relied upon for diagnosis. In fact, a negative IgG titer makes the diagnosis of toxoplasmosis less likely in an immune-compromised patient. Seronegative recipients of solid organ transplants may acquire disseminated infection acutely. In this setting, early antibody levels may either be too low for detection or may be detectable in the absence of clinically significant illness; thus, the use of serology in transplant patients is problematic. In short, although serology may establish a diagnosis of toxoplasmosis in normal hosts, the diagnosis in patients with impaired cell-mediated immunity requires direct evidence of infection via culture, PCR, or histopathology.

Flatworms
Schistosoma *Species (Katayama Fever, Schistosomiasis)*
Katayama fever occurs in a minority of persons with schistosomiasis and reflects acute infection in patients exposed for the first time to *Schistosoma* spp., usually *japonicum* or *mansoni*. Travelers returning from South America, Africa, or Asia are at risk for this serum sickness-like illness (366). The incubation period is between two to eight weeks after exposure to contaminated fresh water. The cornerstone of diagnosis is the visualization of eggs on microscopic examination of stool, urine, or infected tissues. Repeated exams or concentration of specimens may be needed to detect the organisms (367). If stool and urine specimens are negative, biopsies of rectal or bladder mucosa may be positive (366,368).

Serological tests are useful for Katayama Fever because patients, by definition, have not had remote prior exposure to *Schistosoma* antigens. Accordingly, a positive serological test in a symptomatic traveler constitutes strong evidence of disease. EIA is available in some commercial laboratories and is superbly sensitive and specific for exposure to *S. mansoni* (369). However, its sensitivity for *S. japonicum* is <50%. Species-specific IFA or newer EIA and Western blot tests may be requested if infection by non-*mansoni* species of *Schistosoma* infections is suspected despite unrevealing microscopic inspection and EIA serology (370–372).

NONINFECTIOUS INFLAMMATORY CAUSES OF FUO

A variety of inflammatory syndromes occur that have no known infectious etiology. Some are archetypal autoimmune disorders, such as systemic lupus erythematosus. For others, the host response is likely to be appropriate and directed at yet undis-covered infectious agents: Kikuchi-Fujimoto disease is a noteworthy example. Most of the following conditions are diagnosed through a combination of clinical evaluation and judicious use of laboratory tests or pathologic examination of biopsy specimens. Although specific tests that are associated with the following conditions are discussed, their predictive value is limited in the absence of a com-patible clinical syndrome.

IMMUNE MEDIATED
Vasculitis
Temporal Arteritis
Temporal arteritis (TA), also known as giant cell arteritis, is a systemic vasculitis that is an important cause of FUO in the elderly. Some series report that as many as 16% of FUO's in elderly patients are caused by this disorder (373). Diagnostic modalities include erythrocyte sedimentation rate (ESR), ultrasound of the tem-poral arteries and arterial biopsy, all of which have pitfalls. Classically ESR is mark-edly elevated in TA; in fact one of the five American College of Rheumatology criteria for the diagnosis of TA is an elevated ESR (374), which is usually >50. However, there has been a significant minority of well-documented cases with mild or even no elevation in the ESR. In one series, nine of 167 biopsy-confirmed cases had ESR <40 (375). Causes of low ESR in TA include localized disease and impaired serological immune response. Thus, ESR cannot be used to rule out this entity.
    Diagnosis of TA usually depends on pathology. However, the chief diffi-culty with pathologic confirmation of TA is that the vascular abnormalities are discontinuous. Thus sampling error may lead to false-negative results. Although the diagnostic accuracy of ultrasound used alone is controversial (376,377), it may be helpful when used to guide temporal artery biopsy. Some experts advocate bilateral biopsies of large portions of the temporal artery (378). Patho-logic evaluation, when positive, reveals granulomatous and lymphocytic inflam-mation involving the wall of the temporal artery often with characteristic giant cells.

Pauci-Immune or Antineutrophil Cytoplasmic Antibodies-Associated Vasculitides
Antineutrophil cytoplasmic antibodies (ANCA) have been associated with several pauci-immune vasculitides. These conditions are called pauci-immune because no immune complex deposition is visualized on pathologic specimens. ANCA are directed towards antigens in neutrophil cytoplasm and may create either cyto-plasmic or perinuclear patterns on immunofluoroescence stains: hence "c"-ANCA and "p"-ANCA (379). Specific antigens responsible for the staining patterns have been identified. Proteinase 3 (PR-3) is an enzyme present in neutrophil lysosomal granules and is the chief antigen responsible for c-ANCA. On the other hand,

p-ANCA is less specific and may be directed toward multiple antigens, including lactoferrin, elastase, and cathepsin-D. The most specific antibody causing this staining pattern is anti-myeloperoxidase (anti-MPO), which is more helpful than p-ANCA alone for diagnosing pauci-immune vasculitis. Anti-PR-3 and anti-MPO antibodies can be detected using EIA.

Wegener's Granulomatosis
This systemic vasculitis is associated with granulomas (often necrotizing) of small to medium blood vessels and classically involves the sinuses, lungs, or kidneys. The sensitivity of anti-PR-3 antibodies or c-ANCA varies between 63% and 91% and probably depends on the point in the course of disease when the tests are performed (379). Sensitivity increases as the disease progresses. As serological tests have low sensitivity, a negative test should not dissuade further workup. On the other hand, these tests are over 90% specific for Wegener's. Still, the positive predictive value can be quite low if this test is not used judiciously because of the rarity of this illness. In practice, most cases are confirmed pathologically because of the high stakes associated with diagnosis: namely, treatment with powerful immunosuppresants, such as cyclophosphamide.

Churg-Strauss Syndrome
Similar to Wegener's, Churg-Strauss syndrome is a systemic pauci-immune vasculitis associated with granulomatous inflammation. Peripheral eosinophilia, atopy, and asthma are hallmarks of this syndrome. The sinopulmonary involvement is often less destructive when compared with Wegener's. Pathology reveals eosinophil-rich inflammatory lesions both in and outside of vessels, with a predilection for smaller vessels than Wegener's. Anti-MPO are moderately specific for this condition, but are also seen in microscopic polyangiitis (379).

Microscopic Polyangiitis
Microscopic polyangiitis (MPA) is a systemic vasculitis that, similar to Churg-Strauss syndrome, is associated with anti-MPO antibodies in up to 70% of cases (379). Unlike both Wegener's and Churg-Strauss syndrome, MPA is not associated with granulomas. This vasculitis affects small vessels and is often associated with glomerulonephritis or alveolar hemorrhage (380). The diagnosis depends on pathologic findings on lung or kidney biopsy, which reveal necrotizing vasculitis with little or no immune-complex deposition. Unlike periarteritis nodosa (discussed later), MPA has a predilection for the smallest vessels and can involve veins as well as arteries and capillaries.

Periarteritis Nodosa
Periarteritis nodosa (PAN) is another systemic pauci-immune vasculitis but tends to involve larger vessels than does MPA (380). Another contrasting point for PAN is the low prevalence of anti-MPO antibodies when compared to MPA. The diagnosis of PAN is often made via mesenteric angiography, which reveals characteristic microaneurysms, even in the absence of overt gastrointestinal symptoms. In patients with mononeuritis multiplex, biopsies of associated nerves and/or muscles often can lead to a diagnosis as well. Pathologic evaluation reveals segmental vascular lesions, which tend to form at arterial branch points. Granulomas

should be absent and varying degrees of intimal proliferation are seen, sometimes with intraluminal thrombosis. PAN is associated with hepatitis B in up to 10% of cases; so it is reasonable to exclude HBV with routine serological testing when the diagnosis of PAN has been made (381).

Rheumatoid Arthritis

Incomplete or early presentations of rheumatoid arthritis (RA) may lead to a febrile syndrome without a clear cause. Nonspecific markers of inflammation, such as, ESR or C reative protein (CRP), are commonly elevated. Oftentimes clinicians request a rheumatoid factor (RF) in the face of diagnostic uncertainty. RF represents antibodies directed against other antibodies, classically IgM reacting to the Fc portion of IgG (379). Unfortunately, the test characteristics leave something to be desired. Many illnesses marked by systemic inflammation, such as endocarditis, hepatitis, or tuberculosis, are also associated with RF. If applied to an unselected population, the positive predictive value of RF ranges from 20% to 30%. Furthermore, especially early in the course of RA, RF may be absent and therefore cannot be used to exclude this rheumatologic condition.

A newer serological test, anticyclic citrullinated peptide (anti-CCP), has greater diagnostic accuracy than RF (382). Citrulline is an amino acid that is created by enzymatic modification of arginine in synovial fluid. The resultant proteins containing citrulline may be pathologic autoantigens in RA. Its sensitivity, although greater than RF, is still at best 75%. The best feature of this test is its improved specificity, which is at least 98%. Thus, though not diagnostic, a positive test in the right clinical context should encourage careful consideration of RA or other autoimmune conditions, such as Sjogren's. Unlike RF, systemic infections such as hepatitis tend not to produce anti-CCP.

Systemic Lupus Erythematosus

Systemic lupus erythematosus (SLE) is a systemic autoimmune disease with protean manifestations, including fever. One of the diagnostic criteria for SLE, which is, in fact, a hallmark of the disease, is the presence of antinuclear antibodies (ANA) (383,384). These autoantibodies react to components of the cell nucleus (379). They are detected via indirect immunofluorescence using human HEp2 tumor cells. Clinically, significant titers are ≥1:160. Laboratories also report patterns of ANA immunofluorescence. Although speckled and homogenous patterns are nonspecific, a nucleolar pattern is somewhat specific for SLE, but may also be seen in systemic sclerosis or myositis. A peripheral staining pattern correlates with anti-dsDNA antibodies, and thus is suggestive of SLE.

Antinuclear antibodies are almost universally present in SLE, with sensitivity cited as high as 95% to 100%. In fact, controversy exists over whether ANA-negative lupus even exists.

Because of the high sensitivity of ANA for SLE, it is reasonable to check for ANA when evaluating a patient with FUO. If these antibodies are truly absent, one has effectively ruled out SLE, especially if the presentation lacks clinical features suggestive of lupus. The main caveat is that a positive ANA does not establish the diagnosis of SLE in a patient with FUO. Several other rheumatologic conditions as well as infections are well known to induce antinuclear antibodies.

Inflammatory Disorders of Uncertain Etiology

Kikuchi-Fujimoto Disease

Kikuchi disease is a syndrome involving cervical lymphadenopathy (usually posterior) often in association with fever or rash (385). It may be suspected when tests for infectious mononucleosis are negative in young, otherwise healthy adults. Diagnosis relies on pathology and requires an experienced pathologist to exclude lymphoma or adenopathy associated with SLE (386,387). Pathology reveals chronic inflammatory nodules, which may be confluent or patchy, with coagulative necrosis. Neutrophils are seldom seen. Excisional biopsy of a lymph node is ideal, but the diagnosis is made via fine needle aspiration as well (388). An ANA may be helpful if the pathologist cannot exclude SLE through pathologic evaluation alone.

Adult-Onset Still's Disease

Adult-onset Still's disease can cause a prolonged febrile syndrome often with only nonspecific signs and symptoms. Still's disease is a clinical diagnosis because no definitive serological markers or pathologic findings are yet available. Dramatically elevated ferritin levels, however, are suggestive of this disorder.

Inflammatory Bowel Disease (IBD)

Both ulcerative colitis and Crohn's disease may have atypical presentations in which fever and extra-intestinal symptoms predominate. These idiopathic inflammatory disorders should be considered particularly when there is an abnormal abdominal or rectal examination. Radiographic studies may suggest the diagnosis, but direct inspection via endoscopy with biopsy is needed to confirm the clinical impression and exclude other diseases (389,390). Endoscopically, ulcerative colitis usually shows continuous inflammation of the large bowel mucosa, whereas Crohn's disease usually shows discontinuous inflammatory lesions with a predilection for the terminal ileum. Multiple biopsies should be obtained and subjected to both pathologic and microbiologic studies. For example, tuberculosis can affect the terminal ileum, mimicking Crohn's disease; thus, mycobacterial cultures should be done. Other mimics that should be considered include enteric fever, pseudomembranous colitis, radiation colitis, and ischemic colitis.

Traditionally the diagnosis of IBD has been made when a patient has consistent radiographic, endoscopic, and pathologic findings, and other infectious and noninfectious causes of bowel inflammation have been excluded. Autoantibodies are being increasingly used to help diagnose indeterminate colitis (391,392). The most widely used of these are anti-*Saccharomyces cerevisiae* (ASCA) antibodies and atypical p-ANCA. Atypical p-ANCA occurs when the perinuclear staining pattern is detected on immunofluorescence but is due to antigens other than MPO resulting in a negative anti-MPO test (Terjung 2000) (393). Atypical p-ANCA is associated with ulcerative colitis, whereas ASCA is associated with Crohn's disease. The diagnostic utility of autoantibodies to diagnose idiopathic IBD is still under evaluation. These tests have not been studied from the perspective of a FUO evaluation, and so should be reserved to help distinguish ulcerative colitis from Crohn's disease when other etiologies of fever and bowel inflammation have been excluded.

Behçet's Disease

Behçet's disease is an idiopathic systemic illness with protean manifestations of chronic vascular inflammation. A classic presentation (uveitis, arthritis, and marked mucosal ulceration) will suggest the diagnosis (394), but occasionally these patients may undergo evaluations for FUO when more subtle presentations occur. Tests for celiac sprue, SLE, HSV, IBD, cyclic neutropenia, and HIV should be considered early in the evaluation to exclude these entities. Diagnosis relies on careful clinical assessments of skin, mucous membranes, and eyes (395). Pathergy skin tests or biopsy of mucocutaneous lesions may help support the diagnosis.

The pathergy skin test is done on the volar aspect of the forearm using a sterile 20-guage needle. The needle should be inserted obliquely to the skin surface to a depth of half centimeter. It is rotated slightly and removed. A physician then examines the site one to two days later. The test is considered positive if a red papule ($\geq$2 mm) or a pustule is found at the sight of insertion. This test is most sensitive during episodes of increased disease activity. For unknown reasons, patients with Behçet's disease from North America or northern Europe are less likely to have a positive pathergy test (395).

Dermatopathology can also help support the diagnosis and exclude other diseases. Early mucocutaneous lesions show neutrophilic inflammation of blood vessels with edematous changes to the endothelium (396). Extravasation of red blood cells and leukocytotoclasia are also seen. Fully developed lesions may demonstrate leukocytoclastic vasculitis with or without fibrinoid necrosis of the vessels.

Periodic Fever Syndromes

Genetically acquired syndromes associated with recurrent fever have been identified. These disorders should be suspected when there is a chronic history of recurrent fever or FUO coupled with serosal, synovial, or cutaneous inflammation, especially in a patient with a family history of a similar affliction. The diagnostic options for some well-described syndromes are discussed in the following section.

Familial Mediterranean Fever

This autosomal recessive disease occurs in peoples of Mediterranean descent and is marked by sporadic episodes of fever and serosal inflammation (397). The gene mutations responsible affect MEFV, a gene located in chromosome 16p. Genetic testing for all known mutations is available and will often help with the diagnosis. However, as many as 45% of patients diagnosed with this illness in the United States do not harbor a known genetic mutation (398). The diagnosis in these cases is usually made clinically. Dramatic response to a therapeutic trial of colchicine lends support to the clinical impression.

Some other confirmatory diagnostic tests have been explored. In one such test, patients are challenged with metaraminol, a peripheral vasoconstrictor (399). Patients with familial Mediterranean fever (FMF) are much more likely than controls to develop a symptomatic episode. The fact that this disorder is thought by some to be mediated via abnormal catecholamine metabolism provides a plausible rationale for the increased sensitivity of FMF patients to metaraminol provocation.

Plasma level of dopamine beta-hydroxylase is another proposed diagnostic test for FMF that relies on abnormal catecholamine metabolism (400). Dopamine beta-hydroxylase activity was found in one series to be significantly elevated in untreated patients whether or not they were symptomatic. These tests involving catecholamine activity are not standardized nor relied upon in practice to make the diagnosis of FMF. As more genetic mutations are identified, increasingly sensitive genetic testing panels will probably obviate the need for other means of testing.

Hyper-IgD Syndrome
This autosomal recessive disorder occurs in patients of northern European descent and its hallmark is recurrent episodes of fever with lymphadenopathy (397). The mutations responsible have been localized to chromosome 12q and affect the meva-lonate kinase gene. The gene product is an enzyme needed for cholesterol and non-sterol isoprene synthesis. Genetic testing helps establish the diagnosis, but is unnecessary if a patient has a compatible clinical history with a repeatedly elevated IgD. Two abnormal measurements at least one month apart will suffice. Despite the name, not all symptomatic patients with the genetic defect have an elevated IgD. Thus, genetic testing should be pursued when normal IgD levels are found in a patient with a compatible syndrome.

TNF Receptor-Associated Periodic Syndrome
This autosomal dominant disorder may occur in multiple ethnic groups and is characterized by prolonged recurrent episodes of fever often associated with pleur-isy, arthralgias, myalgias, and migratory erythema (397). The disease is caused by mutations in TNFRSF1A, a gene located on chromosome 12p that encodes a TNF receptor. Because of incomplete penetrance and spontaneous disease causing mutations, this illness should be suspected even in the absence of a family history when faced with a suggestive clinical syndrome. Diagnosis relies on the demonstration of a TNFRSF1A mutation in a patient with recurrent episodes of systemic inflammation.

MALIGNANT CAUSES OF FUO

With increasing prevalence in older patients, cancer may present as a FUO. Hema-tologic malignancies (particularly lymphoma), renal cell carcinoma, and hepato-cellular carcinoma are the most prevalent cause of FUO due to undiagnosed malignancies (401,402). Review of peripheral blood and bone marrow smears, radiographic imaging, and biopsy are the modalities used to establish these diagnoses.

Occasionally, patients with known malignancies will undergo evaluation for FUO. Paraneoplastic fever, also known as tumor fever, is often in the differential, but remains a diagnosis of exclusion. Tumor fever is mediated by inflammatory cyto-kines, such as interleukin 6, interleukin 1, tumor necrosis factor, and interferon. These cytokines may be produced by host macrophages or by the tumor itself in patients with advanced cancer. Therapeutic trails with nonsteroidal anti-inflammatory drugs (NSAIDS) are sometimes used to help with the diagnosis. NSAIDS constitute a well-documented treatment option for tumor fever (403–406). One small study of 22 patients with undiagnosed fever in the setting of a known malignancy suggested that a fever that completely and rapidly resolves with naproxen may help distinguish tumor fever from infectious and rheumatologic causes of fever (406,407). In this series, 250 mg of naproxen was used twice daily; a rapid, complete response was judged by absence of fever within 24 hours of the therapeutic trial that persisted while on naproxen. Of note, these patients all had a high pretest probability of tumor fever. It is not known how well this diagnostic test would perform today if subjected to wider use, especially considering all the changes in cancer treatments, nosocomial flora and available diagnostic modalities that have occurred in the last 20 years.

ENDOCRINE CAUSES OF FUO

Because prolonged fever often prompts a search for potential infectious or rheumatologic etiologies, simple testing for endocrine causes of FUO may be overlooked. Adrenal insufficiency, thyrotoxicosis, and, rarely, pheochromocytoma have all been documented to cause FUO.

Adrenal Insufficiency

Adrenal insufficiency should always be in a differential for FUO because it is easily treated and potentially fatal if undiagnosed. Suspicion may be raised even further when a patient has unexplained eosinophilia or a history of prolonged steroid use. Because cortisol deficiency can occur without mineralocorticoid deficiency in secondary adrenal insufficiency, serum chemistries cannot be relied upon to exclude this diagnosis. An elevated random cortisol level makes the diagnosis unlikely. However, if there is any question, a high-dose cosyntropin stimulation test can be done (408). In this test, 250 μg of cosyntropin is given parenterally and a cortisol level is checked between 30 and 60 minutes later. A baseline level is not necessary if a previous random cortisol level has already been checked; an incremental increase in cortisol level is not as accurate as the absolute level post-stimulation. A random or poststimulation cortisol level of at least 18 μg/dL excludes the diagnosis of clinically significant adrenal insufficiency.

Thryotoxicosis

Even as other signs and symptoms of excess thyroid hormone are usually present, fever may be the predominant clinical finding in thyrotoxicosis. A low thyroid-stimulating hormone (TSH) will suggest the diagnosis. However, in the rare case of a thyrotopin-secreting neoplasm, serum levels of thyroid hormones are needed as well (409). Free T4 assays have become widely available and are more accurate and easy to interpret than testing that relies on total thyroxine levels and indirect measurement of thyroxine binding proteins (410). Free T3 should also be checked because of the uncommon syndrome of isolated T3 thyrotoxicosis.

Pheochromocytoma

Although often listed as an endocrine cause of FUO, true persistent fever constitutes a rare presentation of this rare disorder. Still, it is reasonable to screen for this condition if certain other features of pheochromocytoma, such as symptomatic paroxysms (headache, palpitations, diaphoresis, and pallor) or unexplained hypertension or tachycardia, are present. The standard test is a 24-hour urine collection for catecholamines, vanillylmandelic acid (VMA), and metanephrines (411). False positives may occur in the face of severe illness, renal failure, or sympathomimetic medications. Now that plasma-free metanephrines assays have become more widely available, some experts have concluded that this test represents the ideal balance between convenience and accuracy (412).

REFERENCES

1. McNeil MM, Brown JM. The medically important aerobic actinomycetes: epidemiology and microbiology. Clin Microbiol Rev 1994; 7(3):357–417.
2. Lerner PI. Nocardiosis. Clin Infect Dis 1996; 22(6):891–903.

3. Brown JM, McNeil MM. *Nocardia, Rhodococcus, Gordonia, Actinomadura, Streptomyces,* and other aerobic actinomycetes. In: Murray PR, Baron EJ, Jorgensen JH, et al., eds. Manual of Clinical Microbiology, 8th ed. Vol. 1. Washington, DC: ASM Press, 2003:502–531.
4. Simpson GL, Stinson EB, Egger MJ, et al. Nocardial infections in the immunocompromised host: A detailed study in a defined population. Rev Infect Dis 1981; 3(3):492–507.
5. Deem RL, Doughty FA, Beaman BL. Immunologically specific direct T lymphocyte-mediated killing of *Nocardia asteroides.* J Immunol 1983; 130(5):2401–2406.
6. Georghiou PR, Blacklock ZM. Infection with *Nocardia* species in Queensland. A review of 102 cliical isolates. Med J Aust 1992; 156(10):692–697.
7. Beaman BL, Beaman L. *Nocardia* species: host-parasite relationships. Clin Microbiol Rev 1994; 7(2):213–264.
8. Uttamchandani RB, Daikos GL, Reyes RR, et al. Nocardiosis in 30 patients with advanced human immunodeficiency virus infection: clinical features and outcome. Clin Infect Dis 1994; 18(3):348–353.
9. Corti ME, Villafane-Fioti MF. Nocardiosis: a review. Int J Infect Dis 2003; 7(4):243–250.
10. Ashdown LR. An improved screening technique for isolation of *Nocardia* species from sputum specimens. Pathology 1990; 22(3):157–161.
11. Wada R, Itabashi C, Nakayama Y, et al. Chronic granulomatous pleuritis caused by *nocardia*: PCR based diagnosis by nocardial 16S rDNA in pathological specimens. J Clin Pathol 2003; 56(12):966–969.
12. Brown JM, Pham KN, McNeil MM, et al. Rapid identification of *Nocardia farcinica* clinical isolates by a PCR assay targeting a 314-base-pair species-specific DNA fragment. J Clin Microbiol 2004; 42(8):3655–3660.
13. Cloud JL, Conville PS, Croft A, et al. Evaluation of partial 16S ribosomal DNA sequencing for identification of *nocardia* species by using the MicroSeq 500 system with an expanded database. J Clin Microbiol 2004; 42(2):578–584.
14. Breitkopf C, Hammel D, Scheld HH, et al. Impact of a molecular approach to improve the microbiological diagnosis of infective heart valve endocarditis. Circulation 2005; 111(11):1415–1421.
15. Raoult D, Birg ML, La Scola B, et al. Cultivation of the bacillus of Whipple's disease. N Engl J Med 2000; 342(9):620–625.
16. Raoult D, La Cola B, Lecocq P, et al. Culture and immunological detection of *Tropheryma whippelii* from the duodenum of a patient with Whipple disease. JAMA 2001; 285(8):1039–1043.
17. Maiwald M, von Herbay A, Fredricks DN, et al. Cultivation of *Tropheryma whipplei* from cerebrospinal fluid. J Infect Dis 2003; 188(6):801–808.
18. Marth T, Raoult D. Whipple's disease. Lancet 2003; 361(9353):239–246.
19. Durrand DV, Lecomte C, Cathebras P, et al. Whipple Disease. Clinical review of 52 cases. The SNFMI Research Group on Whipple Disease. Medicine (Baltimore) 1997; 76(3):170–184.
20. Lange U, Teichmann J. Whipple arthritis: diagnosis by molecular analysis of synovial fluid—current status of diagnosis and therapy. Rheumatology 2003; 42(3):473–480.
21. Elkins C, Shuman TA, Pirolo JS. Cardiac Whipple's disease without digestive symptoms. Ann Thorac Surg 1999; 67(1):250–251.
22. Mahnel R, Marth T. Progress, problems and perspectives in diagnosis and treatment of Whipple's disease. Clin Exp Med 2004; 4(1):39–43.
23. Gubler JG, Kuster M, Dutly F, et al. Whipple endocarditis without overt gastrointestinal disease: report of four cases. Ann Intern Med 1999; 131(2):112–116.
24. Fenollar F, Lepidi H, Raoult D. Whipple's endocarditis: review of the literature and comparisons with Q fever, *Bartonella* infection, and blood culture-positive endocarditis. Clin Infect Dis 2001; 33(8):1309–1316.
25. Lepidi H, Fenollar F, Dumler JS, et al. Cardiac valves in patients with Whipple endocarditis: microbiological, molecular, quantitiative, histologic, and immunohistochemical studies of 5 patients. J Infect Dis 2004; 190(5):935–945.
26. Muller SA, Vogt P, Altwegg M, et al. Deadly carousel or difficult interpretation of new diagnostic tools for Whipple's disease: case report and review of the literature. Infection 2005; 33(1):39–42.

27. Ramzan NN, Loftus E, Burgart LJ, et al. Diagnosis and monitoring of Whipple disease by polymerase chain reaction. Ann Intern Med 1997; 126(7):520–527.
28. Von Herbay A, Ditton HJ, Maiwald M. Diagnostic application of a polymerase chain reaction assay for the Whipple's disease bacterium to intestinal biopsies. Gastroenterology 1996; 110(6):1735–1743.
29. Pezella FR, Paglia MG, Colosimo C. Cerebrospinal fluid analysis for Whipple's disease in patients with progressive supranuclear palsy. Mov Disord 2004; 19(2):220–222.
30. Von Herbay A, Ditton HJ, Schuhmacher F, et al. Whipple's disease: staging and monitoring by cytology and polymerase chain reaction analysis of cerebrospinal fluid. Gastroenterology 1997; 113(2):434–441.
31. Papadopoulou M, Rentzos M, Nicolaou C, et al. Cerebral Whipple's disease diagnosed using PCR: the first case reported from Greece. Mol Diagn 2003; 7(3–4): 209–211.
32. Krober SM, Kaiserling E, Horny HP, et al. Primary diagnosis of Whipple's disease in bone marrow. Hum Pathol 2004; 35(4):522–525.
33. Lowsky R, Archer GL, Fyles G, et al. Brief report: diagnosis of Whipple's disease by molecular analysis of peripheral blood. N Engl J Med 1994: 331(20):1343–1346.
34. Ehrbar HU, Bauerfeind P, Dutly F, et al. PCR-positive tests for *Tropheryma whippelii* in patients without Whipple's disease. Lancet 1999; 353(9171):2214.
35. Smego RA, Foglia G. Actinomycosis. Clin Infect Dis 1998; 26(6):1255–1261.
36. Barabas J, Suba Z, Szabo G, Nemeth Z, et al. False diagnosis caused by Warthin tumor of the parotid gland combined with actinomycosis. J Craniofac Surg 2003; 14(1):46–50.
37. Rankow RM, Abraham DM. Actinomycosis: a masquerader in the head and neck. Ann Otolaryngol 1978; 87(2 Pt 1):230–237
38. Lerner PI. The lumpy jaw. Cervicofacial actinomycosis. Infect Dis Clin North Am 1988; 2(1):203–220.
39. Burns BV, al-Ayoubi A, Ray J, et al. Actinomycosis of the posterior triangle: a case report and review of the literature. J Laryngol Otol 1997; 111(11):1082–1085.
40. Hilfiker ML. Disseminated actinomycosis presenting as a renal tumor with metastases. J Pediatr Surg 2001; 36(10): 1577–1578.
41. Santos LD, Rogan KA, Kennerson AR. Cytologic diagnosis of suppurative cholecystitis due to *Candida albicans* and *Actinomyces*. A report of 2 cases. Acta Cytologica 2004; 48(3):407–410.
42. Pollock PG, Myers DS, Frable WJ, et al. Rapid diagnosis of actinomycosis by thin-needle aspiration biopsy. Am J Clin Pathol 1978; 70(1):27–30.
43. Lee YC, Min D, Holcomb K, et al. Computed tomography guided core needle biopsy diagnosis of pelvic actinomycosis. Gynecol Oncol 2000; 79(2):318–323.
44. Kinnear W, MacFarlane J. A survey of thoracic actinomycosis. Respir Med 1990; 84(1):57–59.
45. Lee C, Lin M, Tsai Y, et al. Thoracic actinomycosis—Review of 9 cases. Chang Gung Med J 1991; 14(4):246–252.
46. Slack J. The source of infection in actinomycosis. J Bacteriol 1942; 43,193–209.
47. Holmberg K. Diagnostic methods for human actinomycosis. Microbiol Sci 1987; 4(3):72–78.
48. Lewis R, McKenzie D, Bagg J, et al. Experience with a novel selective medium for isolation of *Actinomyces* spp. from medical and dental specimens. J Clin Microbiol 1995; 33(6);1613–1616.
49. Parry CM, Hien TT, Dougan G, et al. Typhoid fever. N Engl J Med 2002; 347(22): 1770–1782.
50. El-Newihi HM, Alamy ME, Reynolds TB. *Salmonella* hepatitis: analysis of 27 cases and comparison with acute viral hepatitis. Hepatology 1996; 24(3):516–519.
51. Klotz SA, Jorgensen JH, Buckwold FJ, et al. Typhoid fever. An epidemic with remarkable few clinical signs or symptoms. Arch Intern Med 1984; 144(3):533–537.
52. Gilman RH, Terminel M, Levine MM, et al. Relative efficacy of blood, urine, rectal swab, bone-marrow, and rose-spot cultures for recovery of *Salmonella typhi* in typhoid fever. Lancet 1975; 1(7918):1211–1213.

53. Hoffman SL, Punjabi NH, Rockhill RC, et al. Duodenal string-capsule culture compared with bone-marrow, blood and rectal-swab cultures for diagnosing typhoid and paratyphoid fever. J Infect Dis 1984; 149(2):157–161.

54. Watson KC. Laboratory and clinical investigation of recovery of *Salmonella typhi* from blood. J Clin Microbiol 1978; 7(2):122–126.

55. Hoffman SL, Edman DC, Punjabi NH, et al. Bone marrow aspirate culture superior to streptokinase clot culture and 8 mL 1:10 blood-to-broth ration blood culture for diagnosis of typhoid fever. Am J Trop Med Hyg 1986; 35(4):836–839.

56. Gasem MH, Domans WM, Isbandrio BB, et al. Culture of *Salmonella typhi* and *Salmonella paratyphi* from blood and bone marrow in suspected typhoid fever. Trop Georgr Med 1995; 47(4):164–167.

57. House D, Wain J, Ho VA, et al. Serology of typhoid fever in an area of endemicity and its relevance to diagnosis. J Clin Microbiol 2001; 39(3):1002–1007.

58. Shukla S, Patel B, Chitnis DS. 100 years of Widal test & its reappraisal in an endemic area. Indian J Med Res 1997; 105:53–57.

59. Ohanu ME, Mbah AU, Okonkwo PO, et al. Interference by malaria in the diagnosis of typhoid using Widal test alone. West Afr J Med 2003; 22(3):250–252.

60. Brenner SA, Rooney JA, Manzewitsch P, et al. Isolation of *Bartonella (Rochalimaea) hensalae*: effects of methods of blood collection and handling. J Clin Microbiol 1997; 35(3):544–547.

61. Agan BK, Dolan MJ. Laboratory diagnosis of *Bartonella* infections. Clin Lab Med 2002; 22(4):937–962.

62. Welch DF, Hensel DM, Pickett DA, et al. Bacteremia due to *Rochalimaea henselae* in a child: Practical identification of isolates in the clinical laboratory. J Clin Microbiol 1993; 31(9):2381–2386.

63. Chenoweth MR, Somerville GA, Krause DC, et al. Growth characteristics of *Bartonella henselae* in a novel liquid medium: primary isolation, growth-phase-dependent phage induction, and metabolic studies. Appl Environ Microbiol 2004; 70 (2):656–663.

64. Fournier PE, Robson J, Zeaiter Z, et al. Improved culture from lymph nodes of patients with cat scratch disease and genotypic characterization of *Bartonella henselae* isolates in Australia. J Clin Microbiol 2002; 40(10):3620–3624.

65. Larson AM, Dougherty MJ, Nowowiejski DJ, et al. Detection of *Bartonella (Rochalimaea) quintana* by routine acridine orange staining of broth blood cultures. J Clin Microbiol 1994; 32(6):1492–1496.

66. Spach DH, Callis KP, Paauw DS, et al. Endocarditis caused by *Rochalimaea quintana* in a patient infected with human immunodeficiency virus. J Clin Microbiol 1993; 31(3): 692–694.

67. Spach DH, Kanter AS, Daniels NA, et al. *Bartonella (Rochalimaea)* species as a cause of apparent "culture-negative" endocarditis. Clin Infect Dis 1995; 20(4):1044–1047.

68. Koehler JE, Quinn FD, Berger TG, et al. Isolation of *Rochalimaea* species from cutaneous and osseous lesions of bacillary angiomatosis. N Eng J Med 1992; 327(23):1625–1631.

69. Drancourt M, Mainardi JL, Brouqui P, et al. *Bartonella (Rochalimaea) quintana* endocarditis in three homeless men. N Eng J Med 1995; 332(7):419–423.

70. Wong MT, Thornton DC, Kennedy RC, et al. A chemically defined liquid medium that supports primary isolation of *Rochalimaea (Bartonella) henselae* from blood and tissue specimens. J Clin Microbiol 1995; 33(3):42–744.

71. Knobloch J, Solano L, Alvarez O, et al. Antibodies to Bartonella bacilliformis as determined by fluorescence antibody test, indirect haemagglutination and ELISA. Trop Med Parasitol 1985; 36(4):183–185.

72. LeBoit PE, Berger TG, Egbert BM, et al. Epithelioid haemangioma-like vascular proliferation in AIDS: manifestation of cat scratch disease bacillus infection? Lancet 1988; 1(8592):960–963.

73. LeBoit PE, Berger TG, Egbert BM, et al. Bacillary angiomatosis. The histopathology and differential diagnosis of a pseudoneoplastic infection in patients with human immunodeficiency virus disease. Am J Surg Pathol 1989; 13(11):909–920.

74. Baorto E, Payne RM, Slater LN, et al. Culture-negative endocarditis due to *Bartonella henselae*. J Pediatr 1998; 132(6):1051–1054.

75. Reed J Brigati DJ, Flynn SD, et al. Immunocytochemical identification of *Rochalimaea henselae* in bacillary (epithelioid) angiomatosis, parenchymal bacillary peliosis, and persistent fever with bacteremia. Am J Surg Pathol 1992; 16(7):650–657.

76. Slater LN, Pitha JV, Herrera L, et al. *Rochalimaea henselae* infection in AIDS causing inflammatory disease without angiomatosis or peliosis: Demonstration by immuno-cytochemistry and corroboration by DNA amplification. Arch Pathol Lab Med 1994; 118(1):33–38.

77. Min KW, Reed JA, Welch DF, et al. Morphologically variable bacilli of cat scratch disease are identified by immunocytochemical labeling with antibodies to *Rochalimaea henselae*. Am J Clin Pathol 1994; 101(5):607–610.

78. Foucault C, Rolain JM, Raoult D, et al. Detection of *Bartonella quintana* by direct immu-nofluroescence examination of blood smears of a patient with acute trench fever. J Clin Microbiol 2004; 42(10):4904–4906.

79. Mallqui V, Speelmon EC, Verastegui M, et al. Sonicated diagnostic immunoblot for bartonellosis. Clin Diagn Lab Immunol 2000; 7(1):1–5.

80. Rolain JM, Lecam C, Raoult D. Simplified serological diagnosis of endocarditis due to *Coxiella burnetii* and *Bartonella*. Clin Diagn Lab Immunol 2003; 10(6):1147–1148.

81. Chamberlin J, Laughlin L, Gordon S, et al. Serodiagnosis of *Bartonella bacilliformis* infection by indirect fluorescence antibody assay: test development and application to a population in an area of bartonellosis endemicity. J Clin Microbiol 2000; 38(11):4269–4271.

82. Giladi M, Kletter Y, Avidor B, et al. Enzyme immunoassay for the diagnosis of cat-scratch disease defined by polymerase chain reaction. Clin Infect Dis 2001; 33(11):1852–1858.

83. Zeaiter Z, Fournier P-E, Greub G, et al. Diagnosis of *Bartonella* endocarditis by a real-time nested PCR assay using serum. J Clin Microbiol 2003; 41(3):919–925.

84. Todd S, Xu J, Moore JE, et al. Culture-negative *Bartonella* endocarditis in a patient with renal failure: the value of molecular methods in diagnosis. Br J Biomed Sci 2004; 61(4):190–193.

85. Podglajen I, Bellery F, Poyart C, et al. Comparative molecular and microbiologic diag-nosis of bacterial endocarditis. Emerg Infect Dis 2003; 9(12):1543–1547.

86. Yagupsky P. Detection of *Brucellae* in blood cultures. J Clin Microbiol 1999; 37(11):3437–3442.

87. Mantur BG, Mangalgi SS. Evaluation of conventional Castaneda and lysis centrifu-gation blood culture techniques for diagnosis of human brucellosis. J Clin Microbiol 2004; 42(9):4227–4328.

88. Gamazo C, Vitas AI, Lopez-Goni I, et al. Factors affecting detection of *Brucella melitensis* by BACTEC NR730, a nonradiometric system for hemocultures. J Clin Microbiol 1993; 31(12):3200–3203.

89. Robichaud S, Libman M, Behr M, et al. Prevention of laboratory-acquired brucellosis. Clin Infect Dis 2004; 38(12):e119–e122.

90. Yagupsky P, Peled N, RiesenbergK, et al. Exposure of hospital personnel to *Brucella melitensis* and occurrence of laboratory-acquired disease in an endemic area. Scand J Infect Dis 2000; 32(1):31–35.

91. Navas E, Guerrero A, Cobo J, et al. Faster isolation of *Brucella* spp. from blood by iso-lator compared with BACTEC NR. Diagn Microbiol Infect Dis 1993; 16(1):79–81.

92. Roiz MP, Peralta FG, Valle R, et al. Microbiological diagnosis of brucellosis. J Clin Microbiol 1998; 36(6):1819.

93. Serra J, Vinas M. Laboratory diagnosis of brucellosis in a rural endemic area in north-eastern Spain. Int Microbiol 2004; 7(1):53–58.

94. Young EJ. Serologic diagnosis of human brucellosis: Analysis of 214 cases by aggluti-nation tests and review of the literature. Rev Infect Dis 1991; 13(3):359–372.

95. Ariza J, Pellicer T, Pallares R, et al. Specific antibody profile in human brucellosis. Clin Infect Dis 1992; 14(1):131–140.

96. Young EJ. An overview of human brucellosis. Clin Infect Dis 1995; 21(2):283–289.

97. Swenson RM, Carmichael LE, Cundy KR. Human infection with *Brucella canis*. Ann Int Med 1972; 76(3):435–438.

98. Vrioni G, Gartzonika C, Kostoula A, et al. Application of a polymerase chain reaction enzyme immunoassay in peripheral whole blood and serum specimens for diagnosis of acute human brucellosis. Eur J Clin Microbiol Infect Dis 2004; 23(3):194–199.

99. Al Dahouk S, Tomaso H, Nockler K, et al. The detection of *Brucella* spp. using PCR-ELISA and real-time PCR assays. Clin Lab 2004; 50(7):387–94.

100. Queipo-Ortuno MI, Garcia-Ordonez MA, Gil R, et al. PCR-DIG ELISA with biotinylated primers is unsuitable for use in whole blood samples from patients with brucellosis. Mol Cell Probes 2004; 19(4):243–250.

101. Navarro E, Cassao MA, Solera J. Diagnosis of human brucellosis using PCR. Expert Rev Mol Diagn 2004; 4(1):115–123.

102. Morata P, Queipo-Ortuno MI, Reguera JM, et al. Development and evaluation of a PCR-enzyme-linked immunosorbent assay for diagnosis of human brucellosis. J Clin Microbiol 2003; 41(1):144–148.

103. Doern GV, Davaro R, George M, et al. Lack of requirement for prolonged incubation of Septi-Chek blood culture bottles in patients with bactermia due to fastidious bacteria. Diagn Microbiol Infect Dis 1996; 24(3):141–143.

104. Das M, Badley AD, Cockerill FR, et al. Infective endocarditis caused by HACEK micro-organisms. Annu Rev Med 1997; 48:25–33.

105. Berbari EF, Cockerill FR, Steckelberg JM. Infective endocarditis due to unusual or fastidious microorganisms. Mayo Clin Proc 1997; 72(6):532–542.

106. Den Boer JW, Yzerman EP. Diagnosis of *Legionella* infection in Legionnaires' disease. Eur J Clin Microbiol Infect Dis 2004; 23(12):871–878.

107. Yu VL, Plouffe JF, Pastoris MC, et al. Distribution of *Legionella* species and serogroups isolated by culture in patients with sporadic community-acquired legionellosis: an international collaborative survey. J Infect Dis 2002; 186(1):127–128.

108. Tompkins LS, Roessler BJ, Redd SC, et al. *Legionella* prosthetic-valve endocarditis. N Engl J Med 1988; 318(9):530–535.

109. Ryan KJ. *Legionella*. In: Ryan KJ, Ray CG, eds. Sherris Medical Microbiology, An Introduction to Infectious Diseases, 4th ed. New York: McGraw-Hill, 2004:415–420.

110. Edelstein PH. Improved semiselective medioum for isolation of *Legionella pneumophila* from contaminated clinical and environmental specimens. J Clin Microbiol 1981; 14(3):298–303.

111. Roig J, Domingo C, Morera J. Legionnaires' disease. Chest 1994; 105(6):1817–1825.

112. Edelstein PH. Legionnaires' disease. State-of-the-art clinical article. Clin Infect Dis 1993; 16(6):741–749.

113. Fields BS, Benson RF, Besser RE. *Legionella* and Legionnaires' disease: 25 years of investigation. Clin Microbiol Rev 2002; 15(3):506–526.

114. Murdoch DR. Diagnosis of *Legionella* infection. Clin Infect Dis 2003; 36(1):64–69.

115. Luck PC, Igel L, Helbig JH, et al. Comparison of commercially available media for the recovery of *Legionella* species. Int J Hyg Environ Health 2004; 207(6):589–593.

116. Morrill WE, Barbaree JM, Fields BS, et al. Increased recovery of *Legionella micadadei* and *Legionella bozemanii* on buffered charcoal yeast extract agar supplemented with albumin. J Clin Microbiol 1991; 28(3):616–618.

117. Lee TC, Vickers RM, Yu VL, et al. Growth of 28 *Legionella* species on selective culture media: a comparative study. J Clin Microbiol 1993; 31(10):2764–2768.

118. Muder RR, Yu VL. Infection due to Legionella species other than *L. pneumophila*. Clin Infect Dis 2002; 35(8):990–998.

119. Benin AL, Benson RF, Besser RE. Trends in Legionnaires' disease, 1980-1998: declining mortality and new patterns of diagnosis. Clin Infect Dis 2002; 35(9):1039–1046.

120. Yzerman EP, den Boer JW, Lettinga KD, et al. Sensitivity of three urinary antigen tests associated with clinical severity in a loarge outbreak of Legionnaires' disease in the Netherlands. J Clin Microbiol 2002; 40(9):3232–3236.

121. Lettinga KD, Verbon A, Weverling GJ, et al. Legionnaires' disease at a Dutch flower show: Prognostic factors and impact of thereapy. Emerg Infect Dis 2002; 8(12):1448–1454.

122. Kazandjian D, Chiew R, Gilbert GL. Rapid diagnosis of *Legionella pneumophila* sergroup 1 infection with the Binax enzyme immunoassay urinary antigen test. J Clin Microbiol 1997; 35(4):954–956.

123. Helbig JH, Uldumm SA, Bernander S, et al. Clinical utility of urinary antigen detection for diagnosis of community-acquired, travel-asociated, and nosocomial Legionnaires' disease. J Clin Microbiol 2003; 41(2):838–840.

124. McWhinney PH, Ragunathan PL, Rowbottham TJ. Failure to produce detectable antibodies to *Legionella pneumophila* by an immunocompetent adult. J Infect 2000; 41(1):91–92.

125. Maltezou HC, La-Scola B, Astra H, et al. *Mycoplasma pneumoniae* and *Legionella pneumophila* in community-acquired lower respiratory tract infections among hospitalized children: diagnosis by real time PCR. Scand J Infect Dis 2004; 36(9):639–642.

126. Herpers BL, de Jongh BM, van der Zwaluw K, et al. Real-time PCR assay targets the 23S-5S spacer for direct detection and differentiation of *Legionella* spp. and *Legionella pneumophila*. J Clin Microbiol 2003; 41(10):4815–4816.

127. Murdoch DR. Molecular genetic methods in the diagnosis of lower respiratory tract infections. APMIS 2004; 112(11):713–727.

128. Rantakokko-Jalava K, Jalava J. Development of conventional and real-time PCR assays for detection of *Legionella* DNA in respiratory specimens. J Clin Microbiol 2001; 39(9):2904–2910.

129. Saslaw S. Chronic meningococcemia: Report of a case. N Engl J Med 1962; 266:605–607.

130. Rompalo AM, Hood EW, Roberts PL, et al. The acute arthritis dermatitis syndrome. The changing importance of *Neisseria gonorrhoeae* and *Neisseria meningitidis*. Arch Intern Med 1987; 147(2):281–283.

131. Densen P. Complement deficiencies and meningococcal disease. Clin Exp Immunol 1991; 86 (suppl 1):57–62.

132. Levin S, Painter MB. The treatment of acute meningococcal infection in adults. A reappraisal. Ann Intern Med 1966; 64(5):1049–1056.

133. Durand ML, Calderwood SB, Weber DJ, et al. Acute bacterial meningitis in adults. A review of 493 episodes. N Engl J Med 1993; 328(1):21–28.

134. Bohr V, Rasmussen N, Hansen B, et al. 875 cases of bacterial meningitis: diagnostic procedures and the impact of preadmission antibiotic therapy. J Infect 1983; 7(3):193–202.

135. Janda WM, Knapp JS. *Neisseria* and *Moraxella catarrhalis*. In: Murray PR, Baron EJ, Jorgensen JH et al, eds. Manual of Clinical Microbiology, 8th ed. Vol. 1. Washington, DC: ASM Press, 2003:585–608.

136. Muller PD, Donald PR, Burger PJ, et al. Detection of bacterial antigens in cerebrospinal fluid by a latex agglutination test in 'septic unknown' meningitis and serogroup B meningococcal meningitis. S Afr Med J 1989; 76(5):214–215.

137. McGraw TP, Bruckner DA. Evaluation of the Directigen and Phadebact agglutination tests. Am J Clin Pathol 1984; 82(1):97–99.

138. Newcombe J, Cartwright K, Palmer WH, et al. PCR of peripheral blood for diagnosis of meningococcal disease. J Clin Microbiol 1996; 34(7):1637–1640.

139. Bryant PA, Ki HY, Zaia A, et al. Prospective study of a real-time PCR that is highly sensitive, specific, and clinically useful for diagnosis of meningococcal disease in children. J Clin Microbiol 2004; 42(7):2919–2925.

140. Ni H, Knight AI, Cartwright K, et al. Polymerase chain reaction for diagnosis of meningococcal meningitis. Lancet 1992; 340(8833):1432–1434.

141. Frans J, Verhaegen J, Van Noyen R. *Streptobacillus moniliformis*: case report and review of the literature. Acta Clin Belg 2001; 56(3):187–190.

142. Gilroy SA, Khan MU. Rat bite fever: case report and review of the literature. Infect Dis Clin Pract 2002; 11(7):403–405.

143. Rupp ME. *Streptobacillus moniliformis* (rat bite fever). In: Yu VL, Weber R, Raoult D, eds. Antimicrobial Therapy and Vaccines, 2nd ed, Vol. 1. Microbes. New York: Apple Tree Productions, LLC, 2002:685–690.

144. Von Graeventitz A, Zbinden R, Mutters R. *Actinobacillus, Capnocytophaga, Eikenella, Kingella, Pasteurella*, and other fastidious or rarely encountered gram-negative rods. In: Murray PR, Baron EJ, Jorgensen JH, et al, eds. Manual of Clinical Microbiology, 8th ed. Vol. 1. Washington, DC: ASM Press, 2003:609–622.

145. Wallet F, Savage C, Loiez C, et al. Molecular diagnosis of arthritis due to *Streptobacillus moniliformis*. Diagn Microbiol Infect Dis 2003; 47(4):623–624.

146. Berger C, Altwegg M, Meyer A, et al. Broad range polymerase chain reaction for diagnosis of rat-bite fever caused by *Streptobacillus moniliformis*. Pediatr Infect Dis J 2001; 20(12):1181–1182.

147. Li D, Vaglenov A, Kim T, et al. High-yield culture and purification of Chlamydiaceae bacteria. Microbiol Meth 2005; 61(1):17–24.

148. Mahony JB, Chernesky MA. Effect of swab type and storage temperatue on the isolation of *Chlamydia trachomatis* from clinical specimens. J Clin Microbiol 1985; 22(51):865–867.

149. Jones RB, Van Der Pol B, Katz BP. Effect of differences in specimen processing and passage technique on recovery of *Chlamydia trachomatis*. J Clin Microbiol 1989; 27(5):894–898.

150. Tuuminen T, Palomaki P, Paavonen J. The use of serologic tests for the diagnosis of chlamydial infections. J Microbiol Methods 2000; 42(3):265–279.

151. Persson K, Treharne J. Diagnosis of infection caused by *Chlamydia pneumoniae* (strain TWAR), in patients with "ornithosis" in southern Sweden 1981–1987. Scand J Infect Dis 1989; 21(6):675–679.

152. Bruu AL, Haukenes G, Aasen S, et al. *Chlamydia pneumoniae* infections in Norway 1981–1987 earlier diagnosed as ornithosis. Scand J Infect Dis 1991; 23(3):299–304.

153. Gaydos CA, Roblin PM, Hammerschlag MR, et al. Diagnostic utility of PCR-enzyme immunoassay, culture and serology for detection of *Chlamydia pneumoniae* in symptomatic and asymptomatic patients. J Clin Microbiol 1994; 32(4):903–905.

154. Nilsson K, Liu A, Pahlson C, et al. Demonstration of intracellular microorganisms (*Rickettsia* spp., *Chlamydia* pneumoniae, *Bartonella* spp.) in pathological human aortic valves by PCR. J Infect 2005; 50(1):46–52.

155. Cochrane M, Pospischill A, Walker P, et al. Discordant detection of *Chlamydia pneumoniae* in patients with carotid artery disease using polymerase chain reaction, immunofluorescence microscopy and serological methods. Pathology 2005; 37(1):69–75.

156. Nebe CT, Rother M, Brechtel I, et al. Detection of *Chlamydophila pneumoniae* in the bone marrow of two patients with unexplained chronic anaemia. Eur J Haematol 2005; 74(1):77–83.

157. Oldach DW, Gaydos CA, Mundy LM, et al. Rapid diagnosis of *Chlamydia psittaci* pneumonia. Clin Infect Dis 1993; 17(3):338–343.

158. Baum SG. *Mycoplasma pneumoniae* and Atypical Pneumonia. In: Mandell GL, Bennett JE, Dolin R, eds. Mandell, Douglas, and Bennett's Principles and Practice of Infectious Diseases, 6th ed. Vol 2. Philadelphia: Elsevier Churchill Livingstone, 2005: 2271–2280.

159. Feizi T. Cold agglutinins, the direct coombs' test and serum immunoglobulins in *Mycoplasma pneumoniae* infection. Ann NY Acad Sci, 1967; 143(1):801–812.

160. Feizi T, Taylor-Robinson D. Cold agglutin anti-I and *Mycoplasma pneumoniae*. Immunology 1967; 13(4):405–409.

161. Cheng JH, Wang HC, Tang RB, et al. A rapid cold agglutinin test in *Mycoplasma pneumoniae* infection. Chin Med J 1990; 46(1):49–52.

162. Rosenfield RE, Schmidt PJ, Calvo RC, et al. Anti-I, a frequent cold agglutinin in infectious mononucleosis. Vox Sang 1965; 10(5):631–634

163. Lind K, Spencer ES, Anderson HK. Cold agglutinin production and cytomegalovirus infection. Scand J Infect Dis 1974; 6(2):109–112.

164. Talkington DF. Shott S, Fallon MT, et al. Analysis of eight commercial enzyme immunoassay tests for detection of antibodies to *Mycoplasma pneumoniae* in human serum. Clin Diagn Lab Immunol 2004; 11(5):862–867.

165. Beersma MF, Dirven K, van Dam AP, et al. Evaluation of 12 commercial tests and the complement fixation test for *Mycoplasma pneumoniae*-specific immunoglobulin G (IgG) and IgM antibodies, with PCR used as the "gold standard". J Clin Microbiol 2005; 43(5):2277–2285.

166. Jacobs E. Serological diagnosis of *Mycoplasma pneumoniae* infections: a critical review of current procedures. Clin Infect Dis 1993; 17(suppl 1):S79–S82.

167. Thacker WL, Talkington DF. Comparison of two rapid commercial tests with complement fixation for serologic diagnosis of *Mycoplasma pneumoniae* infections. J Clin Microbiol 1995; 33(5):1212–1214.

168. Miyashita N, Saito A, Kohno S, et al. Multiplex PCR for the simulteneous detection of *Chlamydia pneumoniae, Mycoplasma pneumoniae* and *Legionella pneumophila* in community-acquired pneumonia. Respir Med 2004; 98(6):542–550.
169. Michelow IC, Olsen K, Lozano J, et al. Diagnostic utility and clinical significance of naso- and oropharyngeal samples used in a PCR assay to diagnose *Mycoplasma pneumoniae* infection in children with community-acquired pneumonia. J Clin Microbiol 2004; 42(7):3339–3341.
170. Pinar A, Bozdemir N, Kocagoz T, et al. Rapid detection of bacterial atypical pneumonia agents by multiplex PCR. Cent Eur J Public Health 2004; 12(1):3–5.
171. Raty R, Ronkko E, Klemola M. Sample type is crucial to the diagnosis of *Mycoplasma pneumoniae* pneumonia by PCR. J Med Microbiol 2005; 54(3):287–291.
172. Blackmore TK, Reznikov M, Gordon DL. Clinical utility of the polymerase chain reaction to diagnose *Mycoplasma pneumoniae* infection. Pathology 1995; 27(2):177–181.
173. Templeton KE, Scheltinga SA, Graffelman AW, et al. Comparison and evaluation of real-time PCR, real-time nucleic acid sequence-based amplification, conventialal PCR, and serology for diagnosis of *Mycoplasma pneumoniae.* J Clin Microbiol 2003; 41(9):4366–4371.
174. Blaskovic D, Barak I. Oligo-chip based detection of tick-borne bacteria. FEMS Microbiol Lett 2005; 243(2):473–478.
175. Hoen B, Selton-Suty C, Lacassin F, et al. Infective endocarditis in patients with negative blood cultures: analysis of 88 cases from a one-year nationwide survey in France. Clin Infect Dis 1995; 20(3):501–506.
176. Muhlemann K, Matter L, Meyer B, et al. Isolation of *Coxiella burnetii* from heart valves of patients treated for Q fever endocarditis. J Clin Microbiol 1995; 33(2):428–431.
177. Brouqui P, Marrie TJ, Raoult D. Coxiella. In: Murray PR, Baron EJ, Jorgensen JH, et al., eds. Manual of Clinical Microbiology, 8th ed. Vol 1. Washington, DC: ASM Press, 1999:1030–1036.
178. Turk WG, Howitt G, Turnberg LA, et al. Chronic Q fever. Q J Med 1976; 45(178):193–217.
179. Dupont HT, Thirion X, Raoult D. Q fever serology: cutoff determination for microimmunofluorescence. Clin Diagn Lab Immunol 1994; 1(2):189–196.
180. Musso D, Raoult D. *Coxiella burnetii* blood cultures from acute and chronic Q-fever patients. J Clin Microbiol 1995; 33(12): 3129–3132.
181. Miller JD, Curns AT, Thompson HA. A growth study of *Coxiella burnetii* Nine Mile Phase I and Phase II in fibroblasts. FEMS Immunol Med Microbiol 2004; 42(3):291–297.
182. Fenollar F, Fournier PE, Raoult D. Molecular detection of *Coxiella burnetii* in the sera of patients with Q fever endocarditis or vascular infection. J Clin Microbiol 2004; 42(11):4919–4924.
183. Fournier PE, Raoult D. Comparison of PCR and serology assays for early diagnosis of acute Q fever. J Clin Microbiol 2003; 41(11):5094–5098.
184. Lepidi H, Houpikian P, Liang Z, et al. Cardiac valves in patients with Q fever endocarditis: microbiological, molecular, and histologic studies. J infect Dis 2003; 187(7):1097–1106.
185. Brouqui P, Dumler JS, Raoult D. Immunohistologic demonstration of *Coxiella burnetii* in the valves of patients with Q fever endocarditis. Am J Med 1994; 97(5):451–458.
186. Dumler JS, Bakken JS. Ehrlichial diseases of humans: emerging tick-borne infections. Clin Infect Dis 1995; 20(5):1102–1110.
187. Drew WL. *Rickettsia, Coxiella, Ehrlichia,* and *Bartonella.* In: Ryan KJ, Ray CG, eds. Sherris Medical Microbiology: An introduction to infectious diseases, 4th ed. New York: McGraw-Hill, 2004:471–479.
188. Bakken JS, Krueth J, Wilson-Nordskog C, et al. Clinical and laboratory characteristics of human granulocytic ehrlichiosis. JAMA 1996; 275(3):199–205.
189. Goodman JL, Nelson C, Vitale B, et al. Direct cultivation of the causative agent of human granulocytic ehrlichiosis. N Eng J Med 1996; 334(4):209–215.
190. Standaert SM, Yu T, Scott MA, et al. Primary isolation of *Ehrlichia chaffeensis* from patients with febrile illnesses: clinical and molecular characteristics. J Infect Dis 2000; 181(3):1082–1088.

191. Bakken JS, Aguero-Rosenfeld ME, Tilden RL, et al. Serial measurements of hematologic counts during the active phase of human granulocytic ehrlichiosis. Clin Infect Dis 2001; 32(6):862–870.
192. Paddock CD, Folk SM, Shore GM, et al. Infections with *Ehrlichia chaffeensis* and *Ehrlichia ewingii* in persons coinfected with human immunodeficiency virus. Clin Infect Dis 2001; 33(9):1586–1594.
193. Dawson JE, Fishbein DB, Eng TR, et al. Diagnosis of human ehrlichiosis with the indirect fluorescent antibody test: kinetics and specificity. J Infect Dis 1990; 162(1):91–95.
194. Massung RF, Slater KG. Comparison of PCR assays for detection of the agent of human granulocytic ehrlichiosis, *Anaplasma phagocytophilum*. J Clin Microbiol 2003; 41(2): 717–722.
195. Fenollar F, Raoult D. Molecular genetic methods for the diagnosis of fastidious microorganisms. APMIS 2004; 112(11):785–807.
196. Sirigireddy DR, Ganta RR. Multiplex detection of *Ehrlichia* and *Anaplasma* species pathogens in peripheral blood by real-time reverse transcriptase-polymerase chain reaction. J Mol Diagn 2005; 7(2):308–316.
197. Dumler JS, Brouqui P. Molecular diagnosis of human granulocytic anaplasmosis. Expert Rev Mol Diagn 2004; 4(4):559–569.
198. Wagner ER, Bremer WG, Rikihisa Y, et al. Development of a p28-based PCR assay for *Ehrlichia chaffeensis*. Mol Cell Probes 2004; 18(2):111–116.
199. Walls JJ, Caturegli P, Bakken JS, et al. Improved sensitivity of PCR for diagnosis of human granulocytic ehrlichiosis using epank1 genes of *Ehrlichia phagocytophila*-group ehrlichiae. J Clin Microbiol 2000; 38(1):354–356.
200. Levett PN. *Leptospira* and *Leptonema*. In: Murray PR, Baron EJ, Jorgensen JH, et al, eds. Manual of Clinical Microbiology, 8th ed. Vol. 1. Washington, DC: ASM Press, 2003: 929–936.
201. Vijayachari P, Sugunan AP, Umapathi T, et al. Evaluation of darkground microscopy as a rapid diagnostic procedure in leptospirosis. Indian J Med Res 2001; 114:54–58.
202. Smythe LD, Smith IL, Smith GA, et al. A quantitative PCR (TaqMan) assay for pathogenic *Leptospira* spp. BMC Infect Dis 2002; 2(1):13.
203. Levett PN, Morey RE, Galloway RL, et al. Detection of pathogenic leptospires by real-time quantitative PCR. J Med Microbiol 2005; 54(1):45–49.
204. Lucchesi PM, Arroyo GH, Etcheverria AI, et al. Recommendations for the detection of *Leptospira* in urine by PCR. Rev Soc Bras Med Trop 2004; 37(2):131–134.
205. Ooteman MC, Vago AR, Koury MC. Potential application of low-stringency single specific primer-PCR in the identification of *Leptospira* in the serum of patients with suspected leptospirosis. Can J Microbiol 2004; 50(12):1073–1079.
206. Palaniappan RU, Chang YF, Chang CF, et al. Evaluation of lig-based conventional and real time PCR for the detection of pathogenic leptospires. Mol Cell Probes 2005; 19(2):111–117.
207. Shukla J, Tuteja U, Batra HV. DNA probes for identification of leptospires and disease diagnosis. Southeast Asian J Trop Med Public Health 2004; 35(2):346–352.
208. Merien F, Baranton G, Perolat P. Comparison of polymerase chain reaction with microagglutination test and culture for diagnosis of leptospirosis. J Infect Dis 1995; 172(1):281–285.
209. Romero EC, Billerbeck AE, Lando VS et al. Detection of *Leptospira* DNA in patients with aseptic meningitis by PCR. J Clin Microbiol 1998; 36(5):1453–1455.
210. Yitzhaki S, Barnea A, Keysary A, et al. New approach for serological testing for leptospirosis by using detection of *Leptospira* agglutination by flow cytometry light scatter analysis. J Clin Microbiol 2004; 42(4):1680–1685.
211. Levett PN, Whittington CU. Evaluation of the indirect hemagglutination assay for diagnosis of acute leptospirosis. J Clin Microbiol 1998; 36(1):11–14.
212. Wagenaar JF, Falke TH, Nam NV, et al. Rapid serological assays for leptospirosis are of limited value in southern Vietnam. Ann Trop Med Parasitiol 2004; 98(8):843–850.
213. Chappel RJ, Goris M, Palmer MF, et al. Impact of proficiency testing on results of the microscopic agglutination test for diagnosis of leptospirosis. J Clin Microbiol 2004; 42(12):5484–5488.

214. Effler PV, Domen HY, Bragg SL, et al. Evaluation of the indirect hemagglutination assay for diagnosis of acute leptospirosis in Hawaii. J Clin Microbiol 2000; 38(3): 1081–1084.
215. Bajani MD, Ashford DA, Bragg SL, et al. Evaluation of four commercially available rapid serologic tests for diagnosis of leptospirosis. J Clin Microbiol 2003; 41(2):803–809.
216. Magnarelli LA, Anderson JF, Johnson RC. Cross-reactivity in serological tests for Lyme disease and other spirochetal infections. J Infect Dis 1987; 156(1):183–188.
217. Vitale G, La Russa C, Galioto A, et al. Evaluation of an IgM-ELISA test for the diagnosis of human leptospirosis. New Microbiol 2004; 27(2):149–154.
218. Winslow WE, Merry DJ, Pirc ML, et al. Evaluation of a commercial enzyme-linked immunosorbent assay for detection of immunoglobulin M antibody in diagnosis of human leptospiral infection. J Clin Microbiol 1997; 35(8):1938–1942.
219. Cumberland P, Everard CO, Levett PN. Assesment of the efficacy of an IgM-ELISA and microscopic agglutination test (MAT) in the diagnosis of acute leptospirosis. Am J Trop Med Hyg 1999; 61(5):731–734.
220. Wilske B, Schriefer ME. *Borrelia*. In: Murray PR, Baron EJ, Jorgensen JH, et al, eds. Manual of Clinical Microbiology, 8th ed. Vol. 1. Washington, DC: ASM Press, 2003:937–954.
221. Goodman RL, Arndt KA, Steigbigel NH. *Borrelia* in Boston. JAMA 1969; 210(4):722.
222. Sciotto CG, Lauer BA, White WL, et al. Detection of *Borrelia* in acridine orange-stained blood smears by fluorescence microscopy. Arch Pathol Lab Med 1983; 107(7):384–386.
223. Stoenner HG, Dodd T, Larsen C. Antigenic variation of *Borrelia hermsii*. J Exp Med 1982; 156(5):1297–1311.
224. Porcella SF, Raffel SJ, Schrumpf ME, et al. Serodiagnosis of louse-borne relapsing fever with glycerophosphodiester phosphodiesterase (GlpQ) from Borrelia recurrentis. J Clin Microbiol 2000; 38(10):3561–3571.
225. Schwan TG, Schrumpf ME, Hinnebusch BJ, et al. GlpQ: an antigen for serological discrimination between relapsing fever and Lyme borreliosis. J Clin Microbiol 1996; 34(10):2483–2492.
226. Pfyffer GE, Brown-Elliott BA, Wallace RJ. *Mycobacterium*: General Characteristics, Isolation, and Staining Procedures. In: Murray PR, Baron EJ, Jorgensen JH, et al, eds. Manual of Clinical Microbiology, 8th ed. Vol. 1. Washington, DC: ASM Press, 2003:532–559.
227. Daloviso JR, Montenegro-James S, Kemmerly SA, et al. Comparison of the amplified *Mycobacterium tuberculosis* (MTB) direct test, Amplicor MTB PCR, and IS6110-PCR for detection of MTB in respiratory specimens. Clin Infect Dis 1996; 23(5):1099–1106.
228. Catanzaro A, Perry S, Clarridge JE, et al. The role of clinical suspicion in evaluation a new diagnostic test for active tuberculosis: results of a multicenter prospective trial. JAMA 2000; 283(5):639–645.
229. Carpentier E, Drouillard B, Dailoux M, et al. Diagnosis of tuberculosis by Amplicor *Mycobacterium tuberculosis* test: a multicenter study. J Clin Microbiol 1995; 33(12): 3106–3110.
230. Barnes PF. Rapid diagnostic tests for tuberculosis—Progress but no gold standard. Am J Resp Crit Care Med 1997; 155(5):1497–1498.
231. Bradley SP, Reed SL, Catanzaro A. Clinical efficacy of the amplified *Mycobacterium tuberculosis* direct test for the diagnosis of pulmonary tuberculosis. Am J Respir Crit Care Med 1996; 153(5):1606–1610.
232. Dilworth JP, Goyal M, Young DB, et al. Comparison of polymerase chain reaction for IS6110 and Amplicor in the diagnosis of tuberculosis. Thorax 1996; 51(3):320–322.
233. American Thoracic Society Workshop. Rapid diagnostic tests for tuberculosis: what is the appropriate use? Am J Respir Crit Care Med 1997; 155(5):1804–1814.
234. Levine H, Metzger W, Lacera D, et al. Diagnosis of tuberculous pleurisy by culture of pleural biopsy specimen. Arch Intern Med 1970; 126(2):269–271.
235. Gill V, Cordero PJ, Greses JV, et al. Pleural tuberculosis in HIV-infected patients. Chest 1995; 107(6):1775–1776.
236. Vlaspolder F, Singer P, Roggeveen C. Diagnostic value of an amplification method (Gen-Probe) compared with that of culture for diagnosis of tuberculosis. J Clin Microbiol 1995; 33(1):2699–2703.

237. Shah S, Miller A, Mastellone A, et al. Rapid diagnosis of tuberculosis in various biopsy and body fluid specimens by the AMPLICOR *Mycobacterium tuberculosis* polymerase chain reaction test. Chest 1998; 113(5):1190–1194.

238. Kayacan O, Karnak D, Delibalta M, et al. Adenosine deaminase activity in bronchoalveolar lavage in Turkish patients with smear negative pulmonary tuberculosis. Respir Med 2002; 96(7):536–541.

239. Koh KK, Kim EJ, Cho CH, et al. Adenosine deaminase and carcinoembryonic antigen in pericardial effusion diagnosis, especially in suspected tuberculous pericarditis. Circulation 1994; 89(6):2728–2735.

240. Maartens G, Willcox PA, Benatar SR. Miliary tuberculosis: rapid diagnosis, hematologic abnormalities, and outcome in 109 treated adults. Am J Med 1990; 89(3): 291–296.

241. Caws M, Wilson SM, Clough, et al. Role of IS6110-targeted PCR, culture, biochemical, clinical, and immunological criteria for diagnosis of tuberculous meningitis. J Clin Microbiol 2000; 38(9):3150–3155.

242. Lopez-Cortes LF, Cruz-Ruiz M, Gomez-Mateos J, et al. Adenosine deaminase activity in the CSF of patients with aseptic meningitis: utility in the diagnosis of tuberculous meningitis or neurobrucellosis. Clin Infect Dis 1995; 20(3):525–530.

243. Kim JH, Langston AA, Gallis HA. Miliary tuberculosis: epidemiology, clinical manifestations, diagnosis, and outcome. Rev Infect Dis 1990; 12(4):583–590.

244. Munt PW. Miliary tuberculosis in the chemotherapy era: With a clinical review in 69 American adults. Medicine (Baltimore) 1972; 51(2):139–155.

245. Salzman SH, Schindel ML, Aranda CP, et al. The role of bronchoscopy in the diagnosis of pulmonary tuberculosis in patients at risk for HIV infection. Chest 1992; 102(1):143–146.

246. Barnes PF, Bloch AB, Davidson PT, et al. Tuberculosis in patients with human immunodeficiency virus infection. N Engl J Med 1991; 324(23):1644–1650.

247. Shafer RW, Kim DS, Weiss JP, et al. Extrapulmonary tuberculosis in patients with human immunodeficiency virus infection. Medicine (Baltimore) 1991; 70(6):384–397.

248. Pacios E, Alcala L, Ruis-Serrano MJ, et al. Evaluation of bone marrow and blood cultures for the recovery of mycobacteria in the diagnosis of disseminated mycobacterial infections. Clin Microbiol Infect 2004; 10(8):734–737.

249. Kilby JM, Marques MB, Yaye DL, et al. The yield of bone marrow biopsy and culture compared with blood culture in the evaluation of HIV-infected patients for mycobacterial and fungal infections. Am J Med 1998; 104(2):123–128.

250. Stone BL, Cohn DL, Dane MS, et al. Utility of paired blood cultures and smears in diagnosis of disseminated *Mycobacterium avium* complex infections in AIDS patients. J Clin Microbiol 1994; 32(3):841–842.

251. Havlir D, Kemper CA, Deresinski SC. Reproducibility of lysis-centrifugation cultures for quantification of *Mycobacterium avium* complex bacteremia. J Clin Microbiol 1993; 31(7):1794–1798.

252. Hussong J, Peterson LR, Warren JR, et al. Detecting disseminated *Mycobacterium avium* complex infections in HIV-postitive patients. The usefulness of bone marrow trephine biopsy specimens, aspirate cultures, and blood cultures. Am J Clin Pathol 1998; 110(6):806–809.

253. Gamboa F, Manterola JM, Lonca J, et al. Detection and identification of mycobacteria by amplification of RNA and DNA in pretreated blood and bone marrow aspirates by a simple lysis method. J Clin Microbiol 1997; 35(8):2124–2128.

254. Park H, Jang H, Song E, et al. Detection and genotyping of *Mycobacterium* species from clinical isolates and specimens by oligonucleotide array. J Clin Microbiol 2005; 43(4):1782–1788.

255. De Francesco MA, Colombrita D, Pinsi G, et al. Detection and identification of *Mycobacterium avium* in the blood of AIDS patients by the polymerase chain reaction. Eur J Clin Microbiol Infect Dis 1996; 15(7):551–555.

256. Sathapatayavongs B, Batteiger BE, Wheat J, et al. Clinical and laboratory features of disseminated histoplasmosis during two large urban outbreaks. Medicine (Baltimore) 1983; 62(5):263–270.

257. Wheat LJ, Connolly-Stringfield PA, Baker RL, et al. Disseminated histoplasmosis in the acquired immune deficiency syndrome: clinical findings, diagnosis and treatment, and review of the literature. Medicine (Baltimore) 1990; 69(6):361–374.

258. Walsh TJ, Larone DH, Schell WA, et al. *Histoplasma, Blastomyces, Coccidioides*, and other dimorphic fungi causing sytstemic mycoses. In: Murray PR, Baron EJ, Jorgensen JH, et al, eds. Manual of Clinical Microbiology, 8th ed. Vol 2. Washington, DC: ASM Press, 2003:1781–1797.

259. Wheat LJ, Musial CE, Jenny-Avital E. Diagnosis and management of central nervous system histoplasmosis. Clin Infect Dis 2005; 50(6):844–852.

260. Wheat LJ. Laboratory diagnosis of histoplasmosis: Update 2000. Semin Respir Infect 2001; 16(2):131–140.

261. Ryan KJ. *Cryptococcus, Histoplasma, Coccidioides*, and other systemic fungal pathogens. In: Ryan KJ, Ray CG, eds. Sherris Medical Microbiology, An Introduction to Infectious Diseases, 4th ed. New York: McGraw-Hill, 2004:669–684.

262. Guimaraes AJ, Pizzini CV, de Matos Guedes, HL, et al. ELISA for early diagnosis of histoplasmosis. J Med Microbiol 2004; 53(6):509–514.

263. Wheat LJ, Garringer T, Brizendine E, et al. Diagnosis of histoplasmosis by antigen detection based upon experience at the histoplasmosis reference laboratory. Diagn Microbiol Infect Dis 2002; 43(1):29–37.

264. Kricka LJ. Human anti-animal antibody interferences in immunological assays. Clin Chem 1999; 45(7):942–956.

265. Wheat LJ, Connolly P, Durkin M, et al. False-positive *Histoplasma* antigenemia caused by antithymocyte globulin antibodies. Transpl Infect Dis 2004; 6(1):23–27.

266. Auwaerter PG. Infectious mononucleosis in middle age. JAMA 1999; 281(5):454–459.

267. Brigden ML, Au S, Thompson S, et al. Infectious mononucleosis in an outpatient population: diagnostic utility of 2 automated hematology analyzers and the sensitivity and specificity of Hoagland's criteria in heterophile-positive patients. Arch Pathol Lab Med 1999; 123(10):875–881.

268. Aronson MD, Komaroff AL, Pass TM, et al. Heterophil antibody in adults with sore throat: frequency and clinical presentation. Ann Intern Med 1982; 96(4):505–508.

269. Obel N, Hoier-Madsen M, Kangro H. Serological and clinical findings in patients with serological evidence of reactivated Epstein-Barr virus infection. APMIS 1996; 104(6):424–428.

270. Feng Z, Li Z, Sui B, et al. Serological diagnosis of infectious mononucleosis by chemiluminescent immunoassay using capsid antigen p18 of Epstein-Barr virus. Clin Chim Acta 2005; 354(1):77–82.

271. Evans AS, Niederman JC, Cenabre LC, et al. A prospective evaluation of heterophile and Epstein-Barr virus-specific IgM antibody tests in clinical and subclinical infectious mononucleosis: Specificity and sensitivity of the tests and persistence of antibody. J Infect Dis 1975; 132(5):546–554.

272. Humar A, Mazzulli T, Moussa G, et al. Clinical utility of cytomegalovirus (CMV) serology testing in high-risk CMV D+/R- transplant recipients. Am J Transplant 2005; 5(5):1065–1070.

273. Hodinka RL. Human cytomegalovirus. In: Murray PR, Baron EJ, Jorgensen JH, et al., eds. Manual of Clinical Microbiology, 8th ed. Vol 2. Washington, DC: ASM Press, 2003:1304–1318.

274. Zurlo JJ, O'Neill D, Polis MA, et al. Lack of clinical utility of cytomegalovirus blood and urine cultures in patients with HIV infection. Ann Intern Med 1993; 118(1):12–17.

275. Schroeder R, Michelon T, Fagundes I, et al. Comparison between RFLP-PCR and antigenemia for pp65 antigen for diagnosis of cytomegalovirus disease after kidney transplant. Transplant Proc 2004; 36(4):891–893.

276. Wohl DA. Zeng D, Stewart P, et al. Cytomegalovirus viremia, mortality, and end-organ disease among patients with AIDS receiving potent antiretroviral therapies. J Acquir Immune Defic Syndr 2005; 38(5):538–544.

277. Skapova D, Racil Z, Dvorakova D, et al. Significance of qualitative PCR detection method for preemptive therapy of cytomegalovirus infection in patients after

allogeneic hematopoietic stem cell transplantation—single-centre experience. Neoplasma 2005; 52(2):137–142.

278. Bek B, Boeckh M, Lepenies J, et al. High-level sensitivity of quantitative pp65 cytomegalovirus (CMV) antigenemia assay for diagnosis of CMV disease in AIDS patients and follow-up. J Clin Microbiol 1996; 34(2):457–459.

279. Van den Berg AP, van der Bij W, van Son WJ, et al. Cytomegalovirus antigenemia as a useful marker of symptomatic cytomegalovirus infection after renal transplantation—a report of 130 consecutive patients. Transplantation 1989; 48(6):991–995.

280. Lesprit P, Scieux C, Lemann M, et al. Use of the cytomegalovirus (CMV) antgenemia assay for the rapid diagnosis of primary CMV infection in hospitalized adults. Clin Infect Dis 1998; 26(3):646–650.

281. Ye Q, Luo G, He X, et al. Prospective study of relationship between cytomegalovirus pneumonia and viral load in renal transplant recipients. Transplant Proc 2004; 36(10):3036–3041.

282. Ljungman P, von Dobeln L, Ringholm L, et al. The value of CMV and fungal PCR for monitoring of acute leukaemia and autologous stem cell transplant patients. Scand J Infect Dis 2005; 37(2):121–126.

283. Schvoerer E, Henriot S, Zachary P, et al. Monitoring low cytomegalovirus viremia in transplanted patients by a real-time PCR on plasma. J Med Virol 2005; 76(1):76–81.

284. Van den Berg AP, Klompmaker IJ, Haagsma EB, et al. Antigenemia in the diagnosis and monitoring of active cytomegalovirus infection after liver transplantation. J Infect Dis 1991;164(2):265–270.

285. Shinkai M, Bozzette SA, Powderly W, et al. Utility of urine and leukocyte cultures and plasma DNA polymerase chain reaction for identification of AIDS patients at risk for developing human cytomegalovirus disease. J Infect Dis 1997; 175(2):301–308.

286. Schacker T, Collier AC, Hughes J, et al. Clinical and epidemiologic features of primary HIV infection. Ann Intern Med 1996; 125(4):257–264.

287. Quinn TC. Acute primary HIV infection. JAMA 1997; 278(1):58–62.

288. Kassutto S, Rosenberg ES. Primary HIV type 1 infection. Clin Infect Dis 2004; 38(10):1447–1453.

289. Sun HY, Chen MJ, Hung CC, et al. Clinical presentations and virologic characteristics of primary human immunodeficiency virus type-1 infection in a university hospital in Taiwan. J Microbiol Immunol Infect 2004; 37(5):271–275.

290. Janssen RS, Satten GA, Stramer SL, et al. New testing strategy to detect early HIV-1 infection for use in incidence estimates and for clinical and prevention purposes. JAMA 1998; 280(1):42–48.

291. Pilcher CD, Price MA, Hoffman IF, et al. Frequent detection of acute primary HIV infection in men in Malawi. AIDS 2004; 18(3):517–524.

292. Daar ES, Little S, Pitt J, et al. Diagnosis of primary HIV-1 infection. Ann Intern Med 2001; 134(1):25–29.

293. Rich JD, Merriman NA, Mylonakis E, et al. Misdiagnosis of HIV infection by HIV-plasma viral load testing: a case series. Ann Intern Med 1999; 130(1):37–39.

294. Filler S, Causer LM, Newman RD, et al. Malaria surveillance—United States 2001. MMWR Surveill Summ 2003; 52(5):1–14.

295. Rogers WO. *Plasmodium* and *Babesia*. In: Murray PR, Baron EJ, Jorgensen JH, et al, eds. Manual of Clinical Microbiology, 8th ed. Vol 2. Washington, DC: ASP Press, 2003:1944–1959.

296. Marx A, Pewsner D, Egger M, et al. Meta-analysis: accuracy of rapid tests for Malaria in travelers returning from endemic areas. Ann Intern Med 2005; 142(10):836–846.

297. Amexo M, Tolhurst R, Barnish G, et al. Malaria misdiagnosis: effects on the poor and vulnerable. Lancet 2004; 364(9448):1896–1898.

298. Singh N, Saxena A. Usefulness of a rapid on-site *Plasmodium falciparum* diagnosis (Paracheck PF) in forest migrants and among the indigenous population at the site of their occupational activities in central India. Am J Trop Med Hyg 2005; 72(1):26–29.

299. Moody A. Rapid diagnostic tests for malaria parasites. Clin Microbiol Rev 2002; 15(1):66–78.

300. Susi B, Whitman T, Blazes DL, et al. Rapid diagnostic test for *Plasmodium falciparum* in 32 Marines medically evacuated from Liberia with a febrile illness. Ann Intern Med 2005; 142(6):476–477.

301. Farcas GA, Zhong KJ, Lovegrove FE, et al. Evaluation of the Binax NOW ICT test versus polymerase chain reaction and microscopy for the detection of malaria in returned travelers. Am J Trop Med Hyg 2003; 69(6):589–592.

302. Jelinek T, Groubusch MP, Schwenke S, et al. Sensitivity and specificity of dipstick tests for rapid diagnosis of malaria in nonimmune travelers. J Clin Microbiol 1999; 37(3):721–723.

303. Iqbal J, Khalid N, Hira PR. Comparison of two commercial assays with expert microscopy for confirmation of symptomatically diagnosed malaria. J Clin Microbiol 2002; 40(12):4675–4678.

304. Coleman RE, Maneechai N, Rachapaew N, et al. Field evaluation of the ICT Malaria Pf/ Pv immunochromatographic test for the detection of asymptomatic malaria in a *Plasmodium falciparum/vivax* endemic area in Thailand. Am J Trop Med Hyg 2002; 66(4):379–383.

305. Quintana M, Piper R, Boling HL, et al. Malaria diagnosis by dipstick assay in a Honduran population with coendemic *Plasmodium falciparum* and *Plasmodium vivax*. Am J Trop Med Hyg 1998; 59(6):868–871.

306. Perandin F, Manca N, Calderaro A, et al. Development of a real-time PCR assay for detection of *Plasmodium falciparum*, *Plasmodium vivax*, and *Plasmodium ovale* for routine clinical diagnosis. J Clin Microbiol 2004; 42(3):1214–1219.

307. Myjak P, Nahorski W, Pieniazek NJ, et al. Usefulness of PCR for diagnosis of imported malaria in Poland. Eur J Clin Microbiol Infect Dis 2002; 21(3):215–218.

308. Tham JM, Lee SH, Tan TM, et al. Detection and species determination of malaria parasites by PCR: comparison with microscopy and with ParaSight-F and ICT malaria Pf tests in a clinical environment. J Clin Microbiol 1999; 37(5):1269–1273.

309. Postigo M, Mendoz-Leon A, Perez HA. Malaria diagnosis by the polymerase chain reaction: a field study in south-eastern Venezuela. Trans R Soc Trop Med Hyg 1998; 92(5):509–511.

310. Aubouy A, Carme B. Plasmodium DNA contamination between blood smears during Giemsa staining and microscopic examination. J Infect Dis 2004; 190(7):1335–1337.

311. Gorenflot A, Moubri K, Precigout E, et al. Human babesiosis. Ann Trop Med Parasitol 1998; 92(4):489–501.

312. Sun T, Tenenbaum MJ, Greenspan J, et al. Morphologic and clinical observations in human infection with *Babesia microti*. J Infect Dis 1983; 148(2):239–248.

313. Krause PJ. Babesiosis diagnosis and treatment. Vector Borne Zoonotic Dis 2003; 3(1):45–51.

314. Chisholm ES, Sulzer AJ, Ruebush TK. Indirect immunofluorescence test for human *Babesia micoti* infection: antigenic specificity. Am J Trop Med Hyg 1986; 35(5):921–925.

315. Krause PJ, Telford SR, Ryan R, et al. Diagnosis of babesiosis: evaluation of a serologic test for the detection of *Babesia microti* antibody. J Infect Dis 1994; 169(4):923–926.

316. Ruebush TK, Chisholm ES, Sulzer AJ, et al. Development and persistence of antibody in persons infected with *Babesia microti*. Am J Trop Med Hyg 1981; 30(1):291–292.

317. Loa CC, Adelson ME, Mordechai E, et al. Serological diagnosis of human babesiosis by IgG enzyme-linked immunosorbent assay. Curr Microbiol 2004; 49(6):385–389.

318. Torres-Velez FJ, Nace EK, Won KY, et al. Development of an immunohistochemical assay for the detection of babesiosis in formalin-fixed, paraffin-embedded tissue samples. Am J Clin Pathol 2003; 120(6):833–838.

319. Krause PJ, Telford S, Spielman A, et al. Comparison of PCR with blood smear and inoculation of small animals for diagnosis of *Babesia microti* parasitemia. J Clin Microbiol 1996; 34(11):2791–2794.

320. Persing DH, Mathiesen D, Marshall WF, et al. Detection of *Babesia microti* by polymerase chain reaction. J Clin Microbiol 1992; 30(8):2097–2103.

321. Berman JD. Human leishmaniasis: clinical, diagnostic, and chemotherapeutic developments in the last 10 years. Clin Infect Dis 1997; 24(4):684–703.

322. Guerin PJ, Olliaro P, Sundar S, et al. Visceral leishmaniasis: current status of control, diagnosis, and treatment, and a proposed research and development agenda. Lancet Infect Dis 2002; 2(8);494–501.
323. Murray HW. Kala-azar—Progress against a neglected disease. Editorial in: N Engl J Med 2002; 347(22):1793–1794.
324. Halsey ES, Bryce LM, Wortmann GW, et al. Visceral leishmaniasis in a soldier returning from Operation Enduring Freedom. Mil Med 2004; 169(9):699–701.
325. Reus M, Garcia B, Vazquez V, et al. Visceral leishmaniasis: diagnosis by ultrasound-guided fine needle aspiration of an axillary node. Br J Radiol 2005; 78(926):158–160.
326. Zijlstra EE, Ali MS, el-Hassan AM, et al. Kala-azar: a comparative study of parasitolo-gical methods and the direct agglutination test in diagnosis. Trans R Soc Trop Med Hyg 1992; 86(5):505–507.
327. Sarker CB, Alam KS, Jamal MF, et al. Sensitivity of splenic and bone marrow aspirate study for diagnosis of kala-azar. Mymensingh Med J 2004; 13(2):130–133.
328. Chulay JD, Brycesson AD. Quantitation of amastigotes of *Leishmania donovani* in smears of splenic aspirates from patients with visceral leishmaniasis. Am J Trop Med Hyg 1983; 32(3):475–479.
329. Limoncu ME, Ozbilgin A, Balcioglu IC, et al. Evaluation of three new culture media for the cultivation and isolation of *Leishmania* parasites. J Basic Microbiol 2004; 44(3):197–202.
330. Bruckner DA, Labarca JA. *Leishmania* and *Trypanosoma*. In: Murray PR, Baron EJ, Jorgensen JH, et al, eds. Manual of Clinical Microbiology, 8th ed. Vol 2. Washington, DC: ASM Press, 2003:1960–1969.
331. Martinez P, de la Vega E, Laguna F, et al. Diagnosis of visceral leishmaniasis in HIV-infected individuals using peripheral blood smears. AIDS 1993; 7(2):227–230.
332. Azazy AA. Detection of circulating antigens in sera from visceral leishmaniasis patients using dot-ELISA. J Egypt Soc Parasitol 2004; 34(1):35–43.
333. Sundar S, Sahu M, Mehta H, et al. Noninvasive management of Indian visceral leishma-niasis: clinical application of diagnosis by K39 antigen strip testing at a kala-azar refer-ral unit. Clin Infect Dis 2002; 35(5):581–586.
334. Zijlstra EE, Ali MS, el-Hassan AM, et al. Direct agglutination test for diagnosis and sero-epidemiological survey of kala-azar in the Sudan. Trans R Soc Trop Med Hyg 1991; 85(4):474–476.
335. Ryan JR, Smithyman AM, Rajasekariah GH, et al. Enzyme-linked immunosorbent assay based on soluble promastigote antigen detects immunoglobulin M (igM and IgG anti-bodies in sera from cases of visceral and cutaneous leishmaniasis. J Clin Microbiol 2002; 40(3):1037–1043.
336. Sinha PK, Pandey K, Bhattacharya SK. Diagnosis & management of *Leishmania*/HIV co-infection. Indian J Med Res 2005; 121(4):407–414.
337. Alvar J, Canavate C, Gutierrez-Solar B, et al. *Leishmania* and human immunodeficiency virus coinfection: the first 10 years. Clin Microbiol Rev 1997; 10(2):298–319.
338. Peters BS, Fish D, Golden R, et al. Visceral leishmaniasis in HIV infection and AIDS: clinical features and response to therapy. Q J Med 1990; 77(283):1101–1111.
339. Riera C, Fis R, Lopez P, et al. Evaluation of a latex agglutination test (KAtex) for detec-tion of *Leishmania* antigen in the urine of patients with HIV-*Leishmania* coinfection: value in diagnosis and post-treatment follow-up. Eur J Clin Microbiol Infect Dis 2004; 23(12):899–904.
340. Islam MZ, Itoh M, Mirza R, et al. Direct agglutination test with urine samples for the diagnosis of visceral leishmaniasis. Am J Trop Med Hyg 2004; 70(1):78–82.
341. Vilaplana C, Blanco S, Dominguez J, et al. Noninvasive method for diagnosis of visceral leishmaniasis by a latex agglutination test for detection of antigens in urine samples. J Clin Microbiol 2004; 42(4):1853–1854.
342. Rijal S, Boelaert M, Regmi S, et al. Evaluation of a urinary antigen-based latex aggluti-nation test in the diagnosis of kala-azar in eastern Nepal. Trop Med Int Health 2004; 9(6):724–729.
343. Piarroux R, Gambarelli F, Dumon H, et al. Comparison of PCR with direct examination of bone marrow aspiration, myeloculture, and serology for diagnosis of visceral leish-maniasis in immunocompromised patients. J Clin Microbiol 1994; 32(3):746–749.

344. Nuzum E, White F, Thakur C, et al. Diagnosis of symptomatic visceral leishmaniasis by use of the polymerase chain reaction on patient blood. J Infect Dis 1995; 171(3):751–754.

345. De Oliveira CI, Bafica A, Oliveira F, et al. Clinical utility of polymerase chain reaction-based detection of *Leishmania* in the diagnosis of American cutaneous leishmaniasis. Clin Infect Dis 2003; 37(11):e149–e154.

346. De Doncker S, Huse V, Abdellati S, et al. A new PCR-ELISA for diagnosis of visceral leishmaniasis in blood of HIV-negative subjects. Trans R Soc Trop Med Hyg 2005; 99(1):25–31.

347. Gatti S, Gramegna M, Klersy C, et al. Diagnosis of visceral leishmaniasis: the sensitivities and specificities of traditional methods and a nested PCR assay. Ann Trop Med Parisitol 2004; 98(7):667–676.

348. Fissore C, Delaunay P, Ferrua B, et al. Convenience of serum for visceral leishmaniasis diagnosis by PCR. J Clin Microbiol 2004; 42(1):5332–5333.

349. Gross U, Holpert M, Goebel S. Impact of stage differentiation on diagnosis of toxoplasmosis. Ann Ist Super Sanita 2004; 40(1):65–70.

350. Wilson M, Jones JJ, McAuley JB. *Toxoplasma.* In: Murray PR, Baron EJ, Jorgensen JH, et al., eds. Manual of Clinical Microbiology, 8th ed. Vol. 8. Washington, DC: ASM Press, 2003:1970–1980.

351. Viguer JM, Jimenez-Heffernan JA, Lopez-Ferrer P, et al. Fine needle aspiration of toxoplasmic (Piringer-Kuchinka) lymphadenitis: a cytohistologic correlation study. Acta Cytologica 2005; 49(2):139–143.

352. Dorfman RF, Remington JS. Value of lymph-node biopsy in the diagnosis of acute acquired toxoplasmosis. N Engl J Med 1973; 289(17):878–881.

353. Bastien P. Molecular diagnosis of toxoplasmosis. Trans R Soc Trop Med Hyg 2002; 96(suppl 1):S205–S215.

354. Okhravi N, Jones CD, Carroll N, et al. Use of PCR to diagnose *Toxoplasma gondii* chorioretinitis in eyes with severe vitritis. Clin Experiment Ophthalmol 2005; 33(2):184–187.

355. Hierl T, Reischl U, Lang P, et al. Preliminary evaluation of one conventional nested and two real-time PCR assays for the detection of *Toxoplasma gondii* in immunocompromised patients. J Med Microbiol 2004; 53(7):629–632.

356. Switaj K, Master A, Skrzypezak M, et al. Recent trends in molecular diagnostics for *Toxoplasma gondii* infections. Clin Microbiol Infect 2005; 11(3):170–176.

357. Contini C, Seraceni S, Cultrera R, et al. Evaluation of a real-time PCR-based assay using the lightcycler system for detection of *Toxoplasma gondii* bradyzoite genes in blood specimens from patients with toxoplasmic retinochoroiditis. Int J Parasitol 2005; 35(3):275–283.

358. Martino R, Bretagne S, Einsele H, et al. Early detection of *Toxoplasma* infection by molecular monitoring of *Toxoplasma gondii* in peripheral blood samples after allogeneic stem cell transplantation. Clin Infect Dis 2005; 40(1):67–78.

359. Chandrasekar PH. Real-time polymerase chain reaction for early diagnosis of toxoplasmosis in stem cell transplant recipients: ready for prime time? Clin Infect Dis 2005; 40(1):79–81.

360. Edvinsson B, Jalal S, Nord CE, et al. DNA extraction and PCR assays for detection of *Toxoplasma gondii.* APMIS 2004; 112(6):342–348.

361. Jalal S, Nord CE, Pappalainen M, et al. Rapid and sensitive diagnosis of *Toxoplasma gondii* infections by PCR. Clin Microbiol Infect 2004; 10(10):937–939.

362. Remington JS, Thulliez P, Montoya JG. Recent developments for diagnosis of toxoplasmosis. J Clin Microbiol 2004; 42(3):941–945.

363. Kaul R, Chen P, Binder SR. Detection of immunoglobulin M antibodies specific for *Toxoplasma gondii* with increased selectivity for recently acquired infections. J Clin Microbiol 2004; 42(12):5705–5709.

364. Lappalainen M, Hedman K. Serodiagnosis of toxoplasmosis. Ann Ist Super Sanita 2004; 40(1):81–88.

365. Montoya JG, Huffman HB, Remington JS. Evaluation of the immunoglobulin G avidity test for the diagnosis of toxoplasmic lymphadenopahy. J Clin Microbiol 2004; 42(10):4627–4631.

366. Lucey DR, Maguire JH. Schistosomiasis. Infect Dis Clin North Am 1993; 7(3):635–653.

367. Berhe N, Medhin G, Erko B, et al. Variations in helminth faecal egg counts in Kato-Katz thick smears and their implications in assessing infection status with Schistosoma mansoni. Acta Tropica 2004 92(3):205–212.

368. Harries AD, Fryatt R, Walker J, et al. Schistosomiasis in expatriates returning to Britain from the tropics: a controlled study. Lancet 1986; 1(8472):86–88.

369. Pinto PL, Kanamura HY, Silva RM, et al. Dot-ELISA for the detection of IgM and IgG antibodies to Schistosoma mansoni worm and egg antigens, associated with egg excretion by patients. Rev Inst Med Trop Sao Paulo 1995; 37(2):109–115.

370. Pardo J, Carranza C, Turrientes C, et al. Utility of Schistosoma bovis adult worm antigens for diagnosis of human schistosomiasis by enzyle-linked immunosorbant assay and electroimmunotransfer blot techniques. Clin Diagn Lab Immunol 2004; 11(6): 1165–1170.

371. Sulahian A, Garin YJ, Izri A, et al. Development and evaluation of a Western blot kit for diagnosis of schistosomiasis. Clin Diagn Lab Immunol 2005; 12(4):548–551.

372. Doenhoff MJ, Chiodini PL, Hamilton JV. Specific and sensitive diagnosis of schistosome infection: can it be done with antibodies? Trends Parasitol 2004; 20(1):35–39.

373. Esposito AL, Gleckman RA. Fever of unknown origin in the elderly. J Am Ger Soc 1978; 26(11):498–505.

374. Hunder GG, Bloch DA, Bicel BA, et al. The American College 1990 criteria for the classification of giant cell arteritis. Arthritis Rheum 1990; 33(8):1122–1128.

375. Salvarani C, Hunder G. Giant cell arteritis with low erythrocyte sedimentation rate: frequency of occurrence in a population-based study. Arthritis Rheum 2001; 45(2):140–145.

376. Schmidt WA, Kraft HE, Vorpahl K, et al. Color duplex ultrasonography in the diagnosis of temporal arteritis. N Engl J Med 1997; 337(19):1336–1342.

377. Salvarani C, Silingardi M, Ghirarduzzi A, et al. Is duplex ultrasonography useful for the diagnosis of giant-cell arteritis? Ann Intern Med 2002, 137(4):232–238.

378. Boyev LR, Miller NR, Green WR. Efficacy of unilateral versus bilateral temporal artery biopsies for the diagnosis of giant cell arteritis. Am J Ophthalmol 1999; 128(2):211–215.

379. Schur PH, Shmerling RH. Laboratory tests in rheumatic disorders. In: Hochberg MC, Silman AJ, Smolen JS, et al., eds. Rheumatology, 3rd ed. Vol 1. Edinburgh: Mosby, 2003:199–213.

380. Jennette J, Falk R, Andrassy K, et al. Nomenclature of systemic vasculitides. Proposal of an international consensus conference. Arthritis Rheum 1994; 37(2):187–192.

381. Guillevin L, Lhote F, Cohen P, et al. Polyarteritis nodosa related to hepatitis B virus. A prospective study with long-term observation of 41 pateints. Medicine (Baltimore)1995; 74(5):238–253.

382. Steiner G. Autoantibodies in rheumatoid arthritis. In: Hochberg MC, Silman AJ, Smolen JS, et al, eds. Rheumatology, 3rd ed. Vol 1. Edinburgh: Mosby, 2003:833–841.

383. Tan EM, Cohen AS, Fries JF, et al. The 1982 revised criteria for the classification of systemic lupus erythematosus (SLE). Arthritis Rheum 1982; 25(11):1271–1277.

384. Hochberg MC. Updating the American College of Rheumatology revised criteria for the classification of systemic lupus erythematosus [letter]. Arthritis Rheum 1997; 40(9):1725.

385. Unger PD, Rappaport KM, Strauchen JA. Necrotizing lymphadenitis (Kikuchi's disease). Report of four cases of an unusual pseudolymphomatous lesion and immunologic marker studies. Arch Pathol Lab Med 1987; 111(11):1031–1034.

386. Tsang WY, Chan JC, Ng CS. Kikuchi's lymphadenitis: A morphologic analysis of 75 cases with special reference to unusual features. Am J Surg Pathol 1995; 18(3): 219–231.

387. Dorfman RF. Histiocytic necrotizing lymphadenitis of Kikuchi and Fujimoto. Arch Pathol Lab Med 1987; 111(11):1026–1029.

388. Tsang WY, Chan JC. Fine needle aspiration cytologic diagnosis of Kikuchi's lymphadenitis. A report of 27 cases. Am J Clin Pathol 1994; 102(4):454–458.

389. Tedesco FJ, Moore S. Infectious diseases mimicking inflammatory bowel disease. Am Surg 1982; 48(6):243–249.

390. Waye JD. Endoscopy in inflammatory bowel disease: indications and differential diagnosis. Med Clin North Am 1990; 74(1):51–56.

391. Joossens S, Reinisch W, Vermeire S, et al. The value of serologic markers in indeterminate colitis: a prospective follow-up study. Gastroenterology 2002; 122(5): 1242–1247.
392. Peeters M, Joossens S, Vermeire S, et al. Diagnostic value of anti-*Saccaromyces cervisiae* and antineutrophil cytoplasmic autoantibodies in inflammatory bowel disease. Am J Gastroenterol 2001; 96(3):730–734.
393. Terjung B, Spengler U, Sauerbruch T, et al. "Atypical p-ANCA" in IBD and hepatobiliary disorders react with a 50-kilodalton nuclear envelope protein of neutrophils and myeloid cell lines. Gastroenterology 2000; 119(2):310–322.
394. International Study Group for Behcet's Disease. Criteria for diagnosis of Behcet's disease. Lancet 1990; 335(8697):1078–1080.
395. Yazici H, Yurdakul S, Hamuryudan V, et al. Behcet's syndrome. In: Hochberg MC, Silman AJ, Smolen JS, et al, eds. Rheumatology, 3rd ed. Vol 2. Edinburgh: Mosby, 2003:1665–1669.
396. Fitzpatrick TB, Johnson RA, Wolff K, et al, eds. Behcet's syndrome. In: Color Atlas and Synopsis of Clinical Dermatology, 3rd ed. New York: McGraw-Hill, 1997:322–324.
397. Grateau G. Clinical and genetic aspects of the hereditary periodic fever syndromes. Rheumatology 2004; 43(4):410–415.
398. Samuels J, Aksentijevich I, Torosyan Y, et al. Familial Mediterranean fever at the millennium. Clinical spectrum, ancient mutations, and a survey of 100 American referrals to the National Institutes of Health. Medicine (Baltimore) 1998; 77(4):268–297.
399. Barakat MH, El-Khawad AO, Gumaa KA, et al. Metaraminol provocative test: a specific diagnostic test for familial Mediterranean fever. Lancet 1983; 1(8378):656–657.
400. Barakat MH, Gumaa KA, Malhas LN, et al. Plasma dopamine beta-hydroxylase: rapid diagnostic test for recurrent hereditary polyserositis. Lancet 1988; 2(8623):1280–1283.
401. Schachter J. Fever in Oncology. In: Isaac B, Kernbaum S, Burke M, eds. Unexplained Fever. Boca Raton: CRC Press, 1991:381–384.
402. Wang C, Armstrong D. Neoplastic Diseases. In: Murray HW, ed. FUO: Fever of Undedermined Origin. Mount Kisco: Futura Publishing Company, Inc., 1983:39–48.
403. Tsavaris N, Ainelis A, Karabelis A, et al. A randomized trial of the effect of three nonsteroid anti-inflammatory agents in ameliorating cancer-induced fever. J Intern Med 1990; 228(5):451–455.
404. Johnson M. Neoplastic fever. Palliat Med 1996; 10(3):217–224.
405. Azeemuddin SK, Vega RA, Kim TH, et al. The effect of naproxen on fever in children with malignancies. Cancer 1987; 59(11):1966–1968.
406. Chang JC, Gross HM. Neoplastic fever responds to the treatment of an adequate dose of naproxen. J Clin Oncol 1985; 3(4):552–558.
407. Chang JC, Gross HM. Utility of naproxen in the differential diagnosis of fever of undetermined origin in patients with cancer. Am J Med 1984; 76(4):597–602.
408. Dorin RI, Qualls CR, Crapo LM. Diagnosis of adrenal insufficiency. Ann Intern Med 2003; 139(3):194–204.
409. Wynne AG, Gharib H, Sceithauer BW, et al. Hyperthyroidism due to inappropriate secretion of thyrotropin in 10 patients. Am J Med 1992; 92(1):15–24.
410. Caldwell G, Kellett HA, Gow SM, et al. A new strategy for thyroid function testing. Lancet 1985; 1(8438):1117–1119.
411. Stein PP, Black HR. A simplified diagnostic approach to pheochromocytoma. A review of the literature and report of one institution's experience. Medicine (Baltimore) 1991; 70(1):46–66.
412. Lenders JWM, Pacak K, Walther MM, et al. Biochemical diagnosis of pheochromocytoma: which test is best? JAMA 2002; 287(11):1427–1434.

16 Imaging in Fever of Unknown Origin

Yogi Trivedi, Elizabeth Yung, and Douglas S. Katz
Department of Radiology, Winthrop-University Hospital, Mineola, New York, U.S.A.

INTRODUCTION

Diagnostic workup of patients with fever of unknown origin (FUO) remains a challenge. The spectrum of diseases traditionally recognized as the causes of FUO are infectious, malignant, inflammatory, and undetermined. A good history and physical examination, and appropriate laboratory testing, are paramount in the assessment of FUO. Deciding on the most appropriate imaging test or tests will be based on one's clinical suspicion. With many different imaging modalities available to clinicians for the workup of FUO, it is useful to know about the different imaging studies available. The literature regarding FUO and computed tomography (CT), magnetic resonance imaging (MRI), and positron emission tomography (PET) is limited. There are very few prospective trials comparing the usefulness and accuracy of these imaging modalities (e.g., whole body MRI versus PET, or whole body CT versus MRI, or any of these techniques compared with more traditional nuclear medicine techniques). In this chapter, we discuss the usefulness of nuclear medicine, CT, ultrasonography, MRI, and PET in the evaluation of patients with FUO.

NUCLEAR MEDICINE: TRADITIONAL IMAGING APPROACHES
Gallium

Historically, gallium-67 citrate was the first agent used for imaging inflammation by scintigraphy (1) and it has been utilized in the detection of infections, tumors, and inflammatory diseases for more than 30 years. Gallium is cyclotron produced with a physical half-life of 78 hours, and decays by electron capture with four main gamma emissions suitable for imaging. ^{67}Ga citrate is an iron analog, which is mainly transported in its ionic form or bound to transferrin, with approximately 90% of circulating ^{67}Ga present in the plasma. Hyperemia and increased vascular membrane permeability at sites of infection and inflammation result in increased delivery and accumulation of radiogallium. ^{67}Ga also binds to lactoferrin, which is secreted in high concentrations by leukocytes at sites of inflammation or infection. In addition, siderophore production by bacteria at sites of infection may play a role in the accumulation and retention of ^{67}Ga citrate, as well as direct uptake by certain bacteria, and direct binding to leukocytes (2,3). Approximately 10% to 25% of ^{67}Ga citrate is excreted by the kidneys in the first 24 hours, followed by excretion in the gastrointestinal tract, and the remainder of the radiopharmaceutical distributing throughout the body, concentrating in the liver, spleen, cortical bone, and bone marrow (Fig. 1A). Imaging is typically performed 24 to 72 hours postinjection of 185 to 370 MBq (5–10 mCi). ^{67}Ga citrate uptake is seen in a wide range of inflammatory, infectious, and neoplastic processes, a sensitive but nonspecific radiopharmaceutical. It is very useful in the evaluation of the chest (Figs. 1B

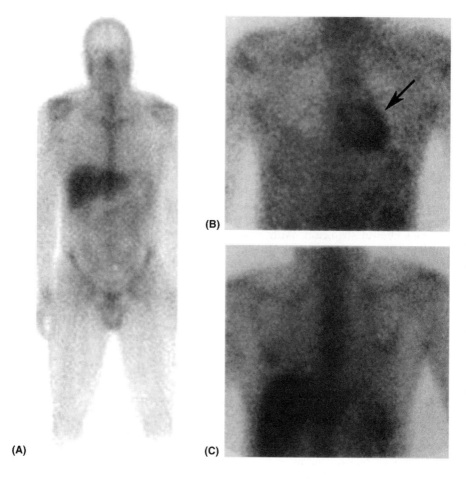

FIGURE 1 (A) Normal gallium scan. (B) Gallium scan of a 28-year-old male with fever of unknown origin reveals abnormal increased cardiac uptake (*black arrow*), which (C) no longer appears following treatment with nonsteroidal anti-inflammatory medication for aseptic myocarditis.

and C). Diffuse gallium uptake in the lungs is commonly seen in bacterial pneumonia, drug reaction (busulfan, cyclophosphamide, amiodorone, bleomycin), adult respiratory distress syndrome, pneumoconiosis (silicosis, asbestosis), pneumocystitis carini, and tuberculosis. The normal excretion of ^{67}Ga citrate in the gastrointestinal and genitourinary tracts diminishes the utility of radiogallium in the evaluation of the abdomen and pelvis, including intra-abdominal abscesses, which comprise approximately 32% of infectious causes of FUO (4). ^{67}Ga imaging also lacks sensitivity for the detection of inflammation involving the pancreas, kidneys, mesentery/omentum, ovaries, spleen, uterus, small and large bowel, and appendix. In a study of 145 patients examined by gallium scintigraphy for FUO, 29% had abnormal gallium scans which were helpful in diagnosis, whereas 49% of abnormal gallium scans were diagnostically noncontributory (5). Prompt diagnosis using ^{67}Ga citrate is limited by the necessity for imaging at 24 and

48 hours postinjection. In addition, the high dosimetry and limited resolution do not favor the frequent use of gallium scintigraphy for infection imaging. Bowel-cleansing preparations, serial imaging, single-photon emission computed tomography (SPECT) imaging, and the development of SPECT/CT coregistration can be used to improve localization (6).

Labeled Leukocytes

Radiolabeled white blood cell scintigraphy is the more commonly used nuclear medicine imaging technique for the evaluation of FUO. White blood cells migrate to sites of infection and inflammation, particularly when the inflammation is acute. In general, labeled leukocytes are not sensitive in the evaluation of viral and parasitic infections. There are fewer false-positive results with labeled leukocyte imaging, which is more specific for infection than gallium scintigraphy. The labeling process requires blood handling, and normally takes about two hours. It can be performed in local pharmacies with pickup and delivery services, or can be accomplished onsite within the laboratory if the proper facilities and personnel are available. FDA-approved radiopharmaceuticals for leukocyte labeling are ^{111}In-oxine or ^{99m}Tc-hexamethylpropylene amine oxine (^{99m}Tc HMPAO). Leukocytes are separated in the buffy coat from the red blood cells by gravity sedimentation and centrifugation before labeling (7). Approximately 50 cc of blood is needed for labeling, and it is recommended that the white blood cell count be at least 3000.

[111]Indium-Labeled Leukocyte Scan

[111]Indium-labeled leukocyte scanning involves a lipophilic metal-chelate complex, [111]indium oxine, which binds and penetrates the cell membrane. Once inside the cell membrane, the indium and oxine dissociate, the oxine freely diffuses out of the cell, and the indium binds to nuclear and cytoplasmic proteins. The normal physiologic distribution of labeled leukocytes is within the liver, spleen, and bone marrow (Fig. 2). [111]In has a physical half-life of 67 hours and decays by electron capture to cadmium-111, with gamma emissions of 172 and 245 keV. The standard injected dose of ^{111}In-oxine labeled autologous white blood cells is 18.5 MBq (500 uCi), a small amount of radioactivity with limited imaging characteristics. The dose is limited because the critical organ is the spleen, which receives an absorbed dose of about 200 mGy/18.5 MBq (20 rad/500 uCi). The whole body dose is 3.7 mGy/18.5 MBq (0.37 rad/500 uCi). Standard, delayed imaging is performed at 24 hours, and early imaging can be performed at four hours. There is no renal or gastrointestinal excretion, allowing evaluation of the abdomen and pelvis, a significant advantage over gallium scintigraphy. Routine evaluation of the spleen is, however, limited, although an additional ^{99m}Tc sulfur colloid liver spleen scan (or a CT or sonogram) can be performed if there is a suspicion of a splenic abscess. The sensitivity of ^{111}In-labeled leukocytes ranges between 45% and 95% and the specificity has been reported between 69% and 86% (8–12).

    ^{111}In-labeled leukocyte scanning is very helpful and accurate for diagnosing vascular graft infections, especially at hemodialysis-access sites, with sensitivities reported greater than 90% and specificity between 85% and 88% (13,14). Morbidity and mortality associated with prosthetic vascular graft infections are high, and infection of prosthetic grafts occurs in approximately 2% of cases. In a study of 30 scans performed in 21 patients with vascular grafts evaluated for infection,

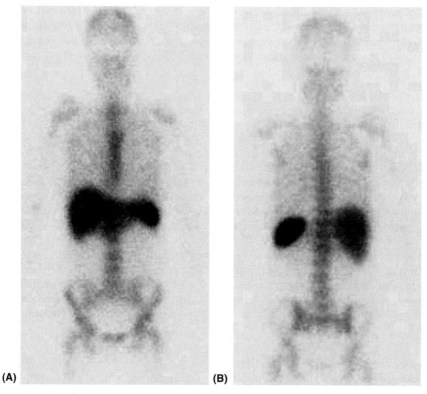

(A)   **(B)**

FIGURE 2 Normal ^{111}In white blood cell scan; **(A)** anterior view, **(B)** posterior view. Note normal uptake in the liver and spleen.

13 were proven to have infected grafts at surgery, and all were positive on ^{111}In-labeled leukocyte scans (14) (Figs. 3 and 4). [111] In-labeled leukocyte scanning is also useful in the evaluation of line sepsis (Figs. 5–7) and abdominal and thoracic infections such as abscess, empyema, and pneumonia (Figs. 8–10). Other potential sources of FUO that can be detected include urinary tract infections (Fig. 11).

[99m]Tc-Hexamethylpropylene Amine Oxine

HMPAO, an agent initially introduced for cerebral imaging, has been used to label leukocytes as well. [99m]Tc HMPAO is lipophilic and penetrates the white blood cell membrane. Once inside, it becomes hydrophilic and is trapped within the cell. [99m]Tc has a half-life of approximately six hours. ^{99m}Tc-HMPAO-labeled imaging utilizes early and delayed imaging obtained at approximately 30 minutes and three hours postreinfusion of the labeled leukocytes, allowing earlier diagnosis compared to ^{111}In-labeled leukocytes. Mountford et al. (12) found that the sensitivity of the ^{99m}Tc HMPAO-labeled leukocyte scan was as high as the 24-hour indium-leukocyte scan for localizing intra-abdominal sepsis. In addition, approximately 1110 MBq (30 mCi) of ^{99m}Tc HMPAO is used to label leukocytes, which is 60 times the ^{111}In-oxine dose. This allows for better imaging characteristics with ^{99m}Tc HMPAO; however the physiologic bowel activity seen with ^{99m}Tc HMPAO reduces the specificity over time (1), and the short half-life limits 24-hour imaging.

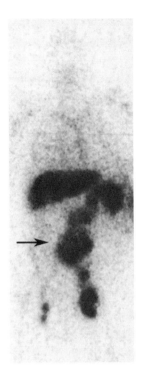

FIGURE 3 ^{111}In white blood cell scan of a 76-year-old man after repair of an abdominal aortic aneurysm, who then developed infection of the aortic graft.

Again, the drawbacks of ^{99m}Tc HMPAO, as with ^{111}In leukocyte imaging, include the need to handle blood for labeling the leukocytes.

In Vivo Leukocyte Labeling

[111]In-oxine- and ^{99m}Tc-HMPAO-labeled leukocytes are in vitro-labeling techniques, which require blood handling and reinfusion, increasing the risks of transmittable diseases and technical errors. Much research has been performed to develop in vivo methods of labeling leukocytes, including labeling antigranulocyte antibodies, antibody fragments, and peptides. NeutroSpec™ (fanolesomab) is a murine monoclonal antigranulocyte antibody that labels leukocytes in vivo. This anti-CD 15 IgM antibody can be labeled easily with 370 to 740 MBq (10–20 mCi) ^{99m}Tc pertechnetate and localizes human polymorphonuclear neutrophils (PMNs) at sites of infection (15). Advantages of this agent are the ability to bind with high affinity and specificity to PMNs in vivo at sites of infection, faster diagnostic interpretation because imaging is performed after one hour, no increased pulmonary uptake, and less exposure to the spleen, which is the dose-limiting organ, an estimated 0.064 mGy/MBq (18 rad/mCi). This radiodiagnostic agent had received FDA approval for the diagnosis of appendicitis in patients ≥5 years with equivocal signs and symptoms; however, it is not currently available for use in the United States at the present time.

Another agent, a murine monoclonal antibody fragment of the IgG1 class that binds to normal cross-reactive antigen-90 present on leukocytes, ^{99m}Tc-labeled anti-NCA-90 FAB fragment (Leukoscan), has been investigated by Becker et al. (16), specifically for the identification of osteomyelitis. The mechanism of uptake of

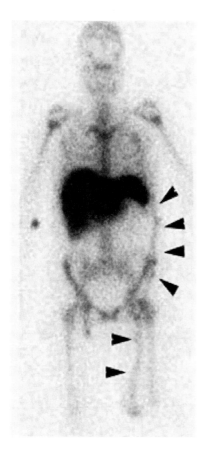

FIGURE 4 ^{111}In-white blood cell scan of a 43-year-old female with an infected left axillary-femoral bypass graft.

radiolabeled monoclonal antigranulocytes can occur by the migration of labeled granulocytes to the site of infection or nonspecific uptake of free antibody due to increased permeability at the site of infection (16). Leukoscan has been approved for use in Europe and Canada; however, it is not available in the United States at the present time.

Other agents, such as ^{99m}Tc BW 250/183 monoclonal antigranulocyte antibody for use in the diagnosis of endocarditis and abdominal abscesses investigated by Meller et al. (17), and a murine monoclonal IgG1 (Granuloscint) that binds to nonspecific cross-reactive antigen-95 on neutrophils, have been investigated; however, they have not gained approval for use in the United States. Much work still remains to find a radiodiagnostic in vivo agent for infection-imaging, which is nontoxic, safe, specific, and rapid acting.

Occult Infection

A modified version of the 1961 Petersdorf and Beeson definition of FUO is an illness at least three weeks duration, with repeatedly documented bouts of fever > 38.3°C and no diagnosis following initial inpatient or outpatient assessment (18). If no localizing signs are present, undetected sites of infection may be present in the abdomen, skeletal system, cardiovascular system, or chest. In this setting, anatomic

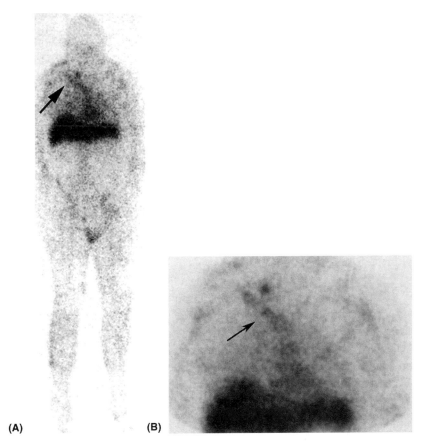

(A)　　　　**(B)**

FIGURE 5 **(A)** ^{111}In-white blood cell scan of a 63-year-old male with cutaneous T-cell lymphoma with an infected right subclavian catheter (*black arrow*). Note increased WBC uptake in the subcutaneous tissues associated with lymphoma. **(B)** Anterior view of the chest.

imaging studies have not proved sensitive or specific. Most hospitalized patients with FUO have a significant past medical or surgical history, and the cause is often due to occult infection (Fig. 12).

Peters described the importance of distinguishing classical fever of unknown origin and occult infection, and the need to select the appropriate imaging modality for patient workup (1). In the case of occult infection, the test of choice is a labeled leukocyte scan. When the source of fever is unknown as in the classical case of FUO, a sensitive but less specific test such as ^{67}Ga scans may be helpful, although ^{67}Ga does not permit differentiation of FUO from tumor or infection, and lacks sensitivity for an abdominal source of infection.

Often, patients with occult infections and FUO are treated with antibiotics before a definite source of infection is determined. Datz et al. (19) reported a sensitivity of 88.7% for ^{111}In-oxine-labeled leukocyte scans in patients treated with antibiotics, compared to 92.1% in patients not on antibiotic therapy, indicating that antibiotic therapy does not significantly affect the sensitivity of

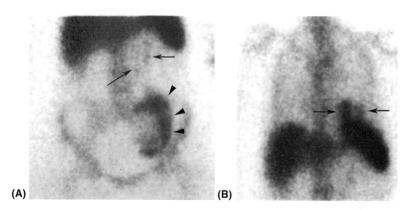

(A)   **(B)**

FIGURE 6   (**A**) [111]In white blood cell scan in a 74-year-old female after automatic implantable cardiac defibrillator battery change (battery in left pelvis) reveals infection of the battery pocket (*black arrowheads*) and infection along the leads (*black arrows*). (**B**) Infected pacing pads around the heart are also seen (*black arrows*).

[111]In-labeled-leukocyte scans (Fig. 13). Similarly, chemotherapy has been found to have no effect on indium-labeled leukocyte scans.

Osteomyelitis

A common cause of occult infection, osteomyelitis often presents as an FUO. Bone infection is commonly caused by hematogenous or contiguous spread of bacteria to bone. Nuclear-medicine bone scans and MRI are two modalities that have high sensitivity for osteomyelitis.

Three-phase bone scan is the classical study for the evaluation of osteomyelitis. The flow phase will reveal increased perfusion due to vasodilation and reactive hyperemia, the blood-pool phase demonstrates the expanded extracellular fluid space related to inflammation, and the delayed images performed at two to four hours after the initial injection demonstrate the chemiadsorption to open bone matrices present at sites of reactive bone turnover. The three-phase bone scan has a sensitivity of >95% for osteomyelitis and is positive within 24 hours of onset (20). However, specificity for osteomyelitis detection decreases when complicated by bone remodeling as a result of fracture, bone contusion, tumor, orthopedic hardware, chronic osteomyelitis, neuropathic joints, or pseudoarthrosis. An ^{111}In-labeled leukocyte scan in conjunction with a three-phase bone scan is helpful in increasing specificity (Fig. 14). Labeled leukocytes do not accumulate in areas of bony turnover in the absence of infection; however, there can be normal uptake in bone marrow, which can be distinguished from uptake secondary to infection by performing concurrently a sulfur colloid bone marrow scan, which demonstrates normal bone marrow.

Evaluation of prosthesis infections can be very difficult. Sensitivity and specificity can be improved with the combination of an ^{111}In-labeled leukocyte scan and a ^{99m}Tc sulfur colloid bone marrow scan (6), which can be performed simultaneously with multiple energy acquisitions (Fig. 15). Labeled leukocyte studies have high false-negative results for vertebral infections, and gallium is more useful for diagnosing vertebral osteomyelitis and discitis (Figs. 9 and 16).

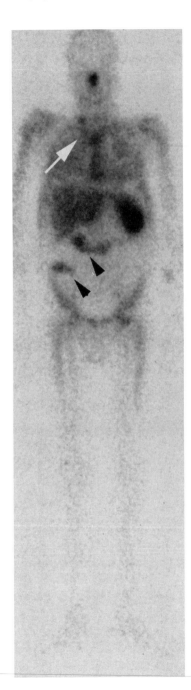

FIGURE 7 ^{111}In-white blood cell scan of an 80-year-old male with end-stage renal disease presenting with fever. Linear uptake in right lower anterior neck (*white arrow*) due to central venous catheter infection. Curvilinear activity in abdomen (*black arrowheads*) may be due to normal swallowed leukocytes, enteritis from any etiology (inflammatory, infectious, or ischemic), active gastrointestinal bleeding, or abscess outside of bowel. Ascites is present, separating the liver and spleen from the ribs laterally.

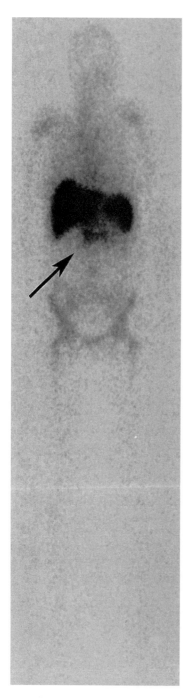

FIGURE 8 ^{111}In-white blood cell scan of a 58-year-old female with a pancreatic abscess (*black arrow*).

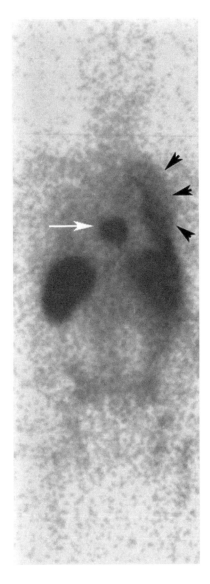

FIGURE 9 Posterior image from ^{111}In-white blood cell scan in an 86 year-old-female with fever demonstrating acute osteomyelitis of T8 and T9 vertebral bodies (*white arrow*) and right empyema (*black arrowheads*).

COMPUTED TOMOGRAPHY, ULTRASOUND, AND MAGNETIC RESONANCE IMAGING

CT has not traditionally been a first-line diagnostic tool in the assessment of FUO. CT has been useful especially in the detection of intra-abdominal and intrapelvic abscesses (Figs. 17 and 18). CT takes advantage of focal change in tissue attenuation related to tumor, inflammation, or infection. CT of the thorax, abdomen and pelvis, as well as of the rest of the body when appropriate (e.g., head and neck), has proven to be useful for detecting occult disease in the critically ill patient (21). Quinn et al. (22) reported a diagnostic yield of only 19% for abdominal CT evaluation of FUO.

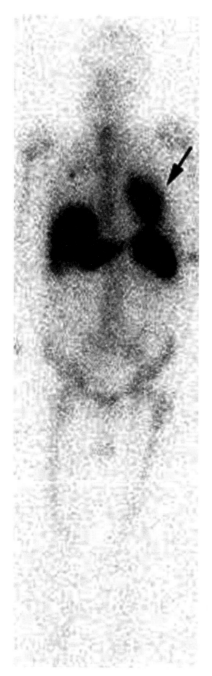

FIGURE 10 ^{111}Indium-labeled white blood cell scan in a 69-year-old male with leukocytosis demonstrates lingular pneumonia (*black arrow*).

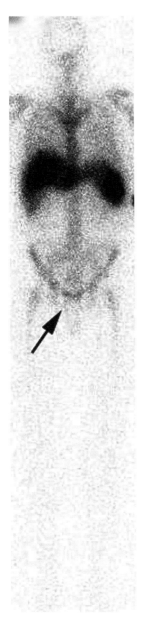

FIGURE 11 A 57-year-old male with fever of unknown origin found to have increased activity in the bladder (*black arrow*) on an ^{111}In-white blood cell scan, consistent with a urinary tract infection.

CT was also not sensitive in evaluation of the chest for FUO according to the study by Quinn et al. (22). However, we believe that multidetector CT of the chest, abdomen, and pelvis is appropriate in the workup of patients with FUO, as thin-section images are sensitive (although not necessarily specific) for findings consistent with infection, especially in immunocompromised patients. CT is not sensitive for osteomyelitis, a well-known but uncommon cause of FUO.

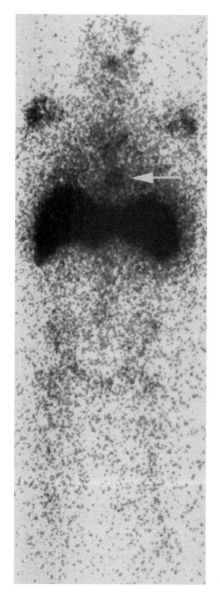

FIGURE 12 ^{111}In-labeled leukocyte scan of 51-year-old diabetic man with a fever and no definite source of sepsis. There is abnormal uptake in the midchest anterior to the heart, consistent with endocarditis (*white arrow*).

Unfortunately, patients with FUO usually do not have localizing signs to direct CT imaging, which, therefore, does not permit overall radiation dose reduction, as large portions of the body need to be imaged.

Sonography is a good alternative without ionizing radiation, for the initial imaging of the abdomen and pelvis in select patients with FUO (i.e., nonobese patients). In comparison to nuclear imaging, it is fast and highly sensitive for the detection of abnormal fluid collections, particularly in the abdomen and pelvis, in experienced hands.

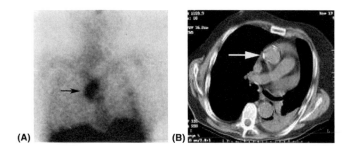

FIGURE 13 (**A**) An ^{111}In-labeled white blood cell scan demonstrates uptake in the upper chest retrosternally, consistent with a mycotic thoracic aortic aneurysm, in a 77-year-old male with staphylococcus bacteremia and pneumococcal sepsis on antibiotics. (**B**) Computed tomography scan shows the aneurysm (*white arrow*); however, it does not clearly demonstrate the site of infection.

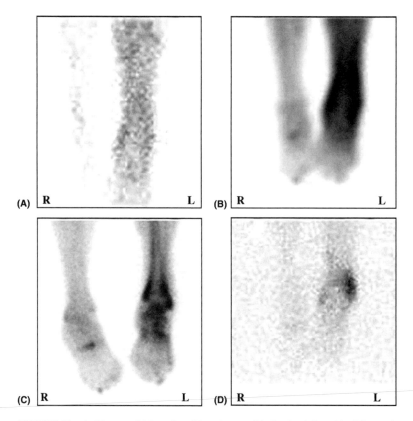

FIGURE 14 A 93-year-old female with osteomyelitis in the left ankle. Three-phase bone scan demonstrates (**A**) increased flow, (**B**) increased soft-tissue uptake in the left lower leg on blood pool image, and (**C**) increased bone uptake in the left lateral malleolus on the delayed image. ^{111}In-labeled WBC scan (**D**) demonstrates increased, labeled leukocyte uptake in the left ankle.

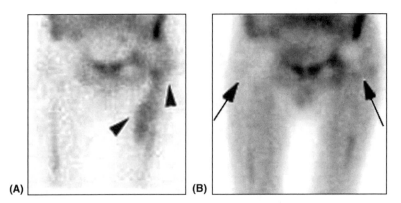

FIGURE 15 85-year-old male with bilateral hip replacements demonstrates (**A**) increased uptake on the ^{111}In-white blood cell scan around the left hip and femur (*black arrowheads*), which is discordant with the (**B**) normal marrow uptake on the ^{99m}Tc sulfur colloid bone-marrow scan compatible with a prosthesis infection. The photopenic defects in both hips (*black arrows*) correlate with the bilateral hip prostheses.

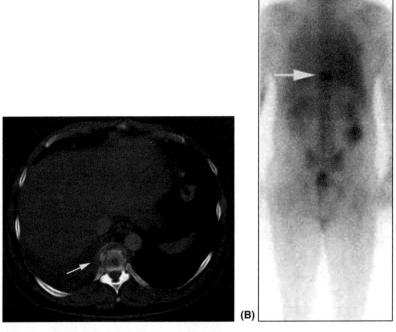

FIGURE 16 (**A**) Computed tomography of the abdomen demonstrates probable osteomyelitis/ discitis (*white arrow*) in a 55-year-old male with back pain involving T9 and T10. (**B**) Posterior view from a gallium scan reveals radiogallium uptake in T9 to T10 (*white arrow*).

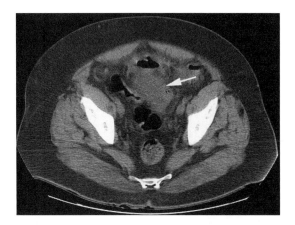

FIGURE 17 A 39-year-old male with fever of unknown origin. Computed tomography reveals a pelvic abscess (*white arrow*).

Interestingly, deep venous thrombosis has been reported to be the cause of FUO in 2% to 6% of cases (6), and venous-duplex Doppler imaging has proven to be useful in such patients (23). However, without a definite regional focus, lower extremity sonography probably should not be the first-line choice when imaging patients with FUO.

A combination of sonography, CT, and ^{111}In-labeled leukocyte imaging (24) can be a particularly effective diagnostic tool. In comparing the utility of CT, sonography, and ^{111}In-leukocyte scans in the assessment of abdominal and pelvic abscesses, it was determined that patients who were not critically ill and who had no localizing signs should be first evaluated with an ^{111}In-labeled leukocyte scan (25). There is no recent literature, to our knowledge, which has prospectively evaluated such a group of patients. Therefore, at present, it is still important to consider whole body nuclear imaging as a first-line technique in patients with FUO

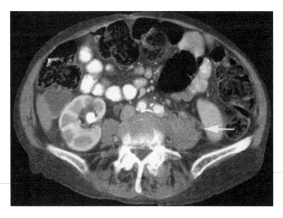

FIGURE 18 A 75-year-old woman presents with occult fever. Computed tomography scan demonstrates a heterogeneous collection in the left psoas, representing an abscess (*white arrow*).

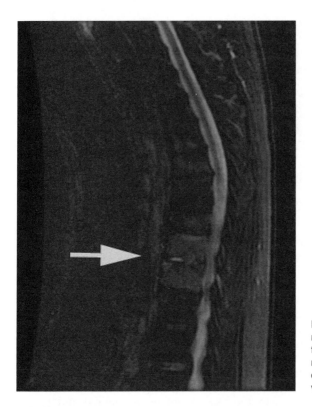

FIGURE 19 Sagittal T2-weighted magnetic resonance imaging of the thoracic spine in a 55-year-old male demonstrates osteomyelitis/ discitis involving the T9 and T10 vertebral bodies (*white arrow*).

without localizing signs or symptoms, followed by CT evaluation if necessary, to focus on a region of interest that may be a potential cause of FUO.

The role of MRI in FUO is not clear. There are limited studies, to our knowledge, which document the sensitivity or specificity of MRI for this purpose. MRI is the study of choice when the central nervous system is suspected as a potential source for FUO. It is an excellent imaging study when evaluating for brain and spinal cord tumors. It has proven to be an effective technique in detecting osteomyelitis (Fig. 19) or for further anatomic evaluation of suspected osteomyelitis initially identified on nuclear medicine studies, as described earlier. Findings of osteomyelitis on MRI typically include low-signal intensity on T1-weighted images and high-signal intensity on T2-weighted images. The role of fast, whole body MR sequences (such as breath-held T2-weighted, gradient-recalled echo, and echo-planar sequences) for the evaluation of patients with FUO has not, to our knowledge, been studied to date.

[18][F]2′-DEOXY-2-FLURO-D-GLUCOSE POSITRON EMISSION TOMOGRAPHY

[18][F]2′-deoxy-2-fluoro-D-glucose positron emission tomography (FDG-PET) appears to be useful in infection imaging. FDG is a positron emitter that accumulates in malignant tissues as well as in inflammatory processes. The spatial resolution of current PET scanners is significantly improved and higher than [67]Ga. Meller et al. performed a prospective study comparing ^{67}Ga scintigraphy versus FDG for the detection of the source of an FUO in 18 patients (26). FDG imaging,

performed on a double-head coincidence camera, demonstrated a sensitivity of 84% and a specificity of 86% in comparison to ^{67}Ga SPECT, which yielded sensitivities and specificities of 67% and 78%, respectively. The positive and negative predictive values were 90% and 75%, respectively, for FDG (28). Zhang et al. (27) evaluated 35 patients with FUO. Their study demonstrated a positive predictive value of 87% and a high negative predictive value of 95%, for FDG-PET imaging. Blockmans et al. (28) compared FDG-PET with gallium scintigraphy in a group of 40 patients with FUO, and found that all abnormal foci of gallium uptake were also detected using PET. With the high sensitivity and specificity of FDG-PET imaging, and the ability to combine PET data with CT anatomical data using the new hybrid PET-CT scanners, we suspect that the diagnostic workup for FUO will be even more accurate and efficient.

CONCLUSION

The diagnosis of FUO should begin with a thorough history and physical examination. The correct sequence of routine noninvasive laboratory studies should then be performed based on potential diagnostic clinical clues (8,29,30). A whole body labeled leukocyte scan has proven to be an effective first-line test to evaluate for occult infection. If there is suspicion of a musculoskeletal or cardiac source of infection, gallium scintigraphy may prove useful. The sensitivity, specificity, and usefulness of gallium scintigraphy are significantly diminished by physiologic radiotracer excretion via the genitourinary and gastrointestinal systems, necessitating further delayed imaging, delaying definitive diagnostic interpretation. In the evaluation of patients with known malignancy and FUO, the fever often results from the tumor or chemotherapy. Labeled leukocytes are more specific for infection, and therefore preferable to gallium scintigraphy in these patients. Further development of new approaches to infection imaging needs to address dosimetry, lack of blood handling, timely definitive interpretation, and improved sensitivity, specificity, and accuracy.

REFERENCES

1. Peters AM. The use of nuclear medicine in infections. Br J Radiol 1998; 71 (843):252–261.
2. Tsan M. Mechanism of gallium-67 accumulation in inflammatory lesions. J Nucl Med 1985; 26(1):88–92.
3. Becker W, Meller J. The role of nuclear medicine in infection and inflammation. Lancet Infect Dis 2001; 1:326–333.
4. Woolery WA, Franco FR. Fever of unknown origin: keys to determining the etiology in older patients. Geriatrics 2004; 59(10):41–45.
5. Knockaert DC, Mortelmans LA, De Roo MC, Bobbaers HJ. Clinical value of gallium-67 scintigraphy in evaluation of fever of unknown origin. Clin Infect Dis 1994; 18:601–605.
6. Yung E, Dey HM. Use of nuclear medicine techniques in the diagnosis and evaluation of sepsis. In: Fein AM, Abraham EM, Balk RA, et al., eds. Sepsis and Multiorgan Failure. Baltimore: Williams and Wilkins, 1997:355–372.
7. Thankur ML, Lavender JP, Arnot RN, Silverster DJ, Segal AW. Indium-111 labeled autologous leukocytes in man. J Nucl Med 1977; 18:1012–1019.
8. Mourad O, Palda V, Detsky AS. A comprehensive evidence-based approach to fever of unknown origin. Arch Intern Med 2003; 163:545–551.
9. Davies SG, Garvie NW. The role of indium-labeled leukocyte imaging in pyrexia of unknown origin. Br J Radiol 1990; 63:850–854.

10. de Kleijn E, Vandenbroucke JP, van der Meer JWM. Fever of unknown origin (FUO): I. A prospective multicenter study of 167 patients with FUO, using fixed epidemiologic entry criteria. Medicine 1997; 76(6):392–400.
11. Schmidt KG, Rasmussen JW, Sorensen PG, Wedebye IM. Indium-111-granulocyte scintigraphy in the evaluation of patients with fever of undetermined origin. Scand J Infect Dis 1987; 19:339–345.
12. Mountford PJ, Kettle AG, O'Doherty MJ, Coakley AJ. Comparison of technetium-99m-HMPAO leukocytes with indium-111-oxine leukocytes for localizing intraabdominal sepsis. J Nucl Med 1990; 31:311–315.
13. Palestro CJ, Vega A, Kim CK, Vallabhajosula S, Goldsmith SJ. Indium-111-labeled leukocyte scintigraphy in hemodialysis access-site infection. J Nucl Med 1990; 31:319–324.
14. Williamson MR, Boyd CM, Read RC, et al. 111in-labeled leukocytes in the detection of prosthetic vascular graft infections. Am J Roentgenol 1986; 147:173–176.
15. Hotze AL, Briele B, Overbeck B, et al. Technetium-99m-labeled anti-granulocyte antibodies in suspected bone infections. J Nucl Med 1992; 33:526–531.
16. Becker W, Bair J, Behr T, Repp R, et al. Detection of soft tissue infections and osteomyelitis using a technetium-99m-labeled anti-granulocyte monoclonal antibody fragment. J Nucl Med 1994; 35(9):1436–1443.
17. Meller J, Ivancevic V, Conrad M, et al. Clinical value of immunoscintigraphy in patients with fever of unknown origin. J Nucl Med 1998; 39(7):1248–1253.
18. Petersdorf RG, Beeson PB. Fever of unexplained origin: report on 100 cases. Medicine 1961; 40:1–30.
19. Datz FL, Thorne DA. Effect of antibiotic therapy on the sensitivity of indium-111-labeled leukocyte scans. J Nucl Med 1986; 27:1849–1853.
20. Thrall JH, Ziessman HA. Nuclear Medicine. The Requisites. St. Louis: Mosby, 1995: 166–167.
21. Mirvis S, Tobin KD, Kostrubiak I, Belzberg H. Thoracic CT in detecting occult disease in critically ill patients. Am J Roentgenol 1987; 148:685–689.
22. Quinn MJ, Sheedy PF, Stephens DH, Hattery RR. Computed tomography of the abdomen in evaluation of patients with fever of unknown origin. Radiology 1980; 136:407–411.
23. Abu Rahma AF, Saiedy S, Robinson PA, Boland JP, Cottrell DJ IV, Stuart C. Role of venous duplex imaging of the lower extremities in patients with fever of unknown origin. Surgery 1997; 121:366–371.
24. Tudor GR, Finlay DB, Belton I. The value of indium-111-labelled leukocyte imaging and ultrasonography in the investigation of pyrexia of unknown origin. Br J Radiol 1997; 70(837):918–922.
25. Knochel JQ, Koehler PR, Lee TG, Welch DM. Diagnosis of abdominal abscesses with computed tomography, ultrasound, and In-111 leukocyte scans. Radiology 1980; 137:425–432.
26. Meller J, Altenvoerde G, Munzel U, et al. Fever of unknown origin: prospective comparison of [18F]FDG imaging with a double-head coincidence camera and gallium-67 citrate SPECT. Eur J Nucl Med 2000; 27(11):1617–1625.
27. Zhang H, Yu JQ, Alavi A. Applications of fluorodeoxyglucose-PET imaging in the detection of infection and inflammation and other benign disorders. Radiol Clin North Am 2005; 43:121–134.
28. Blockmans D, Knockaert D, Maes A, et al. Clinical value of [18F]fluoro-deoxyglucose positron emission tomography for patients with fever of unknown origin. Clin Infect Dis 2001; 32:191–196.
29. Woolery WA, Franco FR. Fever of unknown origin: keys to determining the etiology in older patients. Geriatrics 2004; 59(10):41–45.
30. Roth AR, Basello GM. Approach to the adult patient with fever of unknown origin. Am Fam Physician 2003; 68:2223–2228.

Section IV: Therapy

17 Empiric Therapy in Fever of Unknown Origin: A Cautionary Note

Lucinda M. Elko and Charles S. Bryan
Department of Medicine, University of South Carolina, School of Medicine, Columbia, South Carolina, U.S.A.

> *Better a doubtful remedy than none at all.*
> —Celsus (25 B.C.–A.D. 50)
>
> *Throw out opium . . . a few specifics . . . wine . . . and the vapors which produce the miracle of anesthesia, and I firmly believe that if the whole material medica,* as now used, *could be sunk to the bottom of the sea, it would be all the better for mankind—and all the worse for the fishes.*
> —Oliver Wendell Holmes (1809–1894)

Fever of unknown origin (FUO) amply illustrates the *mot* that "the three most important principles of medicine are diagnosis, diagnosis, and diagnosis." Empiric therapy plays a limited role in FUO, if by FUO we mean *prolonged FUO* (≥3 weeks) (1). Cunha in 1996 recommended empiric therapy for only four situations: antibiotics for culture-negative endocarditis, low-dose corticosteroids for presumed temporal arteritis, antituberculous drugs for suspected military tuberculosis in elderly patients, and naproxen (Naprosyn) for suspected neoplastic fever (2). Our purpose is to review some general principles of empiric therapy and a handful of specific indications. Elsewhere in this volume, various authors discuss empiric therapy for specific subsets of patients with FUO.

The etiologies of FUO are discussed extensively elsewhere in this issue. Infectious diseases, which predominated in early studies and still predominate in the developing world, remain the most common cause in many, but by no means all, recent studies. Infections now explain roughly 30% of cases in developed countries, with the most common ones being intra-abdominal abscess (10%), tuberculosis (5%), and endocarditis (3). Most recent investigators have found the percentage of undiagnosed cases to be much higher than the 7% reported by Petersdorf and Beeson in 1961 (4), presumably because newer imaging, culture, and serologic methods now unmask conditions that were previously much more elusive. In two studies, long-term follow-up of patients with undiagnosed FUO revealed that fever resolved without treatment in the majority of instances, and that only rarely did a serious disorder declare its presence.

PRINCIPLES

Clinicians commonly address three questions: (*i*) What is wrong with the patient? (*ii*) What can I do for the patient? (*iii*) What will be the outcome? Empiric therapy, by definition, compromises the first of these desiderata. Recent studies suggest that patients with FUO for whom no explanation is forthcoming after extensive evaluation and prolonged observation have, in general, a favorable

229

prognosis (5,6). Knockaert et al. reported in 1996 that no cause was established for 10% to 25% of patients evaluated for FUO. In their series of 61 cases, the mortality attributable to FUO was only 3.2% during follow-up periods ranging from one month to 10 years (mean 5.8 years) (6). Thirty-one of 61 patients became symptom-free during the initial hospitalization or within weeks following discharge. One patient was found to have tuberculous meningitis by repeat lumbar puncture within two months of the initial evaluation. No single disease was found to be a frequent cause of prolonged FUO. In another study, Knockaert et al. described episodic FUO as fever meeting the classic FUO criteria defined by Petersdorf and Beeson, but with a fluctuating pattern that included fever-free intervals of at least two weeks. These patients were less eager to undergo extensive testing when the fever subsided. Infections and multisystem diseases were less likely in recurrent FUO as compared to persistent FUO. The infectious etiologies in that series of recurrent FUO were prostatitis, mastoiditis, proteus sepsis without a source, and toxoplasmosis (5).

Criteria for empiric therapy of FUO include a well-formulated hypothesis as to the etiology, an endpoint for the therapeutic trial, an explanation to the patient as to why treatment rather than expectant observation is being recommended, and acknowledgment of the downsides of drugs, including potential toxicity, masking the correct diagnosis, and mistaken diagnosis arising from post hoc, ergo propter hoc, reasoning. This last point—the potential for mistakes—deserves much emphasis. One of us, in preparing a textbook of infectious diseases for primary care physicians, surveyed 600 fellows of the Infectious Diseases Society of America (IDSA) with respect to the diagnoses in which mistakes were most frequently encountered. The survey form asked recipients to check from a list of 23 diagnoses, those in which, in their experience, a mistake by a physician acting in a primary-care capacity led to some combination of death, disability, or litigation (Table 1) (7). We are aware of no similar survey of mistakes made by infectious diseases specialists, nor are we aware of any systematic study of mistakes made during the course of diagnosis and treatment of FUO. A MEDLINE search for the years 1966 through 2004, cross-referencing "fever of unknown origin" and "empiric therapy," disclosed no systematic studies or reviews of this subject. We suspect, however, that many perhaps most, experienced infectious diseases consultants have seen through the years occasional cases of FUO that, had they to do it over, they would manage differently.

Case Report

An elderly retired dentist was seen by one of us (Bryan) in 1975 for evaluation of prolonged FUO. Physical examination was unremarkable except for a systolic murmur. He continued to be febrile with no diagnosis after two months of observation and numerous studies, including liver and bone marrow biopsies. His fever seemed to respond to empiric therapy for cryptic miliary tuberculosis, but recurred. His fever then seemed to respond to empiric therapy for culture-negative endocarditis, only to recur again. Laparotomy revealed Hodgkin's disease.

Empiric therapy of any kind should involve a series of structured questions. What syndrome best describes the patient's likely diagnosis? What are the most likely etiologies? Is the patient at high risk of morbidity and/or mortality? The answers to these questions should form the basis of a decision to treat empirically, or to withhold therapy while observing the patient closely. If one elects to treat, one

TABLE 1 Frequency of Diseases in Which Mistakes Made by Primary Care Physicians Resulted in Serious Consequences[a]

Condition	No. (%) of positive responses	Condition	No. (%) of positive responses
Necrotizing soft tissue infection	112 (64)	Brain abscess	58 (33)
Spinal epidural abscess	96 (55)	Toxic shock syndrome	58 (33)
Sepsis syndrome	95 (54)	Asplenia (failure to vaccinate)	57 (33)
Endocarditis	94 (54)	Rocky Mountain spotted fever	54 (31)
Meningococcal disease	89 (51)	Travel-related problems	54 (31)
Tuberculosis	84 (48)	Acute epiglottitis	35 (20)
Herpes simplex encephalitis	82 (47)	Pelvic inflammatory disease	32 (18)
Antibiotic toxicity	82 (47)	Clostridial syndrome	31 (18)
Pneumonia	80 (46)	Hemophilus influenzae meningitis	29 (17)
Pneumococcal meningitis	80 (46)	Sphenoid sinusitis	22 (13)
Intra-abdominal sepsis	59 (34)	Cavernous sinus thrombosis	21 (12)
AIDS-related problem	58 (33)	Miscellaneous	32 (18)

[a]From a survey sent to 600 fellows of the Infectious Diseases Society of America. The survey instrument listed 23 diagnoses (shown here) and asked the recipients to checkmark those diagnoses in which, in their experience, mistakes made by a physician acting in a primary care capacity had led to death, disability, or litigation. The rate of the response to the survey was 30%. These data do not indicate the actual incidence of mistakes made by primary care (which, some data indicate, is relatively low). Rather, they indicate pitfalls in diagnosis and disease management as seen from the perspective of infectious disease specialists, who are usually consulted on especially difficult cases.
Source: From Ref. 7.

should re-evaluate the patient to determine the presence or absence of an apparent response. With acute infectious diseases, a period of three days generally suffices for the latter purpose, unless one is considering tuberculosis. For most conditions, the patient will begin to show a response after three days if a response is to occur at all. To our knowledge, there are few, if any, systematic data pertaining to what constitutes an adequate therapeutic trial for a condition causing FUO.

SPECIFIC CONDITIONS SOMETIMES CALLING FOR EMPIRIC THERAPY OF FUO
Culture-Negative Endocarditis
In 1996, Cunha stated that empiric antibiotic trials except for culture-negative endocarditis have no place in the management of patients with FUO (2). Through the years, between 2.5% and 31% of cases of infective endocarditis have been culture negative in various series. More recent studies suggest that only about 5% of cases of endocarditis defined by strict criteria are culture negative. Optimum management therapy for these patients, with the exception of injecting drug users, remains controversial. There is, however, general agreement that the regimen should cover enterococci, fastidious gram-negative bacilli of the *Hemophilus, Actinobacillus, Cardiobacterium, Eikenella,* and *Kingella* species (HACEK) group, and nutrient-variant streptococci. Most often recommended is a three-drug regimen comprising penicillin or ampicillin plus gentamicin or streptomycin plus ceftriaxone (8,9). The clinician should, however, weigh carefully the severity of the disease, the risk factors for specific micro-organisms, and the balance between efficacy against the most likely pathogens and the risk of side effects including

drug toxicity and superinfection (2). In making this crucial decision, the clinician would do well to study the insightful review by Broqui and Raoult regarding endocarditis due to rare and fastidious microorganisms (10). Polymerase chain reaction (PCR) technology holds great promise in these cases especially for those that require surgical intervention (11,12). Interestingly, a study of 52 patients with a diagnosis of culture-negative endocarditis showed that 92% of patients who became afebrile within the first week of therapy survived, whereas only 50% survived if fever persisted more than seven days (8).

Culture-Negative Pulmonary Tuberculosis and Cryptic Disseminated Tuberculosis

Recent guidelines issued by the Centers for Disease Control and Prevention (CDC) help clarify the problem of when to use drugs for presumptive tuberculosis in the face of negative studies (13). Moreover, the new CDC recommendations suggest beginning combination drug therapy for patients with a high likelihood of tuberculosis even before the results of acid-fast bacillus (AFB) smears and mycobacterial cultures become available. Approximately 17% of reported new cases of pulmonary tuberculosis have negative cultures (14). A diagnosis of tuberculosis can be strongly inferred by clinical and radiographic response as determined by careful evaluation after two months of therapy (13). If both the clinical suspicion of tuberculosis and the severity of the disease are low, two approaches are acceptable: chemotherapy with a standard four-drug regimen, or close observation without treatment while awaiting the final results of cultures (which usually requires two months) (13).

Disseminated (miliary) tuberculosis is now uncommon in the United States but should be considered in certain situations: elderly patients, in whom the presentation may be that of a wasting illness without fever (15), patients with HIV/AIDS; patients with rheumatoid arthritis treated with corticosteroids, methotrexate, or infliximab (16), and recipients of solid organ transplants (17). The new CDC guidelines are largely silent on the issue of when to treat for presumptive disseminated tuberculosis, and we are unaware of any controlled trials that address this issue. Knockaert et al. found little or no relationship between prolonged FUO and tuberculosis, but it should be noted that the results of their study, which was carried out in Belgium, may not apply directly to certain populations in the United States.

Cunha favored empiric therapy in elderly patients with suspected disseminated tuberculosis (2), and this recommendation should extend to other high-risk populations with suspected severe disease. Drug toxicity and also drug interactions when rifamycin derivatives are used in the regimen must be taken into account. What constitutes an adequate duration of a therapeutic trial in this situation is unclear. However, because the bacillary populations in the individual lesions are substantially lower than those encountered in cavitary pulmonary tuberculosis, a response should nearly always become apparent within two months unless the disease is unusually extensive and/or caused by a multidrug-resistant strain.

Temporal Arteritis (Giant-Cell Arteritis)

As noted elsewhere in this issue, temporal arteritis is an important cause of FUO in elderly persons and can cause permanent disability from cerebrovascular accident or blindness. Treatment initiated after the onset of loss of visual acuity or central visual field rarely restores these deficits, and then only when corticosteroids have been started within three to four days of the onset of visual symptoms (18). Therefore, immediate therapy with steroids is recommended when temporal arteritis with vision loss is suspected. Temporal artery biopsy remains highly desirable. It has become generally accepted among clinicians that temporal artery biopsy should be performed within two weeks from starting steroid treatment. In a recent prospective study of 11 patients with presumed temporal arteritis, six of seven temporal artery biopsies performed after ≥ 4 weeks of steroid therapy revealed characteristic changes of the disease (19). From a retrospective chart review, Nesher et al. concluded that combining steroids with low-dose aspirin reduced cranial ischemic complications (20). Of the 166 patients qualifying for that study, 36 (21%) had already been receiving low-dose aspirin (100 mg/day) for ischemic heart disease. Ischemic complications occurred in 13% of patients receiving only steroids but in only 3% of those receiving both steroids and aspirin ($P = 0.02$) (20). Pending confirmation of these findings, it would seem prudent to add low-dose aspirin to the steroid regimen.

Naproxen Test for Differentiating Between Neoplastic and Other Causes of FUO

In 1984, Chang and Gross reported the apparent usefulness of a "naproxen test" in unexplained fever possibly due to neoplasm. A prompt, complete, sustained lysis of fever occurred within 24 hours of the institution of naproxen, a nonsteroidal anti-inflammatory drug (NSAID), in 14 of 15 cases of fever attributable to neoplasm, but in none of five patients with fever eventually attributed to infection. The case definition of FUO in their study was fever of >1 week as opposed to the usual three weeks, and they required only one temperature reading $\geq 101°F$. Fifteen of the patients had previously received antibiotics, without response. They concluded that "naproxen may be of great value in the differential diagnosis of infectious and neoplastic fever. . . . It is safe and has very few side effects. . . . In addition, our preliminary observation suggests that fever due to infectious disease of nonbacterial origin also does not respond to naproxen" (21).

More recent investigators have questioned the usefulness of the naproxen test (22,23). In 2003, Vanderschuren et al. described the effect of naproxen in 77 patients who met the Petersdorf-Beeson criteria for FUO. They graded responses to naproxen as complete, partial, or none in five categories of patients according to final diagnosis: neoplasms, infections, noninfectious inflammatory disorders, miscellaneous conditions, and cases that remained undiagnosed. The naproxen test was positive in 55% of patients with neoplasms and 38% of patients with other disorders. These investigators determined the naproxen test to be only 55% sensitive and 62% specific for a neoplastic origin of FUO (22). Criticisms of earlier studies of the naproxen test include definitions of FUO and selection bias that favored patients likely to have tumor-associated fever. Moreover, there is still no satisfactory explanation as to why neoplastic fever, but not fever due to other causes, should respond promptly to NSAIDs (23).

CONCLUSIONS

Although the epidemiology of FUO has changed over the past 40 years, the advice concerning empiric therapy has not. In 1963, Sheon and Ommen, after reporting their observations in 60 patients, wrote: "One cannot overemphasize the value of expectant management. Many patients, while waiting for cultures, will become afebrile with rapid return to normal health ... this emphasizes the need for caution in the interpretation of response to therapy .... The use of antibiotics on an empiric basis in a patient with obscure fever may create as well as resolve diagnostic problems .... The best management consists of striving to make a correct diagnosis" (24). In 1983, Hurley similarly concluded: "The patient with classic protracted FUO requires a methodical approach, and precision is of utmost importance. Fortunately, such a patient is rarely desperately ill, so the physician has time to perform the evaluation" (25). We heartily endorse these conclusions. Empiric therapy for FUO should be restricted to highly selected situations, as discussed earlier and also by the authors of other articles in this issue.

REFERENCES

1. Bryan CS. Fever of unknown origin: the evolving definition. Arch Intern Med 2003; 163(9):1003–1004.
2. Cunha BA. Fever of unknown origin. Infect Dis Clin N Am 1996; 10(1):111–127.
3. Arrnstrong W, Kazanjian P. Fever of unknown origin in the general population and in HIV-infected persons. In: Cohen J, Powderly WG, eds. Cohen and Powderly: Infectious Diseases. Vol. 1, ch. 82, 2nd ed. St Louis: Mosby, 2004:871–880.
4. Petersdorf RO, Beeson PB. Fever of unexplained origin: Report on 100 cases. Medicine (Baltimore) 1961; 40:1–30.
5. Knockaert DC, Vanneste LJ, Bobbaers HJ. Recurrent or episodic fever of unknown origin: Review of 45 cases and survey of the literature. Medicine (Baltimore) 1993; 72(3): 184–196.
6. Knockaert DC, Dujardin KS, Bobbaers HJ. Long-term follow-up of patients with undiagnosed fever of unknown origin. Arch Intern Med 1996; 156(6):618–620.
7. Bryan CS. Infectious disease emergencies. In: Bryan CS, ed. Infectious Diseases in Primary Care. Philadelphia: W.B. Saunders Company 2002:111–152.
8. Fowler VG, Scheld WM, Bayer AS. Endocarditis and intravascular infections. In: Mandell GL, Bennett JE, Dolin R, eds. Principles and Practice of Infectious Disease, 5th ed. Vol. 1. Philadelphia: Churchill Livingstone, 2005:975–1022.
9. Moreillon P. Chapter 59: Endocarditis and endarteritis. In: Cohen J, Powderly WG, eds. Cohen and Powderly: Infectious Diseases. Vol. 1, ch. 59, 2nd ed. St Louis: Mosby, 2004:653–668.
10. Brouqui P, Raoult D. Endocarditis due to rare and fastidious bacteria. Clin Microbiol Rev 2001; 14(1):177–207.
11. Qin X, Urdahl KB. PCR and sequencing of independent genetic targets for the diagnosis of culture negative bacterial endocarditis. Diagn Microbiol Infect Dis 2001; 40(4):45–149.
12. Khulordava I, Miller G, Haas D, et al. Identification of the bacterial etiology of culture-negative endocarditis by amplification and sequencing of a small ribosomal RNA gene. Diagn Microbiol Infect Dis 2003; 46(1):9–11.
13. American Thoracic Society, CDC, and Infectious Diseases Society of Americas. Treatment of tuberculosis. MMWR 2003; 52(RR-11):1–77.
14. American Thoracic Society, CDC. Diagnostic standards and classification of tuberculosis in adults and children. Am J Respir Crit Care Med 2000; 161(4):1376–1395.
15. Ozbay B, Uzan K. Extrapulmonary tuberculosis in high prevalence of tuberculosis and low prevalence of HIV. Clin Chest Med 2002; 23(2):351–354.
16. Mayordomo L, Marenco JL, Gomez-Mateos J, et al. Pulmonary military tuberculosis in a patient with anti-TNF-alpha treatment. Scand J Rheumatol 2002; 31(1):44–45.
17. Korner MM, Hirata N, Tenderich G, et al. Tuberculosis in heart transplant recipients. Chest 1997; 111(2):365–369.
18. Hayreh SS, Zimmerman B, Kardon RH. Visual improvement with corticosteroid therapy in giant cell arteritis. Report of a large study and review of literature. Acta Ophthalmol Scand 2002; 80(4):353–367.

19. Ah Kine D, Tijani SO, Parums DV, et al. Effects of prior steroid treatment on temporal artery biopsy findings in giant cell arteritis. Br J Ophthalmol 2002; 86(5):530–532.
20. Nesher G, Berkun Y, Mates M, et al. Low-dose aspirin and prevention of cranial ischemic complications in giant cell arteritis. Arthritis Rheum 2004; 50(4):1332–1337.
21. Chang JC, Gross HM. Utility of naproxen in the differential diagnosis of fever of undetermined origin in patients with cancer. Am J Med 1984; 76(4):597–603.
22. Vandershueren S, Knockaert DC, Peetermans WE, et al. Lack of value of the naproxen test in the differential diagnosis of prolonged fever. Am J Med 2003; 115(7):572–575.
23. Plaisance KI, Mackowiak PA. Antipyretic therapy: physiologic rationale, diagnostic implications, and clinical consequences. Arch Intern Med 2000; 160(4):449–456.
24. Sheon RP, Van Ommen RA. Fever of obscure origin. Am J Med 1963; 34:486–499.
25. Hurley DL. Fever in adults: what to do when the cause is not obvious. Postgrad Med 1983; 74(5):232–244.

Index

About the Editor

BURKE A. CUNHA is Chief, Infectious Disease Division, Winthrop-University Hospital, Mineola, New York, and Professor of Medicine, State University of New York School of Medicine, Stony Brook. Dr. Cunha is the author or coauthor of more than 150 abstracts, 100 electronic publications, 1000 articles, and 150 book chapters. He has edited 20 books on various infectious disease topics and is Editor-in-Chief of the journals *Infectious Disease Practice* and *Antibiotics for Clinicians*. Dr. Cunha is a Fellow of the Infectious Diseases Society of America. Dr. Cunha is internationally recognized as a teacher-clinician and is the recipient of many teaching awards including the prestigious Aesculapius Award. Dr. Cunha is a Master of the American College of Physicians, awarded for lifetime achievement as a master clinician and teacher of infectious diseases. Dr. Cunha received the M.D. degree from Pennsylvania State University College of Medicine, Hershey.

DATE DUE

APR 14 2008			